The Fork Is Mightier Than the Gym

Your Guide to Life-Changing Results

Lisa Cook

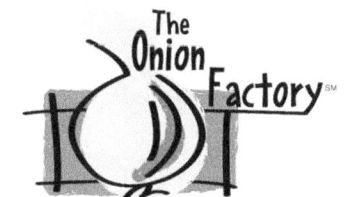

ANDERSON, INDIANA

The Fork Is Mightier Than the Gym, copyright © 2020 by The Onion Factory℠. All rights reserved. An earlier edition of this book was published as *Peeling an Onion: The Complete Guide to Change*, copyright © 2011 by Lisa Lynn Cook.

Cover photo by Richard Wozniak/Shutterstock.com. Illustrations on the following pages are licensed from the sources indicated: p. 33—Cozine/Shutterstock.com; p. 37—Supreeya-Anon/Shutterstock.com; p. 48—bus109/Shutterstock.com; p. 52—bmphotographer/Shutterstock.com; p. 55—Omron/Shutterstock.com and Andrey Popov/Shutterstock.com; p. 57—marekuliasz/Shutterstock.com; p. 67—baldyrgan/Shutterstock.com and Tribalium/Shutterstock.com; p. 74—Nitr/Shutterstock.com/p. 96—Ekaterina Mineava/Shutterstock.com; p. 112—Gayvoronskaya Yana/Shutterstock.com; p. 113—Kei Shooting/Shutterstock.com; p. 121—Callahan/Shutterstock.com; p. 122—John T. Takai/Shutterstock.com; p. 124—mhatzapa/Shutterstock.com; p. 126—Callahan/Shutterstock.com; p. 136—Vulp/Shutterstock.com; p. 137—Konstantin/Shutterstock.com; p. 139—minadezhda/Shutterstock.com; p. 149—Elena Chaykina Photography/Shutterstock.com; p. 159—Gecko Studio/Shutterstock.com; p. 167—Elena Design/Shutterstock.com; p. 175—Dipali 5/Shutterstock.com; p. 185—minadezhda/Shutterstock.com; p. 195—Brent Hofaker/Shutterstock.com; p. 205—Billion Photos/Shutterstock.com; p. 213—Africa Studio/Shutterstock.com; p. 241—New Africa/Shutterstock.com; p. 245—Tetiana Rostopira/Shutterstock.com; p. 248—Blazej Lyjak/Shutterstock.com; p. 252—Golfx/Shutterstock.com; p. 261—Yacobchuk Viacheslav/Shutterstock.com; p. 271—Alexander Raths/Shutterstock.com; p. 273—Didecs/Shutterstock.com; p. 280—Jaroslaw Pawlak/Shutterstock.com

Cover design by Mary Jaracz Design. Interior design by Allison Book Packaging.

No part of this publication may be reproduced, stored in a retrieval system, or transmitted in any form or by any means, electronic, mechanical, photocopying or otherwise without the prior written permission of the publisher.

Notice: This book is not a medical manual. The information given here is intended to help you make informed decisions about your health. It is not intended as a substitute for any treatment that may have been prescribed by your doctor. If you suspect you have a medical problem, we urge you to seek competent medical help. Mention of specific companies, organizations, or authorities in this book does not imply endorsement by the publisher, nor does mention of specific companies, organizations, or authorities imply that they endorse this book.

Direct all editorial inquiries, including requests for permission to reprint material from this book, to this address:

    Publication Dept.
    The Onion Factory
    2700 N 100 W
    Anderson, IN 46011

ISBN: 978-0-578-65379-2

Printed in the United States of America

Dedication

To my boys,
Jake and Gage,
who were very patient while their mom
chased her dreams.

To everyone
who shared their inspiration and support
as we grew this guide.

WHAT'S INSIDE

9 FROM THE AUTHOR

11 HOW IT ALL BEGAN...

13 **1. THE ONION**
Your New Beginning / Vanity / Adversity / Awakenings

19 **2. MY STORY**
My Turning Point / Susan's Results / Body Image / My Mother's Question / "Indiana Wants Me" / My Goal for This Book

25 **3. OUR PROBLEM, OUCH!**
What Is Normal? / Excuses / Chris' Story / This Journey Is about Body Fat / Ann's Story / Why Diet? / Suppress Your Appetite? Not! / Good News for Fluffy People / Body Type and Weight Loss

35 **4. HOW THIS GUIDE DIRECTS YOU**
K.I.S.S. / But Wait... / How Thin Is Thin Enough? / Not a Skinny Fitness Trainer

39 **5. ARE YOU READY TO PEEL?**
Nutritional Formula / Metabolic Formula / Target Heart Rate (THR) / Spending Your Fat Reserve / Using Your Muscles / Eating and Drinking / Peeling / Ruth's Story / Understanding Body Types / Scientific Body Types / The 150-Pound Girl / Anabolic, Catabolic, Metabolic / Catabolic State / Anabolic State / Metabolic State / The Campfire Effect / Making Changes / Body Fat Composition / Hydrostatic Measurement / Electrical Impedance / Calipers / In What Mode Am I? / Peel Mode / Gain Mode / Clean-Up Mode / Out-of-Control Mode / Maintenance Mode

59 **6. FREE SEMINAR**
1. Achieve Target Heart Rate (THR) / 2. Build Muscle / 3. Eat, Don't Starve / Carbohydrates / We Need a New Food Pyramid! / Protein / Start Your Engines! / The Scale / Measurements / Victoria's Secret® / Detoxification / Understanding the Psychology of Change / Stay Fat

71 **7. ADVANCED TOOLS AND TIPS**
"I've Just Got to Go on a Diet!" / Kathy's Story / Denver Bronco Player's Mass / Advanced Protein Theories / Bet You Didn't Know This / Fat Recap / Fiber: Are Beans Okay? / Mom's Sugar Vice / Artificial Sweeteners

85   **8. A SIDE ORDER OF PSYCHOLOGY**
Does Anorexia Have a Mirror Disorder? / Signs / The "It" Girl / Class Reunions / The Root of the Problem / Change Is Good / Weight Loss Versus Weight Gain / Meltdown Fix: Candy / The Cheating Psyche / The Question / "Starving"? / Psychology in Advertising

97   **9. FOOD, FOOD, FOOD**
How You Are Going to Eat / Healthy? / Dressings and Sauces / Salad Dressings / Unlimited Portion Selections / Portion-Control Selections / Do-Not-Touch Selections / Secret Weapons / Sauces / Apologies to Ralph Nader / The Keto Effect / Am I Going to Get Sick of Chicken? / Which Is the Lesser Evil? / Connie's Story / The Intervention / "But I'm Not Hungry" / Read Your Food Labels Carefully / "Gotta Have Milk and Bananas" / Portion Control / The Truth about Healthy Eating

117   **10. EATING OUT**
A Restaurant Plan / Eating Out: Client Specific / Loves to Cook / Fast Food / What I Would Order / Fast Food Favorites: McDonald's / Wendy's / Arby's / Burger King / Taco Bell / Subway / Sit-Down Restaurants: Bob Evans / Cracker Barrel / Applebee's / Red Lobster / Olive Garden / Fine Dining / Can't Cook, But Can Grab at the Grocery / What to Do When You Don't Know What to Do / Trader Joe's Frozen Entrees / An After-Dinner Mint?

137   **11. EAT AWAY!**
Breakfasts / Burgers / Soups / Salads / Dinners / Sides / Snacks / Desserts / Beverages

221   **12. CIRCLE OF INFLUENCE**
Women Set the Pace / All in the Family / Family Influence / Family Influence Continues / Community Influence Spreads / What about the Men? / Man Camp's "Biggest Loser" / Firefighter's Stats / Circle of Influence

231   **13. INSPIRATION TO CHANGE**
Kerrie's Story / Transformations / Medical Stories / Cathy's Story / Sue's Story / Harriet's Story

239   **14. ONION CAMP**
Getting Started / Weight Training Works / WEEK ONE / Beginning Weights and Measures / Computing Your Weekly Weight and Body Composition / WEEK TWO / Making Better Food Choices / The Goods: Complex Carbohydrates (a.k.a. Grass of the Lands) / The Bads: Sugars / The Uglys: Fillers / Muscle Anatomy / Week 2 Training / Basic Onion Routine / It's Test Time / WEEK THREE / Week 3 Training / Abs / X-Tra Credit / It's Test Time / WEEK FOUR / Making Adjustments / Week 4 Training / Emotional

Health / It's Test Time / WEEK FIVE / Week 5 Training / WEEK SIX / Week 6 Training / It's Test Time / WEEK SEVEN / Week 7 Training / WEEK EIGHT / Week 8 Training / Graduation Rant: About Those Filler Carbs / Congratulations! Q and A

269   15. VITAMINS AND MINERALS
Vitamin A / Vitamin D / Vitamin E / Vitamin K / Vitamin C / Potassium / Calcium / Supplements / Essential Fatty Acids / Omega 3 / Omega 6 / Omega 9 / Bodybuilder Friend / Prevention Is the Key / Cruciferous Options

281   16. LIVING IN MAINTENANCE
The Fillers / Cardio Seven Days a Week / Overtraining? / Results Are Typical / Clarification

287   17. FALLEN ONIONS

From the Author

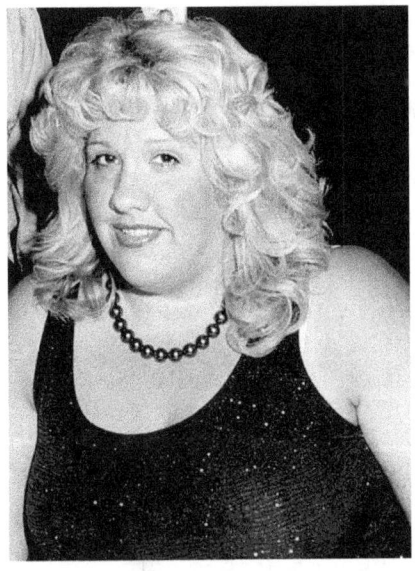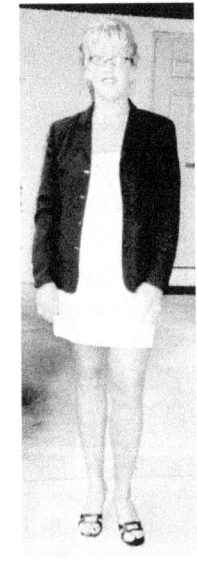

Lisa BEFORE...and AFTER

I'VE SPENT 20 YEARS working with "fluffy" people, including a facility that served 1,500 clients per day, where I watched the same people come in day after day and rarely change. While fit clients maintained their level of fitness, everyone else got frustrated and dropped out. Other trainers never understood why, but I did.

I was an FLUFFY girl working in an industry that promised to make me healthy. So I went to aerobics classes and tried every *regimen de jour* like step aerobics, Pilates, yoga, etc. (Who knows how many pieces of exercise equipment I tried?) If the right exercise equipment and fitness classes had been the secret to good health, I would have become healthy in no time. But it didn't happen.

One day I got mad enough—and motivated enough—to pull all of my knowledge and experience together. That's when I figured out how to lose 100 pounds and keep it off. And here's the irony: It was more about *eating* than not eating. It was more about daily *activity* than weekly gym exercises. Silly me. I had starved myself and shamed myself for so many years, when those things didn't help me at all.

Since then, I've made it my mission to change the way we deal with obesity. Fifteen years into peeling "onions," I found myself having a few more things to share. The first is a little science twist I discovered.

I have said a few times I felt like the Onion Factory has been a mini Eli Lilly research division. We have collected the data on over 1,500 clients that graduated our 8-week course. So I'm proud to say that the information in this guide is evidence based.

As a coach I have been able to weigh and measure that may clients, review their data, and learn the science of weight loss. I did not learn this information I am about to share with you from a book. I learned by rolling up my sleeves, working 12-15 hours per days and made it my mission to figure out how you take someone from 40% fat to 30% fat. Or even better, 50% fat to 40% fat. Has it been easy? HECK NO! But the results are so worth it.

Recently, someone very close to me said he felt I was like Marie Curie, the French-Polish physicist, who put math and science behind the results she observed. Wow, who knew that changing "fluffy" would involve a few math equations and a smidge of balance! Math was certainly not at the top of my favorites in school. But I will share the formulas of weight loss with you and support you with fun stories and inspiration along the way.

In a recent meeting, I learned that three sisters have been working on weight loss. One of the sisters is an "onion," one is a Weight Watchers® girl, and the other sister is somewhere in the middle. Her complaint about the selection of fruit I recommend was this: She was tired of the berries! So

10 /// The Fork Is Mightier Than the Gym

the sister who is an onion suggested she try some melon or maybe a little pineapple. I looked up at her and said, REALLY?

I would like to drive a Ferrari but my checkbook says NO. Likewise, if you have 30%, 40%, or 50% body fat and want to fix that level of "fluffy," you must put the science behind the results you desire. If my checkbook can't afford a Ferrari, then her weight results cannot afford the pineapple.

Weight loss begins in your mind. I've often said I should receive an honorary psychology degree for the past 15 years. In the beginning, I thought if clients had the science to weight loss than that should be enough. I was so wrong.

Change will happen when you understand Y=U. (Ha, another formula!) In other words, the "why" (Y) of weight loss depends entirely on "you" (U). If you desire to fix what is broken, then you must figure out why it's broken and change your behavior accordingly. If you are looking for results, you must ask yourself a few questions....

Are you sabotaging yourself with food?

Do you celebrate with food?

Are you lazy with your nutrition?

Is food your social life?

Do you stress eat?

You will find it difficult to create the "you" that you desire until you find out "why" you allow your life habits to get in the way.

If you simply needed the correct Information and an understanding of the science behind how to get results, then this would be easy. The psychology part might give you a few speed bumps, but you would figure it all out.

Yet knowledge is not enough. You must change your behavior to change your results. When you build great menus and match your level of fitness with the menus, then amazing RESULTS will be typical!

Lisa Cook

How It All Began...

ALL THOSE YEARS WHILE I was trying and failing to lose weight, I chose foods like yogurt and bananas for breakfast when I really wanted pancakes, Belgian waffles, or French toast. On an extra busy day, I might buy a McDonald's® parfait for a quick, healthy meal—or so I thought.

For my $1.49, I received nearly twice the allotted amount of sugar, which would ensure that I'd crave sugar all day. Plus, it wouldn't give me nearly enough protein.

One day, as I was preparing to appear on a local TV program, I compared the nutrition label for McDonald's® parfait to ours. No wonder I was having trouble! Armed with that information, I was able to resist the temptation of those golden arches. Knowledge led to a change of habits, and that led to a striking change of results! The same can be true for you.

Get ready, your life is about to change....

McDonald's® Breakfast Parfait

Nutrition Facts
Serving Size: 1 Parfait, 5.3 oz.

Amount Per Serving
Calories   100
Total Fat   2 grams
Total Carbohydrate   31 grams
Sugars   21 grams
Protein   4 grams

The Onion Factory℠ Breakfast Parfait

Nutrition Facts
Serving Size: 1 Parfait, 12 oz.

Amount Per Serving
Calories   173
Total Fat   1.5 grams
Total Carbohydrate   11 grams
Sugars   8 grams
Protein   27 grams

1. The Onion

YOUR LIFE IS COMPLEX AND MULTI-LAYERED

LIKE AN ONION,

BUT YOU CAN PEEL EACH LAYER AWAY.

SOMEONE ONCE SAID ABOUT me, "One day she'll turn into a diamond." I struggled for years with that imprint and often thought, but what if I desire to be a ruby, or an emerald? And I continued to grow layer after layer of protection, hiding the real me that was underneath my thin skin. Like me, as you peel away layers, you will find a jewel—ruby, emerald, or diamond—within you.

Peeling an Onion is incredibly easy! I am asked frequently, "Do you need to eat a lot of Onions on this program?" The question always makes me chuckle. My original slogan, "The Woman Within," evolved over time as I realized my mission to help overweight people change. The Onion thing just kind of happened.

On Monday, April 25, approximately one month after holding my first seminar, I received the first confirmation that I was on the right track. I had spent a year writing in my journal, praying, and asking God for direction on how to make my dream a reality, my dream of changing the course of obesity. I often thought: *I wish my angels would just send me an email, because it would be so much easier.* I felt confused about where to start. Attempting to enlighten health club owners about how to handle the obese demographic had burnt me out, and I was at bottom. How in the world could I make this all happen?

On that particular Monday, I read a comment that suggested life is complex and multi-layered like an Onion, so we need to peel each complication away in order to accomplish real change. Indeed, my life had been like an Onion. I had learned by experience that changing my health involved peeling away layer after layer of issues that had contributed to my obesity. The metaphor fit perfectly, so this became The Onion Factory[SM].

Your New Beginning

You may have bought this book because you thought it might help you get back into a favorite outfit you keep tucked in the back of your closet. It definitely can help you do that, but it is about so much more. This is a tool you can use to change your life. It will change the way you view so many things: your current health, your overall strength and endurance, the medications you are taking, and the role food plays in your life. As Onions, we are lost behind layers of emotions, trauma, and losses, disappointments, and more. As you peel away layer after layer, you will find a new you.

Finding the center of an Onion is more than just eating right and exercising properly. For me, it was about sorting through emotional garbage to find out why I had allowed myself to grow into a nearly 300-pound woman.

A few summers ago, as I helped a friend in her photography gallery, one of her pictures caught my eye. It was simply a lump of clay being molded. Around this same time, I was reading *The Purpose Driven Life,* by Rick Warren. I'm not sure if this was my time to find myself, or if all women in their mid thirties go through this stream of emotions feeling lost, empty, frustrated, unhappy, incomplete, and out of control. Boy, was I out of control, nearly 300 pounds worth of bad choices. I was frustrated that I had wasted so many years hiding behind layers of incompleteness.

As I look back, I'm beginning to understand the journey I've been on, how I've been molded, and how very lucky I feel now to have the opportunity to help you change your life.

I created The Onion Factory℠ system out of many years of my own trials and errors, but more importantly, I created the system out of other women's experiences. Their weight-loss journeys inspired me and validated that the Onion philosophy did indeed work.

Lots of teenagers try diets, diet pills, or starvation. Many adults have lost 100 pounds. Some of you may have spent a lifetime of gaining and losing weight. My journey has enabled me to share with you how you can lose those pounds for the rest of your life and never diet, or starve, again. The best part is you will regain abilities you may not have even realized you'd lost. Getting up from the couch, crossing your legs, sitting Indian style, or as one Onion shared, sitting in the pew on Sunday with the Bible on your lap instead of on your stomach.

Let me explain how this whole thing happened. When I was 21 and single, Bally Health and Tennis Corporation hired me just prior to opening a new facility. Once we opened, the manager allowed me to select my office. I had two choices. The first office was a half-circle overlooking the women's workout floor. The second was a half-circle overlooking the bodybuilder's training area. Which office do you think I chose? That's right, the guy's side! And I started paying attention.

It didn't take me long to notice that my lunches differed vastly from the guy trainers and bodybuilders. Mine consisted of very small portions of high-fat food like fettuccini alfredo, cheese, pasta, and other comfort foods, or nothing at all. The guys would bring in coolers full of food like baked, or broiled chicken, egg whites, green veggies, and feed-your-muscles kind of protein shakes.

Twenty years later, I get it. I was feeding my fat cells. They were feeding their lean mass.

As you read this guide, you will learn that your body is an engine, that lean mass is muscle, and that muscle drives your metabolism. I've heard over and over again that we women do not want to put on muscle, or bulk up. But do we really want to put on fat instead? Let's face it. Which really looks better when you're standing naked in front of the mirror hard muscle, or flabby fat? When speaking about your engine, remember, one pound of muscle takes up one-third the amount of space as one pound of fat. And your engine, a.k.a. muscle, burns 50 to 100 calories for every pound of muscle each day as opposed to three calories your body burns each day for every pound of fat. Why have we spent so many decades feeding our fat cells? Were we really that uninformed?

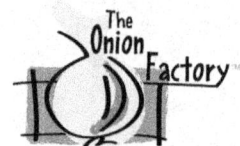 *I was feeding my fat cells, but athletes feed their lean mass.*

I've spent more than two decades calculating people's body compositions. While the American Medical Association has assigned the amount of safe body fat for women at 26 percent, I was in an industry that preached a safe percentage of body fat at 16-20 percent, and bodybuilding competitors needed to go as low as 5-8 percent. No wonder we gave up before we even started.

I was a 46 percent body fat girl working in the fitness industry. What was I thinking? Well, I was not thinking. I was in denial that I had gotten as big as I actually was. I look back at pictures and say, "Oh, my gosh." I even got to the point that I would not let anyone take my picture, so there would be no evidence of reality.

During those years spent calculating body compositions, I saw several changes take place. The composition results went from an occasion high of 30-percent body fat in the 1980's to an average of 40-50 percent in the 2000's.

Today, we seem to be better informed than ever. What happened? If you look back at pictures of your parents, or pictures from the 1950's and 60's, people were not as large as they are today.

Keep in mind that you can fit in a size ten and weigh a decent number on the scale and still be 40 percent fat. So, the scale is not a good way to judge your level of health, or validate that the program you've been following is, or is not, working for you.

Your body's percentage of fat is a realistic guide from which to gauge your results. If you focus on a safe body fat percentage, instead of a number on a scale, you will find that the lost inches will inspire you to finish your weight-loss journey and stop yo-yo dieting forever.

Throughout the past twenty years, I've also watched Type II diabetes explode into epidemic proportions. As I worked with diabetics, I paid attention to the nutrition modifications they had to make.

For instance, a diabetic might be able to eat only eat fourteen grapes. Any more would affect his or her blood sugar level.

I also realized that nearly 100 percent of the client's daily consumption of carbohydrates came from fillers. Foods like white sugar, white flour, and over-processed food, provide very little nutritional value.

Even though I was exposed to these trends, I did not put all of the pieces together until 2003 when I researched obesity for a thirty-page paper I had to write for an undergraduate class. Now I'm glad I had to write that paper! The final piece of the puzzle, which I needed to put The Onion Factory℠ system together, came from the Atkins program, the final "diet" I tried.

Many aspects of the Atkins program made sense and worked for me. It was not about eating less. Smaller portions of junk never worked for me, and starving is overrated. To be honest, I absolutely love to eat! The Atkins program taught me it was not about portion control. I lost 30 pounds, very quickly, while eating a lot of food.

My problem was that the food was very high in fat. I felt yucky, dehydrated, and kind of unclean and incomplete. I missed a lot of natural foods that God created for us to eat in order to be healthy. Although Atkins permitted particular vegetables, I really missed my fruits and vegetables. In addition, I really believe that unlimited fat is not the best option for long-term health.

At this point, I realized that losing weight was not about unlimited fat, nor was it about eating fat-free. Rather, it was about finding a level of fat grams to allow for the proper digestion of vitamins and to help me feel satiated. A little fat in a recipe goes a long way to help you feel satisfied. I decided to find a way of eating that would be realistic for the rest of my life.

Once I put these ideas together, along with the other three steps of the Onion system, I lost 100 pounds in nine months, but more importantly, I kept them off. I did not find a short-term solution for an age-old problem; I found a way of eating that I could live with for the rest of my life.

Am I saying you will never eat bread, pizza, or fried chicken again? Absolutely not. Just during the peeling process, since you already know what this stuff tastes like, you might as well put it aside and get rid of your storage tank as fast as possible. Then, once you're in a safe body-fat percentage and have found a new you, you will have developed new behaviors and gained a new awareness of what you want to eat. This will empower you to maintain the results you have achieved while enjoying a limited, selected amount of your favorite foods.

So this guide is a journey of setting the record straight, empowering you with knowledge, and changing the course of obesity.

Think of this journey as giving birth. You deserve to give yourself the best nine months of development, so you can spend the rest of your life with more energy and feeling great, rather than becoming an early morbidity statistic.

I'm thankful I have lived this journey because I can share with you from personal experience. I'm also thankful that I've made most of the mistakes possible, so you don't have to! I'm also thankful for the past few years having the opportunity to practice and develop the Onion system with so many incredible people.

Vanity

The desire to diet, to lose weight, may begin with vanity. We want to fit into a smaller size, or see a lower number on the scale. As Onions, we all dream of fitting into a size eight, or smaller. At some point, the weight loss desire turns into a yearning for better health and longevity.

Onion campers who are in their 20's and 30's have proven to be the most difficult group to lead all the way through to completion of the Onion system. I am not sure why. However, I found it difficult to collect case studies and data from this demographic to include in this guide. As you turn the corner into your 40's, things seem to change. Maybe you wake up one day and desire better health, and in return you automatically get a better and smaller version of you. At 40, we just seem to get it.

I thought the most difficult part of helping Onions reach their goal and collecting data for this guide would be getting them to commit to burning 400 calories per day on the beast (elliptical), or any other type of cardiovascular training. I felt certain this segment of society wouldn't want to work out. Wow, did they ever prove me wrong; especially, when I watched women even up to 400 pounds continue working hard for an hour. It was, and is, amazing!

I thought teaching and inspiring clients to lift free weights would be difficult for this client base. I was wrong! Not only did they do a great job lifting in camp, progressing from three-pound weights to five pounds and on up to eight pounds and more; they went out and purchased their own sets to use at home, so they could work harder on the routine to obtain better results.

Now I know that the most difficult part of finishing Onions is the psychology of understanding their relationship with food and helping them to change it. They truly need to peel back each layer of themselves.

Adversity

While attending the school of hard knocks, I have discovered that adversity may be the best- kept secret into finding your way. A few years back, my marriage and my job ended. I found myself starting over. If I'd had a million dollars, I would have created a totally different Onion Factory. With that kind of money, I could have equipped my factory with all the same types of machines that other facilities use. For example, I would have never started clients on the beast, the elliptical trainer. I thought those machines were only for fit people, and they were always located in parts of the facility where fit people trained. I would have pointed a fluffy client toward something more passive like aquatics, or a line of equipment that had them working out while sitting down. But haven't we sat long enough?

We in the fitness industry would have started out-of-shape patrons on a stationary bike, or a treadmill. Onions hate this stuff. Beginners wouldn't have been introduced to free weights. Free weights can be intimidating; you must learn to get comfortable with lifting them, and you need a guide, or coach, to teach you proper form.

Remember, Onions do not love working out. If we did, we would not be Onions. Why in the world would we invest in a trainer when working out is not something we want to do? Aren't there pills, or a drink, or something that would just make getting in shape easy?

Through adversity, I found a better, more-user-friendly method for getting my clients to work out and lift weights: one primary piece of equipment, the elliptical, along with simple hand weights. What a blessing in disguise!

Awakenings

If you decide to take the Onion journey, you need to dig deep in your soul and identify your urgency factors, the reasons that will keep you going during the most difficult days. You see, you might feel anger as you learn to replace your emotional voids with something besides food. The reward at the end of this journey will be exposing the real you inside. As you peel back the beginning layers, and people begin to notice it, you will receive some immediate gratification. But that may not be enough to guide you through tough days and you will tend to go back to old habits. So when I speak of urgency factors, the obvious ones are easy: divorce, a class reunion, or a wedding. Or a doctor has told you if you don't change the way you're eating and lose weight, you will die. Even worse, you've already had a medical emergency that might have been prevented if you'd had better nutrition and less fat.

I once read a poem online by Sonny Carroll titled "Awakening." I love these lines,

AWAKENING

A time comes in your life when, in the midst of all your fears and the insanity you're living with, you stop dead in your tracks and a voice inside your head cries out, 'Enough!' Through the fighting, crying, and struggling to hang on despite your despair, you know that now is the time to change. And like a child quieting down after a blind tantrum, your sobs begin to subside, you shudder once or twice, you blink back your tears, and you begin to look at the world through new eyes. This is your awakening. You realize it's time to stop hoping and waiting for something to change; to stop looking for happiness, safety, and security to come galloping over the next horizon. You come to terms with the fact that you are not Cinderella or Prince Charming. In the real world there aren't always fairy tale endings (or beginnings, for that matter) and any guarantee of 'happily ever after' must begin and end with you. And in the process a sense of serenity, of acceptance, is born.—Sonny Carroll, "Acceptance"

2. My Story

**I ALWAYS WONDERED WHY,
AS THE CLOTHES GOT LARGER,
THEY GREW FLOWERS.**

WHEN I WAS IN the ninth grade, I stood 5'10". I was taller than most of the boys and bigger than most of the girls. I hated the label of "big girl" and of feeling like I was not small enough, good enough, pretty enough... I'm sure you understand and perhaps remember the imprints and emotions of a teenager. If you have a teenager, you know the kind of pressure we put on ourselves at that point to fit in. I desperately wanted to be 5'2" and a size two; however, God did not make me that way.

I remember looking for my first prom dress. It was so frustrating trying to find a size fourteen that would fit right and look good. When I was preparing to have my senior pictures taken, I couldn't find the right clothes, and I felt so fat. I look back at those pictures now and think: Wow, I looked pretty good back then. At 300 pounds, I really thought I looked good back in high school! Why did I allow myself to grow into a 300-pound woman, when I was dissatisfied with my appearance as a 175-pound teen?

At least today a plus-sized person has many more options for clothes. During my "heavy" journey, I always wondered why, as the clothes got larger, they grew flowers and looked like something my grandmother would wear. I spent a large part of my life just wanting the cute clothes to be a little larger. Thank goodness for Lane Bryant and Delta Burke fashions, because they gave the plus-sized woman options. On the flip side, I have said so many times that stretch pants and sweat pants were the worst thing to happen to us, Onions. They enabled us to keep growing and growing. We lost the accountability factor of having to zip up our jeans.

In ninth grade, I picked up my first calorie-counting book and tried all of the diets in vogue back then. I went on the egg diet. I tried Dexatrim. Oh, and do you remember the Aids Chocolate Chews diet? I tried it too.

My senior year, I decided to join a fitness facility. A Vic Tanny gym was just down the street from my house. As I walked in, a petite thing with wads of energy greeted me. She seemed so excited to meet me until she looked at the guest register and realized I was too young to sign the contract to join. Since she would make no money on me, she gave me a polite, "Come back when you are eighteen."

After my eighteenth birthday, I returned to the facility. The honeymoon experience was fun. They seemed to take a real interest in my fitness goals and assured me that this was how you do it. After I signed up, I went in for my first workout and encountered a "there is the equipment, help yourself" attitude. This experience proved to be the place where I first caught the bug to make a difference in the fitness industry.

Later, I went to work for this same corporation and several others. At one point, my husband was hired to play for the Denver Broncos, and we moved to Colorado where I continued working in the fitness industry. Some of the facilities I've worked with include the following:

- Scandinavian Health Clubs, Indianapolis
- Holiday Health Clubs, Denver
- Consultant for 19 fitness facilities, Midwest
- Owner/operator of private fitness facility, Anderson, IN
- President, The Onion Factory℠
- Creator, Eat2Lose℠

Even though I worked in the industry, one day when I was thirty-five, I looked in the mirror, jumped on the scales, and found I had grown into the obese category. I was a 300-pound woman attempting to make fitness facilities user-friendly for beginners. While I was trying to help everyone else, I had lost myself.

How in the world had I spent almost twenty years in the fitness industry as a 300-pound woman? I must have been insane! I wanted support. I wanted to be thin so badly, I spent my young-adult lifetime making sure the information and facilities would be there for me like when I was eighteen. In all those years, I hadn't been motivated to change.

An Onion must have motivation. I believe you would not have invested in this book unless when you get up in the morning and look in the mirror butt-naked, you see fat.
One of the most profound statements I've ever heard while working in the fitness industry, was from a senior client who never really had a weight issue. She shared with me that she always worried about the extra five pounds that kept trying to creep up, so she would never need to worry about an extra 50 pounds. It was her way of keeping herself accountable. What a great idea!

Unfortunately, most of us form either false, or temporary motivations such as weddings, anniversaries, or class reunions, and we want results right here, right now. Those are external motivation. Instead, we need an internal process of understanding that our health and our lives are at risk.

Over the past few years, I've learned that one of the primary elements that has been missing from fitness programs is accountability. Yes, we need the right information. But even more, we need a reason to take care of ourselves, an urgency as well as some form of accountability, both of which have been missing.

My Turning Point

One day I conducted a photo shoot to benchmark my friend Susan's success of losing 80 pounds in five months. I kidded her that she was targeted to be a "Calendar Girl." ("Calendar Girl" was the nickname I gave someone when I spotlighted their success stories in the local newspaper. They reminded me of the movie, "The Calendar Girl." You know the one, where all the British girls—very large British Onions—come together to create a calendar for a charitable cause.) Making it as a "Calendar Girl" had become a fun goal at The Onion Factory℠, encouraging the girls to reach their health goals. They received validation through being spotlighted and telling their stories.

All that day, I recalled Susan's statement from the photo shoot: "A picture is worth a thousand words." It made me recall when I was a little girl. In all my childhood pictures, I was not chunky, heavy, or overweight. So what changed? What had been the turning point in my life?

Allow me to share an emotional truth I have never shared before. As I looked back that day, I realized that the trauma of my parent's divorce had been a turning point for me. From

Susan's Results

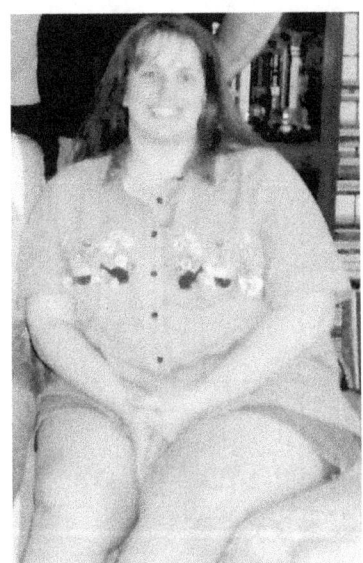

Susan BEFORE

DATE	5/6/07	12/12/07	4/9/08	FINAL
R. ARM	15"	11"	10.5"	-9"
BUST	47.5"	34.5"	34.5"	-13"
WAIST	41.5"	30"	29.5"	-12"
ABS	56.5"	37"	36"	-20.5"
HIP	56.5"	37"	37"	-19.5"
THIGH	28"	22"	22"	-12"
WEIGHT	256	155	152	-104
FAT MASS	116.7	42	40.4	
LEAN MASS	139.3	113	111.6	
FAT TO GO	91.7	17	15.4	
Lbs. Lost			104	
Inches Lost			86	
% Lost			19	

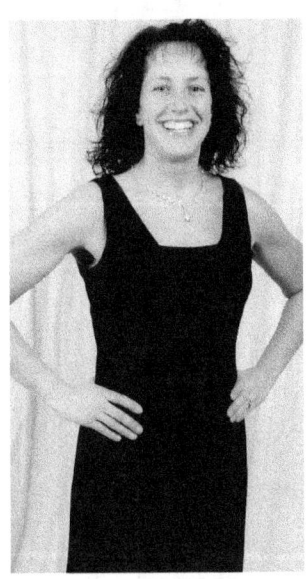

Susan AFTER

---

that point on, I found my refuge from pain and loss in food.

Mom was British, extremely gorgeous, and an incredible musician. As a matter of fact, the big band, for which she played saxophone, is still spotlighted in the Albert and Victoria Museum in London, England. She married my father when he was a sergeant major for the United States Army. Then they relocated to America from Germany and adopted me. Prior to the divorce, I felt pampered, indulged, and always accepted. As an only child, I was probably even a little spoiled. That all changed when I was eight and my parents' marriage ended.

At some point before the divorce, my mom got a little chunky and a neighbor said something to her about her weight. (At times, women can be so brutal to one another.) Whatever was said motivated my mother to regain her incredible figure. It was her urgency factor.

Shortly thereafter, her relationship with my father fell apart. I do not think the divorce was about weight gain or loss; I'm sure it had to do with other factors. But as a child, I could not understand why this was happening. I felt detached from reality and just learned to cope. I coped with food.

There was another factor in my childhood weight gain. As far as I can remember, while my mother was not escaping in food, she allowed me to. So one of us was always enjoying a food experience.

Have you ever had something similar happen to you? The moment you decide to modify your nutrition, to make healthy changes, it seems like everyone around you attempts to sabotage your efforts. They invite you to lunch and suggest, "One bite won't hurt." They say you look fine, just as you are.

As I grew up, my mother was still beautiful and dressed stylishly. Her alluring British accent would make any man swoon, at least

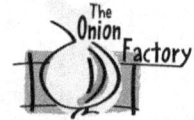 *Every time I lost weight through starvation, I was increasing the number of my fat cells, as well as increasing my percentage of fat.*

that's how I saw it as a young girl. How could I ever live up to that standard?

I was bigger than all the girls, taller than all the boys, and never felt like I fit in. Part of that lack of self-esteem and my insecurities probably stemmed from the divorce and the loss of the emotional stability. Plus, I think every tall girl feels some degree of alienation.

(At this point, as I was writing this manuscript, my editor asked me to explain "different." Well, here goes.)

My feeling different, even peculiar, stems from my beginnings. You see, I spent the first nine months of my life in an orphanage. I am not complaining. I was well cared for and my mom and dad adopted me when I was only nine months old.

Many orphaned children are not adopted at all. The older an orphan child becomes, chances of being adopted lessen. So I have no regrets or sad stories; however, I believe much of the initial nurturing a child needs in order to develop was missing. I am sure there were lots of babies, and surely not all of us could be snuggled, held, and coddled like a newborn would experience with that child's birth parents.

Very early in my development, I learned to hold my bottle and feed myself. So when my parents brought me home and wanted to feed me, I was not used to this. However, hungry for the emotional nourishment they were offering me, I gave in. After a few months of my mom's feeding me, she said that she was ready for me to feed myself. I would not. I had grown accustomed to her feeding me. I was expressing my first sense of independence. Again, I feel like I had a void in my emotional development.

When I add my lack of emotional attachment at birth to the loss of security when my parents divorced, I think I know why I turned to food to fill the void, the loss.

Body Image

I believe I had the first glimpse of "that feeling" when I was about fifteen. I was still taller than all the boys and bigger then the girls, but I must have been finding my way.

I visited my father for the summer and met my four stepbrothers. As I recollect, the first statement I made to my new stepmother was, "I am a vegetarian!" I am not sure if this statement was for shock value, or if it was the current "diet" I was attempting in order to come out of my chunky stage.

That summer, teenage boys first started to really pay attention to me. As they did, I wanted more attention. I found that dieting and starving made me feel in. And thin was in.

(An Onion recently said to me, "You know the fastest way to become invisible?" I said "No." She said, "Gain a hundred pounds." Suppose that means that if you lose a hundred pounds you become visible again?)

That summer of my fifteenth year, I learned that the thinner I became, the more attention I got. All for the wrong reasons, silly me! That summer, I also found the first benchmark of success in my weight-loss journey. I equated that success to a pair of Levis size 26 in the waist with a 36-inch length. I can remember thinking I had made it, because girls back in those days looked at the label other girls had on their jeans. You may not remember, but Levis had a leather tag on the right rear, which announced to the world your waist and length. So we kept those tags on!

Finally, I was not buying clothes in the "big girl" or "chunky" section. For my height, I was really too small and had a hard time finding a pair of jeans that would fit. You know, kind of like finding a 34 DD bra, or needing a size eight top and sixteen bottom. Nonetheless, I liked feeling in control. Being overweight was definitely being out of control.

But the short burst of being in control, using the methods of starvation and deprivation, turned out to be one of the most detrimental choices I could have ever made. I didn't even realize that every time I lost weight through starvation, I was increasing the number of my fat cells, as well as increasing my percentage of fat.

It took another twenty years before I could take control again and fix the engine I'd spent a lifetime destroying. I believe I have been like a lump of clay being molded and prepared to write the Onion guide.

My Mother's Question

I am thankful that I grew up differently. I am different. My differences played a large role in allowing me to visualize this incredible Onion system. If I can peel away my layers to find the source of my eating habits, I know that you can too.

After nearly two decades in the fitness industry, I remember a day that I wish would fade into deep memory. My mother (you know, the one with all the looks that I never thought I could measure up to) said, "Lisa can I ask you a question?"

I said, "Sure."

She said, "How can you be in the fitness industry and look like you do?"

I thought to myself: *That is exactly why I am in the fitness industry.* I was attempting to show club owners what someone like me needed.

As Onions, we need direction, education, support, and grace. We need to be inspired to change, motivated to change, and have a reason to change. (I do not care what reason, just find one!)

At some point after my mother's question, the table shifted. I figured it out. I put together the pieces of the puzzle and I lost more than 100 pounds. Even though I had often lost 25, 40, or 50 pounds, I had never changed my imprints and behaviors. I went on many short term fixes but never got to the root of the evil! I was not properly informed.

I found my purpose. I needed to learn how to put the puzzle together, not just for me, but so that you, too, could achieve results. As I got smaller, my mother was growing older and larger. I invested in several fitness center memberships for her in Florida. I attempted to teach her what I had discovered. But it felt like time and time again she would still ask me, "Can I eat x, y, z food?" The question would drive me crazy. You know, it seems like you have more patience for a perfect stranger than you do at times for someone very near and dear to your heart.

The Onion system is not so much about what you can or cannot eat as it is about understanding what will be stored if you eat too much of it. And understanding that you already have a storage tank and need to spend the reserve rather than add to it. If I had a dollar for every time I have shared the Onion formula with my mother, I would already be retired.

"Indiana Wants Me"

Some of the best ideas in this guide have come from my clients in Indiana. It's real life. We are not some reality show where all one has to do is worry about eating and working out. The women, who have helped me by sharing their bodies, emotions, and experiences along the way, not only had to change their workout and eating behaviors, but they had to continue to take care of the kids, go to work, and live in the real world. Their efforts and desired changes required knowledge, yes, but the changes also took desire and discipline. When the excitement of the first week expired, discipline and desire had to kick in.

A few years ago when I started working with Onion Campers, I had one elliptical machine, a few free weights, and a dream. I never imagined I would end up with a 7,000-square-foot base for The Onion Factory℠, a retail food store, a beautiful retreat to house women for weekend camps, and a book well on its way. In fact, as I think back to my childhood the song lyrics, "Indiana wants me,/ Lord, I can't go back there...," haunt me every time I hear them.

I felt very torn between the relationship I had with my mom and the relationship I desired with my dad who lived in Indiana. I think God has a sense of humor, because I thought I would be the girl living in a Manhattan high rise. Instead, I look out of my bedroom window into a cornfield! Who would have known I would be placed in Indiana to empower women with the knowledge to change?

From the beginning, Onion Campers did not all finish. Some went back to their old ways and found that their old results came back really fast. I decided to offer past campers an opportunity for a refresher course.

A lot has changed over the past few years. We've learned a few short cuts and had many new ideas. Our new facility has a full food division, so if a client is stuck, we can eliminate the margin for error by placing them in our food box.

The formula to lose fat is easy. The discipline to stay in the box and do the basics takes commitment. I have shared over and over: You must find your urgency factor. You must desire the new you more than you want the old one. Weight loss is more about finding yourself than it is about getting rid of the fat.

My Goal for This Book

While I want this guide to impress the medical community and be respected by the professional fitness community, my ultimate goal is that this book will inspire the average Joe or Jane. I want this to be a complete guide that will teach people in Boise, Omaha, or anywhere else in the U.S. how to peel themselves to a safe body composition of 26 percent fat.

I repeat: *My mission is to get as many people as I possibly can to 26 percent body fat*, because exercise alone, or changing your nutrition, or increasing your activity are simply not enough.

Twenty-six percent body fat is a benchmark for good health. That number should motivate you and toward a safe body composition that will prevent premature death. It is scary to think that 58 percent of the American population is dying from heart disease. Yes, there are some factors that we cannot control, like age and heredity; however, there are plenty of risk factors that we can control. One of them happens to be the percentage of fat that our bodies are carrying. Call it my obsession.

In one of my early case studies, I was warming up a client on the elliptical for her personal training session. We were exchanging a little banter about how sore she had gotten from her last training session.

I said, "Your soreness is a rumor."

She kept whining, so I blurted out, "Look, I am not an exercise kinesiologist. I am simply a writer committed to gathering data to finish this guide."

Then she shot back at me, "Have you ever considered that you may be a trainer who's faking being a writer?"

Her statement made me laugh. Truth be told, I'm not a kinesiologist or a professional writer. I am just a girl with a mission to change the course of obesity.

3. Our Problem, Ouch!

WILL WE SPEND OUR TIME ACHIEVING OUR GOALS OR MAKING EXCUSES?

TODAY, I SHOPPED AT one of my favorite organic grocery stores. My mindset has been if fit people go to fitness centers, healthy people must go to health-food grocery stores. My journey has been about trying to figure out the secrets of weight loss, specifically, fat loss.

Back in 2002, I was tired of being a fat girl. I assumed I would find a bunch of thin people at the health-food grocery stores. I quickly realized that vegetarians are not always thin. I watched to see what people were putting in their carts. Many of the foods they selected were full of grains and "natural" sugar. But I noticed their carts were often missing meats and other proteins. Eating organically and healthy may be wonderful, nutritionally, but I am not sure it is weight-loss worthy, or is fixing the problem of obesity.

As I was eating my organic lunch, I watched the checkout lane. I saw a very large, apple-shaped Onion paying for a basketful of high quality, very expensive food. I thought to myself: *This woman is making a large investment in her health, but she is missing the basics, and she is over fat.*

I know from experience when I was attempting to change, I bought into many beliefs that were not necessarily weight-loss worthy. There might have been some great "healthy" benefits from these beliefs, but changing the percentage of fat was not necessarily one of them. So the passion of changing the course of obesity brews within me. I believe this mission of mine started very early in life.

Have you ever seen the movie "Working Girl"? She—Melanie Griffin, you know, Antonio Banderas' wife and Don Johnson's ex wife—has this fire in her belly about a broadcasting idea, but she could not get anyone to listen. She keeps gathering newspaper articles and formulating her idea. Because she did not have the proper credentials, or a high enough position, she could not get anyone to pay attention. She gets really creative and finds a way to make the fire in her belly a reality. She gets bumped and bruised along the way, but she never gives up. If art imitates life, or visa versa, then the "Working Girl" movie might be the best way for you to really understand the fire in my belly.

What Is Normal?

Currently, the average American woman wears a size 14. In past decades, normal looked like a size 8. Throughout the years, I have seen so many women desperate to be able to shop in the regular size clothes. We went from never being able to find clothes that would fit to having plus-size clothing stores readily available. Now we've made a full circle to this place of desperation to regain a sense of normalcy.

Our problem? We don't know where are our numbers are supposed to be. Where are you? Let's start with some beginning benchmarks (chart below). These benchmarks were gathered by the American Heart Association.

Excuses

I need to talk to you about excuses, and we all use 'em. I laugh when I think back to when I believed having a child was the demise of my successful weight loss. At some point, probably when my children were out of diapers (definitely when they started school, and most certainly when they became teenagers), the concept of my extra weight being linked to my being a mom was worn out!

After more than twenty years in the fitness industry, I've observed these top three excuses as to why someone has allowed himself, or herself, to grow into an Onion.

Excuse Number One: You have no time. Okay, do you really have time to feel lousy, or to be sick? After all, an ounce of prevention is worth a pound of cure.

Excuse Number Two: You have no money. I hope you are really angry when you complete this guide and decide to let nothing prevent you from changing your life. How many thousands of dollars have we spent per year on stuff that does not work? And for goodness sake, do you realize the latest surgery craze can cost as much as $30,000, and an endless amount of people are dying for the results? To think this guide, which you purchased for less than $100, is the complete guide to change. That is, if you really want to change, and you are truly are ready, you can.

Excuse Number Three: You are going to start tomorrow, next week, next month, or the beginning of the year. Do you realize the present, right now, is all the time you have? You cannot change the past, but you can most certainly steer your future. You decide. Check off if you would not want to:

1. Have more energy
2. Feel better
3. Sleep better
4. Relieve stress
5. Prevent premature death

When a client really wants to change and really wants the results, The Onion Factory is where *life-changing results are typical.*

Normal Numbers

Body Fat

Competitive	Lean	Safe	Obese
5–8%	16–20%	26%	30%+

Body Mass Index

Low	Normal	High
<18.5	18.5–24.5	25+

Cholesterol / LDL (Artery Blocking) / Women to Men

Low (Good)	Borderline High	High (Bad)	Ouch! (Very Bad)
100–129	130–159	160–189	190+

Cholesterol / HDL (Artery Maintaining) / Women to Men

Low	Normal (OK)	High (Best)
40–50	50–60	60+

3. Our Problem, Ouch! /// 27

Chris' Story

For several years now, Chris has been an angel on my shoulder. She will tell you that she was led to The Onion Factory℠. The Factory's newspaper ad was the first one of its kind to catch her eye, because the picture captured women of all shapes and sizes. She thought it was strange, because most fitness ads pictured people who were in great shape.

Six months earlier, Chris had been to her doctor. For the first time, she heard and read the diagnosis. Obese. Surely she was not obese. Maybe a little chunky. Maybe her blood pressure was a little high. And even though her blood sugar was high, she told me that she certainly was not obese.

I laugh every time I hear her tell this story, because she goes on to say that it took her another six months to digest the reality of her obesity diagnosis before she made the call. You know—the one you make when you first accept that you may need to change, and you get the nerve to dial the number.

For Chris, weight loss had not been the roller-coaster journey most of us experience. This was her first attempt to change after realizing that perhaps the doctor's notes were her call to action to improve her current level of health.

When Chris called, I went through the normal half-dozen questions to find out the caller's needs. "Have you ever been on a diet? How many? Are you currently working out? Do you have any medical limitations?"

Then I asked Chris, "How much weight would you like to lose?" Chris answered that she thought she needed to lose 50 to 60 pounds. I continued, "What size are you now, and what size would you like to be?" She replied that she wore a size 24 and thought it would be great to be an 18.

I replied, "What about a size 16, or a 14?"

With this banter, Chris and I began a journey together. Look at her results so far...

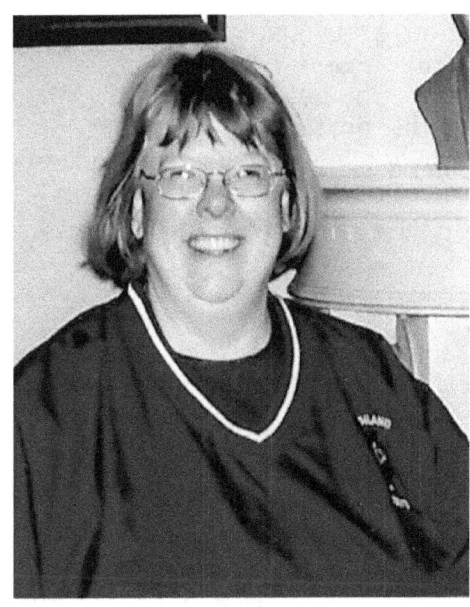

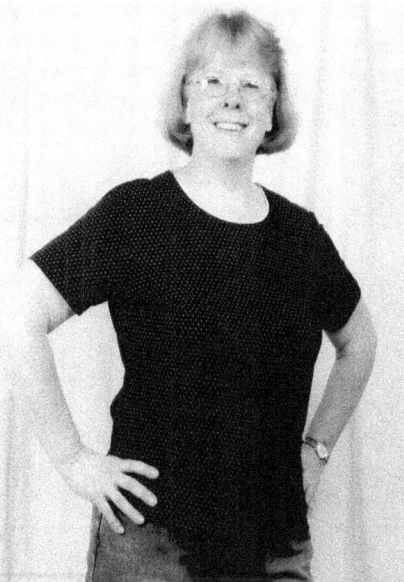

DATE	12/9/04	3/30/05	6/23/05	FINAL
R. ARM	13"	12"	11"	-6"
BUST	53"	44"	40"	-15.5"
WAIST	44.25"	36"	33"	-15.25"
ABS	53.5"	46"	40.5"	-15.5"
HIP	52.75"	46"	41"	-15.75"
THIGH	25.5"	23.5"	23"	-9"
WEIGHT	253	202	178	
FAT MASS	121	82	65	
LEAN MASS	132	120	113	
FAT TO GO	96	57	40	
Lbs. Lost			102	
Inches Lost			77	
% Lost			17.5	

Chris BEFORE   Chris AFTER   Chris' RESULTS

It took her six months to make the call.

The Onion Factory℠ is available 24 hours a day, 7 days a week. Throughout our 8-week Onion Camp, we feed our Onions many of the same recipes we give you in this book. We provide one-on-one training. As a result, our little community is empowered with the knowlewdge to change. This guide gives you The Onion Factory℠ between two covers. Additional help is available through our online community at www.onioncamp.com. If you really want to change, do it. Everything you need is right at your fingertips.

When I first began planning to implement the Onion system, I was only looking to help change the lives of 100-pound overweight girls. I thought: *Who cares if I, only one person, lost 100 pounds? But how incredible would it be if a system could be created documenting numerous 100-pound losses, presenting a track record powerful enough to influence our society and change the course of obesity?* Not a diet, not a short-term fix for a deeper issue, but a lifetime solution and a sustainable system.

Knowledge is power. And unfortunately, with old dieting systems we only learned how to starve and deprive our engines, rather than how to take care of them. I thought, *If 100 girls from a small community lost 100 pounds, then their success would certainly debunk some old habits, old beliefs, and old behaviors.* I call Chris "the angel on my shoulder," because she believed in my vision. She committed to improve her health, but more so, she took a bigger leap of faith and committed to contribute in validating the Onion system by losing 100 pounds, rather than 60. And she lost it in nine months, just like I did.

Originally, my plan was to work with women who wanted to lose 100 pounds or more. My goal has always been to help as many people as I could to reach the safe body composition rate of 26 percent. When an Onion reaches that safe percentage, I feel I have done my job and made a difference. I recently watched the movie "Walk that Line." It is the story about Johnny Cash and June Carter-Cash. I found my favorite line at one point in the movie when she states, "I just wanna matter." For me, changing the course of obesity is my way of mattering.

Through your weight-loss journey—no, not your weight-loss journey, but your journey to find yourself—you need to keep in mind that 26 percent is only the first benchmark. In the fitness world, 16–20 percent is considered the desired range.

The strategies that work to peel away layers of unwanted fat are much different than the strategies to fine-tune or sculpt a body style. I am really good at peeling Onions. Sculpting an Onion is not at this point in time my specialty, or passion.

This Journey Is about Body Fat

In the fall of 2006, I had a few openings in an eight-week camp, so I offered a three-for-one opportunity. A group consisting of a mom, a daughter, and a sister-in-law signed up. Two of the three were not much more than 30 percent body fat. They were around 33 to 34 percent. I am so thankful I had the opportunity to work with girls who were close to reaching their goals, because in eight weeks the two girls reached their 26 percent benchmark.

Finishing a client, in this case two clients, in eight weeks is very exciting. At this stage of the game, we had about six girls who had reached their 26 percent. Speaking of 26 percent successes, I really need to share Ann's story with you.

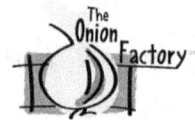 *With old dieting systems we only learned how to starve and deprive our engines, rather than how to take care of them.*

> *Ann went below 26% fat. In fact, she's the first Onion to go below 19%!*

DATE	7/11/07	10/15/07	12/20/07	FINAL
R. ARM	11.75"	10"	9"	-5.5"
BUST	35.5"	31.5"	30.5"	-5"
WAIST	27.5"	23.5"	22.5"	-10"
ABS	39"	34"	32"	-7"
HIP	41"	36"	34"	-7"
THIGH	23.5"	20"	19"	-9"
WEIGHT	148	125	116	
FAT MASS	49.43	32.6	21.9	
LEAN MASS	98.5	92.5	94.1	
FAT TO GO	24.4	7.6	-3	
		Lbs. Lost	32	
		Inches Lost	43.5	
		% Lost	8.2	

Ann's RESULTS

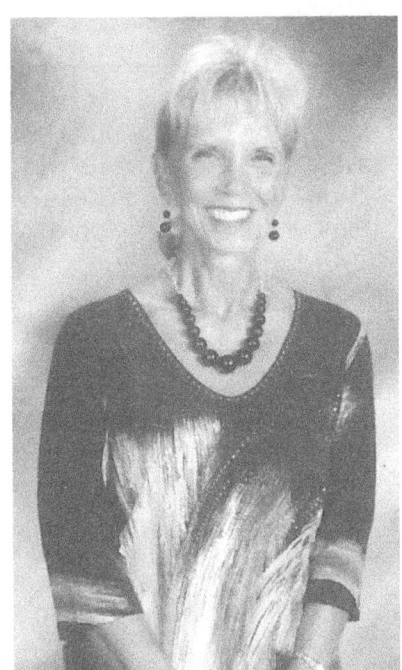

Ann AFTER

Ann's Story

Ann was not really an Onion, or as least she didn't look like a typical Onion. By all visual accounts, many women looked at her and wondered why she was attending an eight-week camp. When she came to camp, Anne wore a size 14 and her body fat was 34 percent. She had been on a few short-term diets, and she had a knee injury, which had impeded her cardiovascular training.

What the other women didn't know was that Ann had just left her plastic surgeon. She was a gorgeous 59-year-old, but she had come to a point in her life when she wanted to look a little better. She had planned to go in for a $9,000 liposuction procedure. However, it had been put on hold due to an abnormal reading on one of her pre-surgical tests.

That same day, Ann bumped into her neighbor, Cathy, who had just graduated from Onion Camp, going from a 33 percent body fat composition to 27 percent. Ann looked at her in amazement and said, "What have you done?"

Cathy told her, "I'm an Onion."

Having been turned down for the surgery and seeing Cathy's new shape, Ann (a teacher who wanted to make these changes over summer break) decided she had to get into an Onion Camp soon. So she asked Cathy for help.

Cathy told her, "Lisa is starting a new camp soon, but I believe it is full."

Nonetheless, Ann convinced Cathy to call the Factory and try to get a spot in the next camp. Ann was a girl on a mission. By the way, Cathy and Ann happen to live one street away from the Factory.

I well remember what happened next. As I was talking on my cell phone with Cathy about squeezing another girl into the next camp, I pulled into my driveway and parked. The instant I hung up the phone, Ann pulled in right behind me. I grinned, got out of the truck, and said, "Hi, you must be Ann."

Ann was an amazing Onion Camper. She stayed in the box, eating healthy and working out, during her entire journey. She started as a size 14 and is currently in a size 2. She went from 34 percent body fat to less than 19 percent in five months and a few days.

Ann is the most disciplined Onion I've ever had. Perhaps 25 years of teaching first graders had conditioned her to build good habits.

Why Diet?

Everyone knows the first week of a "diet" means a large amount of pounds lost on the scale. We love it. The numbers are validation, a feeling we all love. As the diet process continues, the large numbers usually slow down.

We need to go back to the evolution of dieting and learn how we were lead down a wrong path. We dieters never really knew what weight we were losing: water, muscle, or fat? We were just so excited to see the numbers on the scale go down; we assumed we were on the right track. We could take a water pill today and on the scale tomorrow be five pounds lighter. And then, we would believe we'd won a victory. The water loss was just a short-term psychological solution for a bigger problem, which was to change your percentage of fat and overall health.

We have all heard that to keep weight off you need to lose weight slowly, about two pounds per week. Diets of the past were based on calorie restriction. A person usually cut back what they ate, or started to exercise, seldom both. As Onions, we never really loved the exercise part, so we usually tried the latest diet solution.

Whoever thought eating more and getting proper hydration would play such an important role in changing our bodies and our level of health?

You may be wondering how many pounds of fat reserve a body can spend per week. How much of your reserve tank can you really burn? Keep reading and the answers will become obvious.

In the reality-television world of weight loss, you'll see some crazy weekly weight-loss numbers, as much as 28 pounds lost in a week. You have also seen a week where contestants did all the work and lost nothing. How can either of these scenarios be true? Keep in mind with both of these situations, the individuals are thinking, living, and breathing physical workouts, which is not exactly life in the real world!

So let me explain why diets do not work. The first clue is the first three letters of the word, D I E. Diets are about deprivation and starvation. That's why they don't work. The only people who are winning with diets are all the diet centers that keep us coming back for more of their products.

Here's why we come back for more. A diet is a short-term fix for a lifelong problem. It is an eight-week commitment, maybe longer, to drastically reduce your caloric intake. In some cases, you drink a certain number of shakes—without real food value—until you et into a target weight range.

Let's say that you weigh 250 pounds, of which 45 percent is fat. Are you aware that you could lose 100 pounds and still be 45 percent fat? You've not really improved your level of health. In fact, a large portion of the weight you lost could have just been water, or worse, muscle!

Let's take it one step further. You wake up at the beginning of the week, which also happens to be the beginning of the month New Years Day. You've tried on a few outfits, gotten a reality check, and realized you'd better do something about your weight. So, you go to the phone book, or watch the TV commercials, and you select your current favorite diet program. In most cases, these programs restrict your calorie intake to 1,000 calories or maybe as low as 800 calories. Even though the American Dietary Association suggests that it is very difficult to get proper nutrition, even if you are eating good food that has value, below 1,200 calories. We do it anyway. We are desperate. That class reunion is coming up.

Let's say you start with a 1,500-calorie metabolic rate and you have 30 pounds that you need to get off. The diet plan of choice lowers your caloric intake. In some cases, the caloric intake is so low that they may recommend you don't exercise. You lose 30 pounds. But what did you lose? Yes, you lost some fat, maybe some water. But I will bet that you also sacrificed some of your lean mass. And if you did, you just lowered your metabolic rate.

So you started with a metabolic rate of 1.500 calories per day and now it's 1,300. If you couldn't maintain your weight when you had a metabolic rate of 1,500, how in the world are you going to maintain your loss with a lower metabolic rate?

I will assume that while you were on x, y, or z program, you did not learn how to change what you ate, why you ate, or the nutritional value of what you ate. A smaller portion of junk food never really made any sense to me. Everyone wants us to learn how to eat a restricted amount of food for a period of time. And then we go back to our old ways, because we really never learned how to eat or for what reason. Food was meant to fulfill our nutritional needs. You know, vitamins and minerals. Food cannot feed our souls, bolster our emotions, or fill our relational needs!

I am an eater. Show me what I *can* eat, not what I cannot. Measuring my lettuce, or cutting an apple in half never really worked for me. I wanted to find a way I could eat for the rest of my life. More importantly, a plan that would take off the extra weight, lower the risk factors, and keep the pounds off. No more short-term fixes for a problem I had been struggling with since I was a teen.

I have a question for you. This is my favorite part of the seminar. I want you to imagine you are in the front row totally engaged in learning this Onion stuff, and I pop the million-dollar question on you. Remember this is a trick question. Which weighs more, five pounds of fat or five pounds of muscle?

We are so programmed to believe muscle weighs more. Maybe it's the extra pounds, or the numbers on the scale that make us think it's okay if we believe muscle weighs more. The truth is they both weigh five pounds. The misconception is, simply, a five-pound pot roast might be the size of a football, but five pounds of feathers might take up the space of a pillowcase. Which item would you rather have on your tushie? I hope you said the pot roast. At least the roast is solid and takes up less space.

The best part about the difference between fat and muscle is that *muscle mass is your engine.* Muscle can increase or decrease your metabolic rate. Every pound of muscle requires 50–100 calories per day to maintain itself. Fat only needs three calories per pound each day. Fat is literally dead weight.

We are Onions because we allowed ourselves to grow larger than a safe body-fat composition. Anything over 30 percent is morbidly obese. Anything over the 25 pounds of fat that we need to insulate our bodies from cold temperatures will cause risk factors.

When we are morbidly obese, we risk dying from heart disease or developing Type II diabetes. That much fat lowers our quality of life, leaving us with no energy, lethargic, and short of breath.

Remember, lean mass is your metabolic engine. Lean mass includes muscle, bone density, organs, and water. There is not one type of risk factor associated with lean mass. We know that we do not want to lose bone density, yet that happens naturally as we get older. Your organs are vital and water is essential. And, oh yes, muscle has wonderful aesthetic values.

Suppress Your Appetite? Not!

A few times a year, advertisers try to inspire a mad dash for appetite suppressants. Usually this blitz is at the beginning of the new year or the beginning of another holiday season. Time and time again, we are told that we can achieve weight loss by suppressing our appetites. In reality, slowing our appetite could actually slow down our metabolic rate. Our bodies learn and adjust to perform on less food. If we were going to suppress something, it should be our cravings. It is our cravings that tempt us to make bad choices.

The horrible truth about cravings is once you have opened the box such as sugar it is very

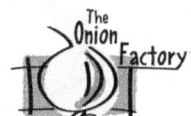

Muscle mass is your engine.

It can increase or decrease

your metabolic rate.

32 /// The Fork Is Mightier Than the Gym

difficult to shut down again. If you can lean on the foods that will not feed your fat cells, or be stored as fat and not open the craving box, you will be able to make better choices. With food, we need to rethink the way we eat and why we eat.

Good News for Fluffy People

If you have a 100 pounds or more to lose, you may be luckier than you realize. You see, you have been carrying around a hundred-pound dumbbell all day long. Pick up a bag of your water softener salt, carry it down your driveway, and tell me how exhausted you are. Now, think of two, or three, of them and carrying them all day long. You have been building muscle, and you did not even realize it! Bravo, save the engine, feed the engine, and burn the fat!

With a calorie restrictive mindset, when you reduce your intake below 1,200 per day, it is very difficult to get enough of the essential vitamins and minerals your body requires. Even with the lower calorie amount, you may not lose weight. Your body simply adjusts. If you are tired and do not feel good, this may be a warning sign that your body is not getting enough proper nutrition to function. We have larger bodies than past generations, but we are malnourished. Calories (sigh)! When I started counting them thirty years ago, I thought I could consume a mere 500 calories per day and lose. My Brainiac

Eating Sugar

- Regardless of your level of activity, the human body cannot process more than about 24 sugar grams a day.

- If your activity level is not great enough, your body will store your surplus food calories as fat. This was the reason for the sugar-free dieting concept. However...

- There are destructive long-term effects from eating foods with little to no nutritional value.

- Ice cream is almost entirely fat and sugar. When you open the door to this temptation, you will want to dive in farther!

- When you do not feed your body adequately, it will burn your lean mass (muscle). This reduces your body's metabolic rate, so that your body cannot utilize the same amount of food. The surplus is then stored as fat.

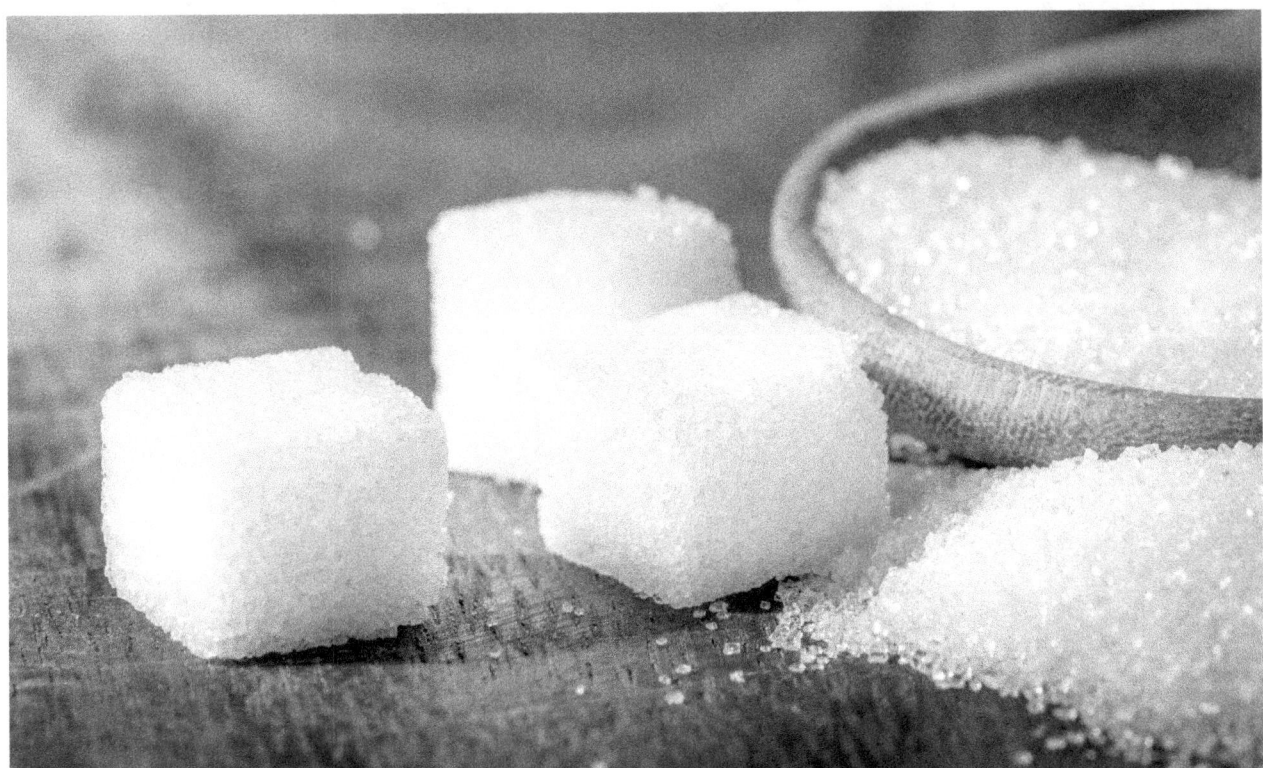

idea was if I used the 500 calories from my favorite foods like pumpkin or cheesecake ice cream from Mothers Ice Cream in Wisconsin (Yum!), then I could have what I wanted to eat and still lose. Silly girl. At that point, I did not understand a few essential things about how the human body works, such as the body's relationship with sugar.

Body Type and Weight Loss

Here is another piece of the changing-your-life puzzle. As you transform your body, you must accept the fact that your body type is your body type. That is what your parents gave you. No matter how lean you get, if your weight is currently held in your butt, your hips, or your chest as you lose and change, those areas are still going to be fuller parts of your figure. You will need to accept the new you with sexy hips, a Jay Lo butt, or a Marilyn Monroe figure.

Recently, I sat down for a client's weigh and measure. The Onion in front of me looked discouraged. She was looking down, her shoulders drooping, and wearing not even a hint of a smile. The scale said she had lost three pounds.

It is amazing how we can make poor food choices or remain inactive for years, but the moment we make a few changes, we want to wave a magic wand and have that 100 pounds disappear right here and right now. Perhaps that is why bariatric surgery has become so popular. We all are looking for that magic pill, potion, or wand to fix us.

I have a secret for you: There is no magic pill or magic formula out there; however, there is a safe way to eat and lose 15–20 pounds per month. There is a way to fix your blood sugar levels. There is a way to strengthen your heart and prevent premature death caused by heart disease and other weight related diseases.

Imagine this: Three pounds of fat lost per week is 12 pounds per month. In nine months, that would add up to 108 pounds. So you see, the secret to weight loss is not in a pill, a surgery, or a potion. It's in you.

The secret is to change your bad choices, bad behaviors, and old beliefs and then finish the journey. Instant gratification never really worked, and we have all heard that "slow and steady wins the race." Everyone is so impressed when they hear the weight loss stories of my clients who have lost 50, 75, or 100 pounds, two or three pounds at a time.

34 /// The Fork Is Mightier Than the Gym

Losing three pounds per week, or more, is not difficult. Staying focused and committed for nine months is the secret.

This process is about knowledge; yes, but the change is just as much about acceptance and understanding.

4. How This Guide Directs You

THIS GUIDE IS ABOUT your journey toward better health, particularly your relationship with food. Once a person changes their relationship with food, he or she will never need to "diet" again.

This program is not about being thin or heavy; it is about eliminating, or improving the health risk factors caused by the food you are eating. This journey is also about becoming empowered with the correct information, so you can increase your activity at an accountable rate.

You will learn how to build additional lean mass, feed your engine, and understand the emotions, which may interfere with your choices, thereby, creating the new you. No more ups and downs; just a journey of peeling and inventing a new you. As you read Chapter Five of this guide, I will share four principles with you on how to change your current life path and find that woman or man who is hiding behind the layers, or maybe even walls, of fat.

Chapter Six is the Free Seminar. You will learn the same materia that I have been teaching for more than two decades in fitness facilities and hospital wellness centers. As you read through this section, you will come to a point where I will ask you to stop and reflect on what you've learned and decide if you are really ready to make this change. You may even need to put this guide away until you really know that you are ready.

Then I'll walk you through a chapter to help your realize the psychology of an Onion and how to change your thinking.

Of course, we will explore food. I'll suggest what foods you will throw in your grocery cart and how to eat out. I'll also give you some great recipes the entire family will enjoy.

Once you know in your heart and soul that you're ready to begin, I will take you step-by-step through an eight-week journey. I've heard that it takes twenty-one days to make or break a new habit. I'm giving you an extra seven days, and then doubling it to help guarantee your new lifestyle behaviors and support the new you!

We'll cross the finish line together and learn how to live in healthy maintenance for the rest of your life.

K.I.S.S.

For a number of years, I taught a Nutrition 101 class in privately owned fitness facilities and hospital wellness centers. I created a KISS (keep it simple, stupid) approach to the factors that were needed to change one's weight and level of health. Frequently, at the end of the one-hour class people would feel empowered with knowledge and the answers, yet still felt confused about where to begin. What is a carb, which are the correct carbs, what are the unlimited ones, which ones do I need to pay attention to, and which ones are going straight to my butt?

Using all the information I'd learned and experienced, I developed a four-step course to elaborate on the information I provided in my free seminar.

This guide is set up with the same format. I will share the four factors you need to change your life. I will take each topic and give you more guidance and knowledge with which to support your journey and to inspire you for eight weeks, just like I do in camp. I will give you a topic for the week, which I will ask you to read on Sunday. I will include tips and ideas to help support you until your next Sunday read.

From my experience in my workshops, you should see between 10 and 20 pounds of fat loss in your first month. The variable is whether, or not, you apply all four of the factors. In my own experience, I've found that my weekly results motivated me to get to the next level. Low, or no results can give you more drive to change the numbers for next week—if you really want it.

The Onion Factory℠ is about feeding yourself in a way that does not leave you hungry. It is about balance and good nutrition. You should see added benefits such as more energy, a better complexion, and a better mental attitude. And it is about finding yourself. Each day you do, you become a little more powerful and purposeful.

But Wait...

Let's put on the brakes for a moment to emphasize that *the journey begins by accepting the body you were given*. Yes, you can learn how to peel an Onion; however, your body style is your body style. You can create a healthier you and a better you. But if you are top-heavy or bottom-heavy at size 24, you will still have that proportion at a size 10. You cannot change the structure of you. Visually, you can make your good points better and hide the imperfections, but butt naked in the mirror, my goal for you is to start loving you. Inside out. We are never going to be Angelina Jolie, Halle Berry, or Marilyn Monroe; however, we can certainly do better than bodies that are 30 plus percentage of fat.

In the psychology of the Onion world, you need to accept yourself. You are not starting

---

"Keep It Simple, Silly!"

(X) Amount of Protein
Depending on Weight and Activity Level

10 Cups "Grass of the Lands"

30 Grams of Fat
or less

24 Grams of Sugar
Choose wisely!

yet another diet, you are not going to starve yourself anymore, and you are not going to start something again that you'll blow by the end of the week. You are going to make small adjustments and continue to cultivate better results. This is not a decision to diet, sabotage, or starve; this is a decision to get well.

You are going to change that attachment you have with the scale. The scale tells us absolutely nothing as far as health risk factors are concerned. The scale is simply a measure of how many pounds you weigh—pounds of good mass and pounds of not-so-good mass. My goal is to reinforce healthy levels of body fat percentages for a better quality of LIFE.

How Thin Is Thin Enough?

For a few years, I dated a guy I called Richard Gere. He was not *the* Richard Gere, but his looks resembled the real one in Hollywood. At one point, I thought he might be the perfect match for me. He was great looking, spiritually mature, we shared wonderful dinners out together, and he was into fitness.

At the point I met him, I was in my size eight Ann Taylor little black dress. (I know this because I have two black dresses, one is a size eight, and the other is a 10. The second one is the back-up plan when I have not been on my best game nutritionally or consistent enough with my exercise efforts. Those two black dresses are a benchmark of my body image.)

One day, he suggested we train for the Indianapolis Mini-Marathon. I am not a runner, but I thought the idea was very cool, and I love a challenge. He would come to my town on his days off and we would walk/run six miles in the park. I got up to three miles straight running. I never really fell in love with running; you know chesty girls and running are not the greatest mix. I soon figured out the reason Richard wanted me to run was he wanted me leaner.

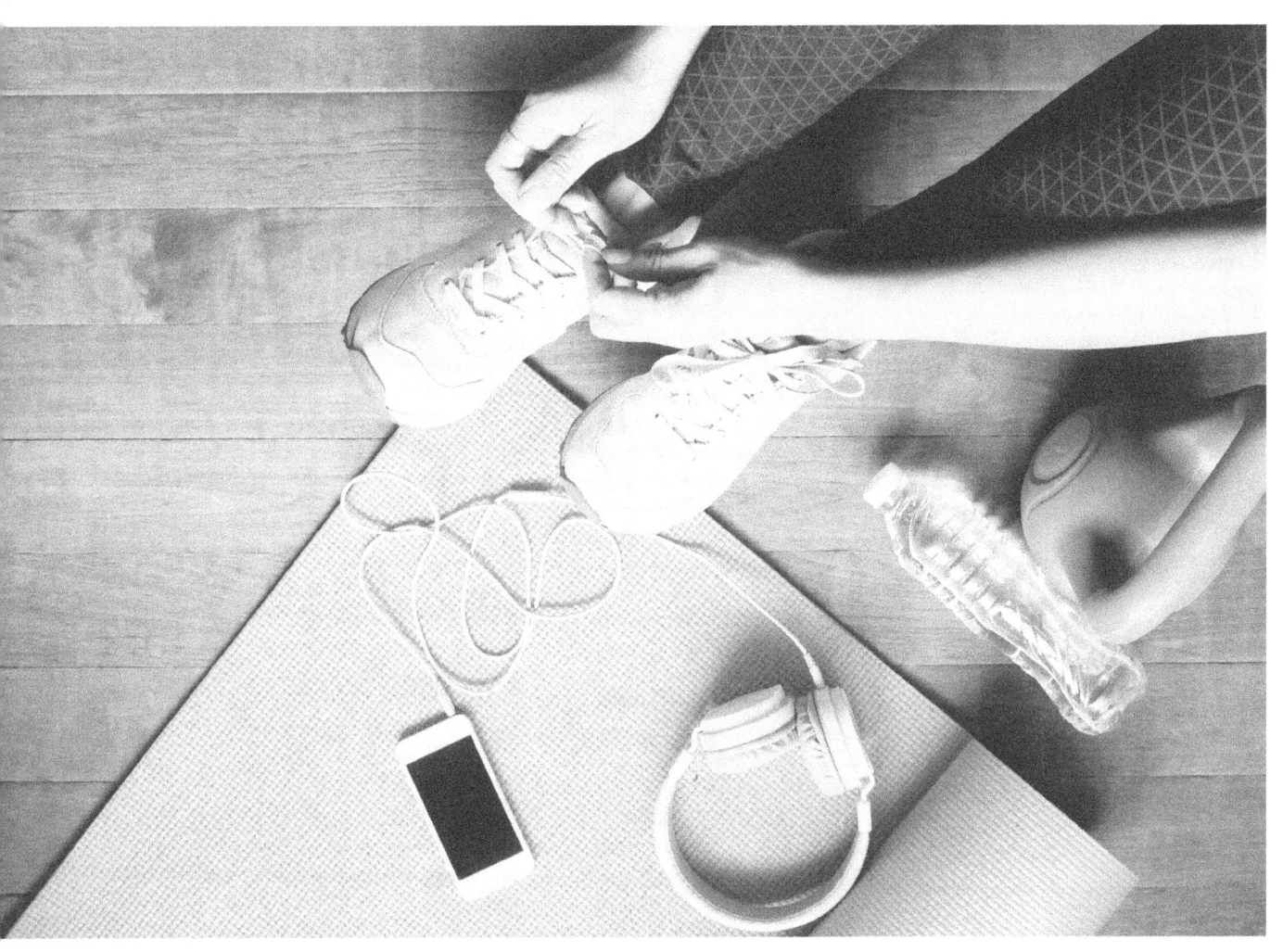

I had already accepted the fact that God did not make me 5'2" and a size 2, and I understood also that God did not create me to be a 300-pound girl. For me, size 8 was good enough, but Richard wanted me to wear the classic size 2.

Once I had worn size six Ralph Lauren jeans, but a size six was really tough for me. Yes, I felt I looked thin; however, there was absolutely no wiggle room with my nutrition and exercise. At size eight, I am on my game. At size ten, I am still comfortable, but by size twelve, I realize it is time to put on the brakes. It's time to get in the box and be accountable.

Richard went on and found his size 2, and I went on and continued to find myself.

Not a Skinny Fitness Trainer

If another fitness professional were to look at me, they might say I still could be leaner. They are correct. There is a huge difference between 26 percent body fat and the fitness standard of 16–20 percent for females. In my size 6 outfit, I have 18 percent body fat, which is a far cry from the 46 percent I started from, but it is very difficult for me to maintain.

To put it simply, I believe I don't need to have a skinny body image to change the course of obesity.

Neither did Richard Simmons. He wasn't trying to make the cover of *Muscle and Fitness Magazine*, but he was passionate and dedicated to helping change the course of obesity. You have to love his high energy and his desire to help women and men like us.

Obesity is not a joke anymore; it is crippling our nation, but proper health choices will enable us to change. This book will help you make those choices every day.

5. Are You Ready to Peel?

AT THE VERY BEGINNING of this book, I mentioned that peeling an Onion is incredibly easy. Once you understand the tools you will need, you will literally peel away layer after layer from your body. In fact, each week as I administer weigh-ins and measurements, I am amazed at how consistently the body truly peels. If clients lose five inches off their chest area, most likely the loss will be seen proportionately in their abdomens and hips.

Let me briefly review how you will safely spend 3–5 pounds of fat and lose 3–5 inches per week. Keep in mind I did not say "diet" them off. I referred to the process as spending. Those extra pounds are just a storage tank of stocked-up calories. These are the five ways you will burn fat as you peel away (spend away) your layers.

The Calorie Spending Chart on this page shows that you will be able to burn 1,700 calories of stored fat every day by changing your eating and exercise habits. Multiply that by seven and it equals 11,900 calories spent from your reserve tank each week. Divide 11,900 by 3,500 calories, which is one pound of fat, and there you have it: a

5 Calorie Spending Areas

1. Metabolic Change	500 Calorie reduction per day
2. THR—Cardiovascular training	400 Calorie reduction per day
3. Weight bearing/strength training	400 Calorie reduction per day
4. Proper hydration	200 Calorie utilization per day
5. Digestion	200 Calorie utilization per day

minimum of three and a half pounds of fat spent per week!

Throughout this guide, you will read personal journeys of clients who experienced even bigger reductions of fat than the projected three and a half pounds.

Nutritional Formula

Before you go any further, I want to give you the basic formula, the nutritional guide, that allowed me to take off more than 100 pounds in nine months, and how others have taken off 100 pounds in as little as six months. I want to give you just the portion of the formula I think needs time to percolate in your brain. I've learned a few tricks along the way, so I think you will have an advantage over me.
I will go over this formula several times throughout this guide. Brainwashing works! We have spent so many years eating the wrong things that it will take repetition for the Onion formula to soak in. Here is the basic formula to the nutrition plan. I will teach you a few adjustments along the way as your cardiovascular, strength training, and activity levels increase.

The chart below will make it easy for you to see how many carbohydrates, proteins, and fats your body requires for your daily caloric intake.

If you can manage to keep an eye on only one part of this chart, remember this: *Not all carbohydrates are created equal.* Yes, they are all processed as sugar, and if your activity level is not active enough to burn them off, then all of the sugar you consume will turn into fat. However, your body does not process all carbohydrates in the same way. Some burn off fast, some slow. If you learn to eat carbohydrates that burn off quickly, you will not fill your fat storage tank.

I'm sure you have heard of the glycemic index, which ranks carbohydrate foods on the basis of how they affect blood sugar (glucose). This is important for many people, because, eating a lot of foods that rank high on the glycemic index will produce spikes in blood sugar that can lead to loss of sensitivity to insulin, the hormone needed to allow blood sugar to enter cells for use as fuel. Insulin resistance is associated with obesity, high blood pressure, elevated blood fats, and an increased risk of Type II diabetes. Knowing the sugar and carbohydrate content of the foods you eat is important in peeling an Onion. If you look at food labels, you will always be able to distinguish between the goodies and the uglies. Here we go.

Nutritional Guide

Caloric Intake: 1,200/Day
Carbohydrates: 720 cal/189g
Protein: 240 cal/60g
Fat: 240 cal/24g

Caloric Intake: 1,300/Day
Carbohydrates: 780 cal/195g
Protein: 260 cal/65g
Fat: 260 cal/26g

Caloric Intake: 1,400/Day
Carbohydrates: 840 cal/210g
Protein: 280 cal/70g
Fat: 280 cal/28g

Caloric Intake: 1,500/Day
Carbohydrates: 900 cal/210g
Protein: 300 cal/75g
Fat: 300 cal/24g

Caloric Intake: 1,600/Day
Carbohydrates: 960 cal/240g
Protein: 320 cal/80g
Fat: 320 cal/32g

Caloric Intake: 1,700/Day
Carbohydrates: 1,020 cal/225g
Protein: 340 cal/84g
Fat: 340 cal/34g

Caloric Intake: 1,800/Day
Carbohydrates: 1,080 Cal/270g
Protein: 360 cal/90g
Fat: 360 Cal/36g

Caloric Intake: 1,900/Day
Carbohydrates: 1,100 Cal/289g
Protein: 380 cal/95g
Fat: 380 Cal/38g

Caloric Intake: 2,000/Day
Carbohydrates: 1,200 Cal/300g
Protein: 400 cal/100g
Fat: 400 Cal/40g

*NOTE: We have rounded these numbers to the nearest 10 for ease of comparison.

CARBOHYDRATES		
THE BADS	**THE UGLIES**	**THE GOODS**
Refined Sugars	Starches	Whole Fruits and Veggies
Table Sugar	Bread and Pasta	Green Leafy Vegetables
Brown Sugar	Potatoes	Cruciferous Vegetables
	Corn	"Grass of the Lands"
	Bananas	Berries

Simple carbohydrates are refined sugars. Consume no more than 24 sugar grams; any more will go straight to your butt. Unless, of course, your activity level is high enough to burn off the extra carbs you ate. One tablespoon of sugar is equal to four grams of simple carbohydrates. Sugars contains no nutritional value, but boy do we crave them! And once you indulge, it is tough to stop.

Next are the *starches*. If you are at, or below 26 percent body fat, you may consume no more than 20 percent, or 46 grams of starch carbs. If your percentage is higher, then leave these carbohydrates alone. You need to spend your storage tank. Starches burn off really slowly and make you feel really tired, and they will make you crave more. Don't do it.

The *complex carbohydrates* are next. You will need to get the majority of your carbohydrates from fruits and veggies. This guide will teach you which ones are unlimited and which ones you need to pay attention to. The best part of leaving starches out of your plan will be week one, when you have more energy. Week two, you will begin to feel better. Week three, you may hit a brief plateau as your body adjusts. Week four, you should be down a dress size!

I am amazed that we have more caffeine products, energy drinks, available to us than ever before, yet we have no more energy. We have grown into a society that is under-oxygenated, under-hydrated, and over-caffeinated! We have a Java store on every street corner, yet our society is tired.

Have you ever noticed after a major holiday feast that everyone wants to sleep? We eat our way into a comatose state from all the white flour and white sugar carbohydrates. If we begin to think of our bodies as an engine and treat it like our cars, then we might change our mindset on how we take care of ourselves. Most of us would not dream of going without an oil change in our cars. However, 75 percent of Americans live in a state of dehydration, which slows down our metabolic rate. We are, currently, a society that has 101 million people at an obese level. We need to stop making choices that impede weight loss. How difficult can it be to drink proper amounts of water and eat proper foods?

Metabolic Formula

The first component is to understand your metabolism. Metabolism converts the fuel in the food we eat into the energy needed to power everything we do, from moving to thinking to growing. Basal metabolism is the amount of calories your body requires while at rest. You can use the formulas below to find the amount of calories your body requires when at rest. The chart below uses kilograms rather than pounds. You can exchange kilograms to pounds by dividing pounds by 2.2. For example, 250 kg = 113.6 pounds.

A few years ago, I read that former wrestler and the governor of Minnesota, Jessie Ventura, stated that the only problem with our nation's weight problem was what we had at the end of our fork. I was a little offended by his statement because at that point in my journey I was all about starvation and glimpses

Metabolic Rates (at rest)

Female	Kilograms (lbs divided by 2.2)	Male	Kilograms (lbs divided by 2.2)
10–18 yrs old	(12.2 x kg wt) = 749	10–18 yrs old	(17.5 x kg wt) = 651
18–30 yrs old	(14.7 x kg wt) = 496	18–30 yrs old	(15.3 x kg wt) = 679
20–60 yrs old	(8.7 x kg wt) = 596	20–60 yrs old	(11.6 x kg wt) = 897
60+	(10.7 x kg wt) = 596	60+	(13.5 x kg wt) = 487

of over-indulgence. I thought: *How can I be any more deprived than I already am? And how are so many other people able to eat and not be overweight. Surely it must be my thyroid or low metabolism.*

Wrong. In fact, I had a metabolic rate of 1,998 calories when I started the Onion system. I knew from more than twenty years in the industry that dietary research has found that our body needs at least 1,200 calories per day to get the proper amounts of vitamins and minerals.

I simply decided I wanted to learn how to eat somewhere in the middle. I selected 1500 daily calories. I wanted my journey to be about learning how to feed the engine versus starving it. I had already wasted way too much time starving it.

Using information I've learned from all the diets I'd tried in the past and from working in the fitness industry, I added some basic nutritional guidelines to formulate proper eating percentages. I took the daily caloric need of 1,500 and divided it according to the percentages above, resulting in the following breakdown:

American Dietary Assn. Guidelines

1,500 calories per day
55–60% from carbohydrates
12–15% from protein
25–30% from fat

Here is a simple formula for calculating caloric content:

- 1 gram fat = 9 calories
- 1 gram protein = 4 calories
- 1 gram carbs = 4 calories
- 1 gram alcohol = 7 calories

Target Heart Rate (THR)

It is important that you train at a cardio-vascular rate that will allow you to obtain results, specifically, to burn fat. If you train at too high a rate, you might sacrifice muscle. If you train too low, you may be just burning up time. There are differing approaches you can use to assess your heart rate. The two I will share are Cooper's Formula and Perceived Execution.

Cooper's Formula is great for Onions, because the numbers allow us to have a guide for where we should perform and how we can improve. In beginning, you will most likely have to stay closer to the 70 percent benchmark. As your conditioning level gets stronger, you will be able to train at the 85 percent level, burning more calories per minute.

Challenge yourself. Your heart is a muscle, and it will gain in strength and endurance. You will be able to push hard and get faster results.

Cooper's Formula

220 - your age = THR _____

Use your THR to compute your low cardio rate 70%_____ and high cardio rate 85%_____

If you are taking medication for high blood pressure or a beta-blocker, you will need to follow the Perceived Execution method. This is a subjective view of how hard you are training. Pick a number that represents how hard you think you are training, fifteen being over the top and one being a breeze.

Perceived Execution

Circle the number that best reflects your level of exertion (15 = highest)

15 13 12 11 10 9 8 7 6 5 4 4 3 1

To attain the best results, attempt to train at a level between 10 and 13. Your medicine is controlling your heart rate to stay at a safe rate; therefore, the Coopers Formula will not work for you. Train carefully. You want to burn fat, but you do not want to overdo it and put yourself at any risk.

To take your heart rate, place two fingers on the side of your neck, or the inside of your wrist where you can feel your pulse. Count beats for 10 seconds, and multiply that number by six to get your heart rate per minute.

Spending Your Fat Reserve

The next step is to work toward burning 400 calories per day through your cardiovascular training. I love the "Beast" (exercise on the elliptical trainer). In a week or two, I have been able to teach every client how to go for 30 minutes and how to burn 10-12 calories per minute. Other cardiovascular options such as walking, riding a bike, or swimming just do not burn like the Beast. It does not matter if the client is 74-years-old, or if the client weighs 440 pounds, or if the client has two knee replacements. The Beast works for everyone. With a little patience and perseverance, you can burn calories on the elliptical machine like you are running six miles per hour.

Household chores (vacuuming, scrubbing)	225 per hr
Yoga (breaking a sweat)	230 per hr
Gardening	230 per hr
Brisk walking	250 per hr
Mowing the lawn (push mower)	295 per hr
Playing golf (walking w/ bag)	300 per hr
Lifting weights	300 per hr
Hiking	390 per hr
Shoveling snow	400 per hr
Power walking	400 per hr
Tennis	510 per hr
Swimming	520 per hr
Bicycling (fast pace)	530 per hr
Circuit weight training	540 per hr
Stairclimber in gym	600 per hr
Jogging (5 MPH)	600 per hr
Running	700 per hr
Water aerobics	710 per hr
Step aerobics	720 per hr
Elliptical or rowing machine	750 per hr
Jump rope	850 per hr
Running	900 per hr

Look At This!

44 /// The Fork Is Mightier Than the Gym

Your heart is your most important muscle. You will keep it strong, as well as burn calories, through daily cardiovascular training. Speaking of muscles...

Using Your Muscles

The great news about strength training is that it gives you a two-for-one investment. Strength training prevents atrophy, which is the deterioration of muscles. Deterioration is also referred to as aging, and no one desires to, willingly, get old. Muscle is the fountain of youth. Muscle takes up less space. Muscle is the key to burning off unwanted fat.

You will burn approximately 400 calories when you learn the entire Onion strength-training routine. You may be thinking, *How do you know that?* Well, as I was putting this system together, I asked a few clients to wear heart-rate monitors. I took them through the routine and I read how many calories they burned.

Spending Your Fat Reserve

- One pound of muscle burns 50–100 calories per day.
- One pound of fat burns only 3 calories per day.
- Fat occupies three times as much space as muscle.
- One pound of fat is 3,500 calories stored.

In The Onion Factory℠, a very special sign hangs over our workout floor. It is a message from bodybuilder Monica Brant. I met Monica in Las Vegas at the first Olympia bodybuilding show I attended. A friend of mine, who competed in bodybuilding, had been opening my eyes to this whole new world. I'd already learned a lot about the benefits of bodybuilder's nutrition for weight loss and good muscle mass.

I had seen Monica's ads in fitness magazines. She was 40-something, about my age, and her fantastic body mesmerized me. I respected the incredible work it took to get a body to look like hers with sleek, full muscles. Not that I ever thought I could go to her level, but I wanted to learn as much as I could to help peel my Onions.

Waiting for my turn to get an autographed photo, I ended up being the last person in line before she left to prepare for her competition. I leaned over and said, "I am on a mission to change the course of obesity. I think you look amazing. Would you share something inspirational to help keep my girls motivated to stay in the box?" She wrote:

To the Onion Factory Ladies,
You only get one shot!!
Make it a good day everyday.
I believe in all of you!!!
                 Monica

The note and photo of her spectacular body encouraged me, and now it inspires everyone in the Factory.

Eating and Drinking

The next two steps are easy, sort of. Who would have thought the two most difficult pieces of this peeling puzzle would be to eat enough food and drink enough water?

Water is so important for a variety of reasons. Dehydration slows down your metabolism.

The body cannot determine the difference between hunger and thirst, so you might be mindless eating when you are really thirsty. Good hydration increases fat loss. Your hydration formula is simple:

Hydration Formula

- ☐ Current body weight divided by 2 = minimum ounces of water needed daily.
- ☐ For every cup of caffeine, add 8 oz. of water.
- ☐ For every 30 minutes of exercise, add 8 oz. of water.

HYDRATION FACTS

- The human body is 80% water.
- At least 75% of the American population is chronically dehydrated.
- About 37% of the American population mistakes thirst for hunger.

Water...
- Regulates the temperature of the human body.
- Carries nutrients and oxygen to body cells.
- Cushions joints.
- Protects organs and tissues from illness and injury.
- Removes wastes from the body.
- Lack of water slows down the body's metabolism.

The final piece of the puzzle is to eat! (Obviously, *not* eating has not worked.)

Imagine your body like the engine of a car. If you forget oil, or neglect a tune up, then all the spark plugs will not fire properly. Our bodies react in much the same way. When you are on your game using the Onion formula, you can change the percentage of fat by one percent per week.

I need you to wrap your brain around the concept that this peeling thing is not about weight loss; it is about fat loss. You see, if you lose 40 pounds, but 20 are from fat and 20 are from lean, then you would be no healthier than when you started at 30, 40, or 50 percent fat levels.

Focus on obtaining a percentage of fat less than 26 percent, so you can avoid the risk factors for heart disease, or diabetes. A simple mistake such as not consuming enough water could prohibit your engine from performing properly.

If you desire that one percent reduction per week, you must work the five basics per week: proper metabolism, cardio, weight bearing, hydration, and a little psychology.

Peeling

I know a couple of things about peeling. To obtain results you must get *mad*, or get *motivated*, or get a combination of both emotions.

When I refer to the mad emotion, it reminds me of clients who are extremely focused on results due to a divorce, loss, or maybe even some form of rejection. It is in our behaviors to fix issues by being out of control and eating everything in sight, or we can choose to be in-control and make some changes in our lives. Rejection can be a wake-up call. There is no better feeling then reinventing yourself, then taking your place in the world you once knew.

I also see people change because they are motivated by an upcoming event such as a class reunion, a vacation, or a medical urgency. Something external gives them the kick in the pants to make improvements.

As an Onion, you may begin your journey due to an external stimulation like I mentioned above. Yet, as you make behavioral changes, they become a lifelong pattern.

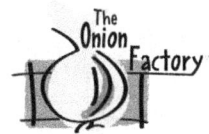

This peeling thing is not about weight loss,

it is about fat loss.

Ruth's Story

I remember the exact moment Ruth told me she had experienced a meltdown. She confessed she blew it with a Pop-Tart®. "A Pop-Tart®?" I asked her. I could understand blowing it for a glass of red wine, or a crème brulee, but a Pop-Tart®? I was perplexed. Ruth went on to say she had also added a smear of butter to her Pop-Tart®. Might she have added a glass of milk into the mix?

In the moment, I think clients lose sight of their goals. That temptation was more important than the larger goal of looking and feeling great. I wanted to know why she ate that Pop-Tart®. Ruth shared she was bored and procrastinating getting her housework done, so she escaped with a Pop-Tart®. I guess I get it. Life can get away from us, and there are times when you just need a moment.

It's not always fun making great food choices. Especially if you have been nurtured with food in childhood. We want to escape to that happy place.

Ruth's journey of 101 pounds lost is not the fastest story I will share with you. What I enjoy about her journey is her commitment to finish. Ruth realizes transitions in her life may derail her, but she now has the tools to make better choices and feel better any time.

How do you change the course of obesity? By not looking at the big picture, but by breaking down the desired results into manageable pieces.

Imagine this. With the onset of the New Year, what if you learned and implemented a few techniques, taking off one pound in January, two pounds in February, and three pounds in March? And you continued each month changing behaviors like learning how to drink more water and feeding your muscle instead of your fat. You begin to walk the park. You pick up a workout DVD and try it. You notice little free-weights and pick them up. You decide to try 20 sit-ups each morning after you brush your teeth.

Your results might unfold like the chart on the following page.

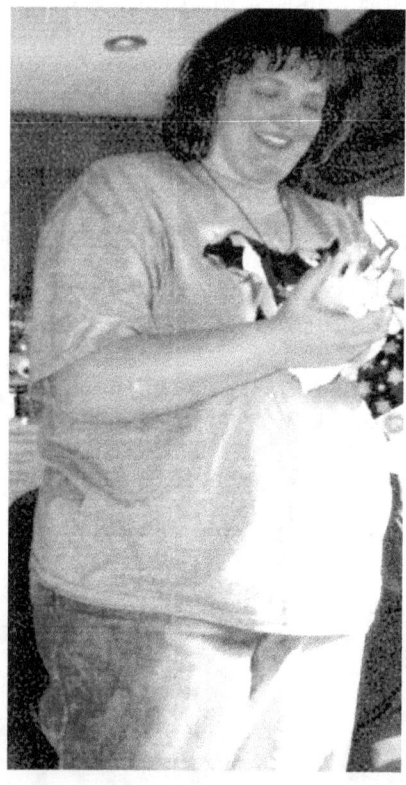

Ruth BEFORE

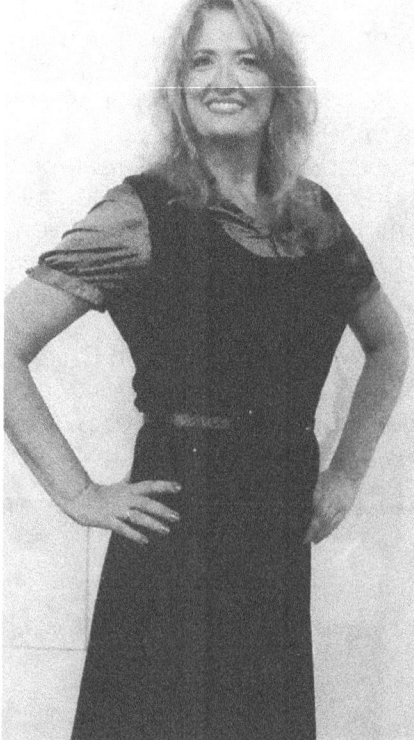

Ruth AFTER

DATE	1/7/07	2/1/08	10/9/08	FINAL
R. ARM	15.5"	12"	11.5"	-8"
BUST	53.5"	43"	40"	-13.5"
WAIST	45"	35"	30.5"	-14.5"
ABS	54"	45"	41"	-13"
HIP	54"	44"	40"	-14"
THIGH	30"	24"	23"	-26"
WEIGHT	288	218	187	-101
FAT MASS	127	79.3	59.8	
LEAN MASS	161	138.7	127.5	
FAT TO GO	102	54.3	34.8	
		Lbs. Lost	101	
		Inches Lost	89	
		% Lost	12.2	

Ruth's RESULTS

Minor Alterations Soon Add Up!

January	1 pound
February	2 pounds
March	3 pounds
April	4 pounds
May	5 pounds
June	6 pounds
July	7 pounds
August	8 pounds
September	9 pounds
October	10 pounds
November	11 pounds
December	12 pounds
TOTAL	**78 pounds**

Understanding Body Types

As a 5'10" girl, I never really knew where I was supposed to land. In what size should I fit? How much should I weigh? What should I be when I grow up? These are emotions and questions I imagine all girls struggle with; however, when you add the feelings of being big and inadequate in the equation well, I spent a lifetime struggling with unwanted emotions, expectations, and imprints.

My first benchmark, which I analyzed over and over again, was the Metropolitan Life height and weight chart. For me, it was the first visual that I could begin having a guide of what was normal and acceptable weight for a bigger girl.

The second benchmark was the Victoria's Secret® size chart. At almost 300 pounds I would sit and calculate how far I had to go, how much I had to lose until I could order something from the catalog. In my mind, I was okay once I could shop at Victoria's Secret®.

Both of these benchmarks were based on pounds on a scale or a size in a catalog. Throughout this entire guide, I will attempt to lead you down a new path of acceptance called body fat percentage. Not to be confused with Body Mass Index. You see, at the end of the day BMI is still based on a girth premise. Not on a how much of your body is good mass (lean mass) and how much is not good mass (fat). And fat is known as the primary risk factor crippling our nation.

I hope you are pondering, "Where is my landing spot"? What do you want? Well it starts here: Twenty six percent fat, or less. That is the new benchmark of accountability. Very much like in the fashion industry when you hear grey is the new black. You now have a new paradigm, a new target, and most importantly, a target that will lead you in the right direction.

Remember at 5'10" in my teens, my self-esteem was an issue. It was tough being taller than most other kids. Sure, girls with straight hair desired curly, blondes wondered what it would be like to be a brunette, and tall girls wished they were 5'2" and a size 2.

Accepting yourself and your body type will be a tremendous psychological journey for you. I have a few thoughts and examples, which might help you design and understand the new you.

First, you need a visual understanding. There are said to be bean, pear, apple and hourglass body styles. You can be any one of these at any size. And yes, bean body styles can grow into Onions. (Drive through McDonald's® often enough and see what happens!)

Here's what we mean by these visual body types. If you were a lean **string bean** in your youth, then you could grow yourself into a filled-out bean, which is more than 30 percent fat. You probably would still not have curvaceous hips or breasts; you'd just be a bigger version of the old you.

Pear body styles carry their weight in their hips. Because of this weight distribution, they are more likely to have a higher risk of certain types of cancer. If I were a pear, from a prevention angle, I would make sure my daily nutrition was full of cruciferous vegetables. **Apples** carry their weight primarily in the

48 /// The Fork Is Mightier Than the Gym

middle. As they grow into Onions, their weight gain is hidden easily. Great legs and great arms go a long way in distracting from an apple's real size. The downside to this body style is all the weight is distributed around the middle, around the organs, around the heart— the most important muscle of all. If you think you might be an apple, make sure cardiovascular training is in your daily plan.

Hourglass figures are said to be the most desirable body styles. They are known to be the most proportioned of all the body types. They gain gracefully. Hourglass body styles seldom see the initial weight gain or loss, until one day they wake up and realize what happened. You begin to look like an apple instead of an hourglass.

Scientific Body Types

We can take the body style thought to the next level of understanding, the scientific approach. The terms go like this; are you a mesomorph, an endomorph, or an ectomorph? Once you decide which one you are, then it might explain why you have, or have not, struggled at certain times of your life with weight management. Or better yet, why someone else appears to eat and never gain, and you look at food and feel like you packed on five pounds.

Mesomorphs are called the gifted ones. They are predisposed to great muscular gains. They are usually athletic looking

Well-Known Mesomorphs
- Oprah Winfrey
- Mariah Carey
- Bruce Willis
- Alicia Keys

and very symmetrical, like an hourglass. Mesomorphs build muscle faster then others and are able to lose fat quickly when their nutrition is online. This is due to their naturally higher muscle base, which, in turn, computes to a higher metabolic rate. Mesomorphs should avoid weight fluctuations so not to sacrifice their lean mass. They need to eat clean to sustain their energy level and learn to utilize fat strategically to satisfy their cravings.

Endomorphs are predisposed to a higher body fat percentage. They are known to have a soft look. Since endomorphs carry higher body fat, cardiovascular training must be very regular. If I were going to place any of the veggie images anywhere, I would place apples and pears in this segment. All body types should eat 5-6 smaller, frequent meals, but especially, if you see yourself as an endomorph.

Ectomorphs are the beans of the world, long and lean. They burn calories rapidly, have have long legs and arms, and have a

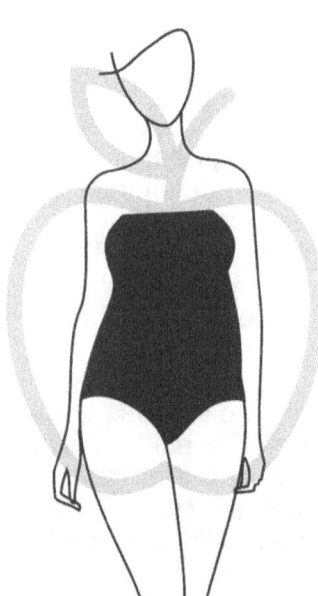
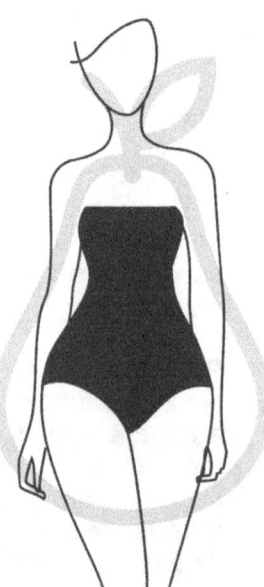
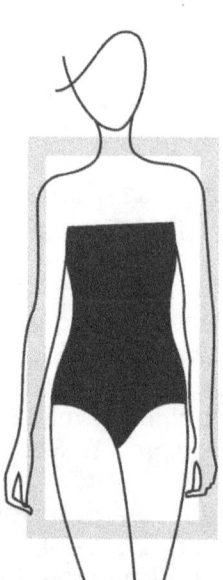
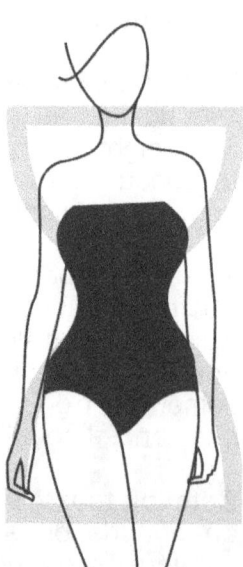

Well-Known Endomorphs
- Catherine Zeta Jones
- Jack Black
- Meatloaf (the singer)
- Sarah Michelle Gellar

Well-Known Ectomorphs
- Angelina Jolie
- Brad Pitt
- Kate Moss

lower body fat percentage. Their muscles are small and require heavy weight training to build them up. Most women would love to be an ectomorph; however, it might be very frustrating to be a male ectomorph.

Let's put this body image, body style, and body fat percentage all together. I hope that after reviewing all three you will have a light bulb moment. Remember, as you peel back the layers and find the real you, whatever your trouble spot is, or was, no matter what size you are, or become, you may still have a trouble spot.

Perfect bodies are rare and take incredible amounts of discipline and work. Sure, you can create a better you. But perfect? I am not so sure. Your mindset needs to be more like finding what body type are you? What are you predisposed to, genetically? Where can you improve? How much time can you find to work on you? And what might happen if you do not make the time?

The piece of understanding that I hope will speak most persuasively to you is the body fat percentage. You must detach yourself from the old measure of success—the number on the bathroom weight scale. It truly means nothing. Allow me to show you my thinking.

Most weight charts base their numbers on an average woman weighing 150 pounds. Most of us realize that it has been a very long time since we have seen 150 pounds, and I am fairly confident that number is no longer the average American woman. I am going to show you 150 pounds on a scale, but I am also going to show you what happens as we change the percentage of fat that correlates to the 150-pound benchmark.

The 150-Pound Girl

They say the average woman weights 150 pounds. I'm not sure where "they" live; however, I am pretty sure that in the Midwest this is not true. Let's consider how the fat percentage numbers look on a 150-pound person at 20%, 30%, and 40% body fat. The scale might tell you that 150-pound bodies are all alike, but a body looks quite different at the same scale weight as the body-fat percentage changes.

One hundred and fifty pounds with 20 percent fat looks like the first column of the chart (see next page). You only have 30 pounds of fat. You need 25 pounds of fat to protect your skeletal system. That leaves you with a five-pound muffin top and a 120-pound engine, from which your metabolic rate is computed. In other words, 120 pounds of you is lean mass. That means you have a pretty strong metabolism. You are probably about a size six and you can eat quite a bit without gaining weight.

However, you are not happy with the little muffin top, so you go on your first diet, which is probably based on some sort of deprivation, skipping or eliminating a meal. Over time, you grow yourself into a 30-percent-fat girl.

So now at 30 percent fat, you have 45 pounds of fat. You need 25 pounds to protect your skeletal system. Now your muffin top is 20 pounds and your engine (metabolic rate) is computed from 105 pounds. You have a lower metabolic rate.

At this point, you might be getting a little frustrated. The scale stills shows you weigh 150 pounds, but your clothes are not fitting the way they use to. By now, you are probably buying a size 10. You can't eat like you used to, and you can't understand

They Say the Average Woman Weighs 150 Lbs.
Here's How That Looks at...

	20% Body Fat	30% Body Fat	40% Body Fat
Total lbs. Fat	30	45	60
Needed for Insulation	25	25	25
Fat Reserve	5	20	35+
Lean Mass ("Engine")	120	105	90
Approx. Dress Size	6	10	14

why you're not losing weight like you did in the past. Yet again, you jump on the diet bandwagon and starve your engine, losing more muscle mass.

The third column of the chart shows what 150 pounds with 40 percent body fat looks like this. You have 60 pounds of fat. You need 25 pounds to protect your skeletal system. Your muffin top is now 35 pounds, your metabolic rate is based on a 90-pound engine, and you are truly frustrated. The scale must be lying! You've gained no weight, but your clothes no longer fit. Your 150 pounds barely squeeze into a size 14, and you only eat once a day. What happened?

You get the picture. This is why we must stop focusing on a number on the bathroom scale and start watching the percentage of fat that we we have. The body is truly amazing when you regulate the needs of the body. I have seen the body lose one percentage of fat per week. This journey is about learning how we can have the power to change and the power to peel fat like peeling an Onion.

I want to help you get to a place where you are okay with who you are, and then, create a healthier version of yourself. "Why?" You may be thinking. Well, because this life is about preventing heart disease, reducing the risk of Type II diabetes and preventing premature death, in addition to improving your quality of life. What size you pick off the rack is simply your choice. By the way, if a guy ever asks how much you weigh, just giggle to yourself because he has no idea about how this works. A truly informed question would be, "What size are you?" When he asks *that* question, we know he is going shopping for us!

Anabolic, Catabolic, Metabolic

You need a solid understanding of the next three terms: *anabolic, catabolic,* and *metabolic*. I hope you have your next "Aha!" moment here.

Catabolic State

The catabolic state is one in which your body stores fat and sleeps or goes into reserve mode. It's just like what the first three letters suggest—like a cat. A cat mainly eats, sleeps, and occasionally catches a mouse.

This state can occur when the body is underfed and you ask it to overperform. I have grounded many of my obsessive-compulsive Onions for a weekend to allow their bodies to rest and recover from a catabolic stint. If you overtrain or underfeed your body, you will not obtain the fat-loss results you are looking for.

Anabolic State

This is the state in which you are consuming the correct amount of fats, not too many sugars, and your protein intake is in line. You are not overtraining. But most importantly, you are consuming enough low glycemic "grass of the lands" (complex carbohydrates) to ignite your fire. In an anabolic state, you will burn fat like crazy. Frequently, I ask clients who are burning five pounds of fat per week if they can feel it when they are in anabolic. This state of fat burning is difficult to put into words; however, the easiest way for me to explain it is this. When your three hours of non-eating are up, you are very ready to eat.

Metabolic State

The last term is *metabolic state*. This is where calorie-counters spend most of their time. All of us have been taught that if we eat fewer calories, we will lose weight. Hmm, I wish it were that simple. If you eat only a few calories but they are from a source like sugar, your body will store the sugar as fat. (This assumes you are not burning the sugar grams off with intense activity such as running or swimming.)

We think we can trick our bodies by manipulating the number of calories we put into them.

I say over and over in an 8-week course. If you are not thirsty, you are not drinking enough water. And if you are not hungry, you are not eating enough of the kind of food that will ignite your fat-burning campfire. So, once you have fed your fat cells and your sugar cravings, you no longer crave food that has real nutritional value and helps you burn fat—food such as clean proteins and "grass of the lands." My favorite choice is broccoli.

You may ask, "Lisa, why broccoli?"

I would answer: "You may not realize it, but broccoli has the same amount of protein as an egg with zero fat, and it helps to prevent cancer."

Notice that broccoli tastes really good when you are ready to eat, but it doesn't sound very good when you are full of fats and carbs. When we think about desserts, it usually does not matter if we are hungry or not. Desserts always seem to sound good.

Let's stop fooling ourselves. If you have invested in this guide, it is because you have a reserve tank of fat that you need to deplete. You are learning that the only weight that's healthy to lose is fat weight. Any other loss, such as water or muscle, will not help you go where you want to go.

So forget calorie counting. Stop buying into the calorie counting mindset. You cannot trick your body into metabolizing everything in the same way. Eating 1,000 calories from fat or sugar, even though it is only 1,000 calories, will not allow you to lose weight.

Let's face it. What happens when you see the 100-calorie snack pack? I imagine this thought crosses your mind: *This is safe*, or, *This is a good choice*. But is it really? Are those 100-calorie snack packs of sugar-free cookies truly as innocent as they appear? What do you get for 100 calories? What is the nutritional value? Will this selection feed your fat cells, or will it be valuable for your lean muscle mass and metabolic rate?

I want you to start thinking in this way, so you will be able to make great decisions in the future and change the relationship you have had, and still have, with food.

For most of us, a product advertised at 100 calories or less says, "Eat me!" In fact, most individuals who struggle with weight cannot just stop at one snack pack.

Imagine what would happen if you ate only 1,500 calories today, but ate them in 15

Nabisco Chips Ahoy!® Chocolate Chip Cookies

Serving Size	1 Package
Calories	100
Fat	5 grams
Carbohydrates	15 grams
Sugars	7 grams

Nabisco Chips Ahoy!® snack packs. (You love Chips Ahoy!® and do not really like broccoli anyway.) The nutritional label shows how that 100-calorie-snack-pack day looks. (See previous page.)

You would get 105 grams of sugar, a four-day supply. Aside from the contents listed above, you are left with 120 grams of fillers. Where are the calories coming from? That's the nutritional missing link. You get 120 grams of fillers—certainly not "grass of the lands"—with no nutritional value.

This is why counting calories never worked and never will. The sooner you understand what your body can and cannot process and what will be stored as fat, the sooner you will be able to change your current level of health and your fat mass to lean mass ratios.

We might call this the Suzi Orman approach to nutrition. Your debt to asset ratio is off balance, and you need to learn to feed the good stuff and stop feeding the bad. You must understand how much of each category your body can process. If it's not processed, and if you don't have additional activity to burn off the extra calories, the difference will be stored as fat, regardless of how many calories are consumed.

Food plays such a large role in our world. We celebrate with it, we stress with it, and we sabotage ourselves with it. Those of us who have been on the dieting roller coaster may be eaters or non-eaters (just as bad), but essentially we are cheaters. We indulge ourselves with food or we escape with food. I challenge you to deep into your soul and understand the physical cards you have been dealt. Realize you have an opportunity to change, regardless of your body type or metabolism. Then use the tools I'm giving you to design the rest of your life the way you decide. If you arrive at a safe body-fat percentage, the rest of the puzzle will fall in place.

I often say the worse thing that ever happened to women was the invention of stretch pants, because we lost our health accountability. We stopped paying attention to how tight our non-stretching clothes had become and kept over-indulging. Sometimes we thought we were making a good

> **Your body has to burn fat like a campfire, slow and steady all day long.**

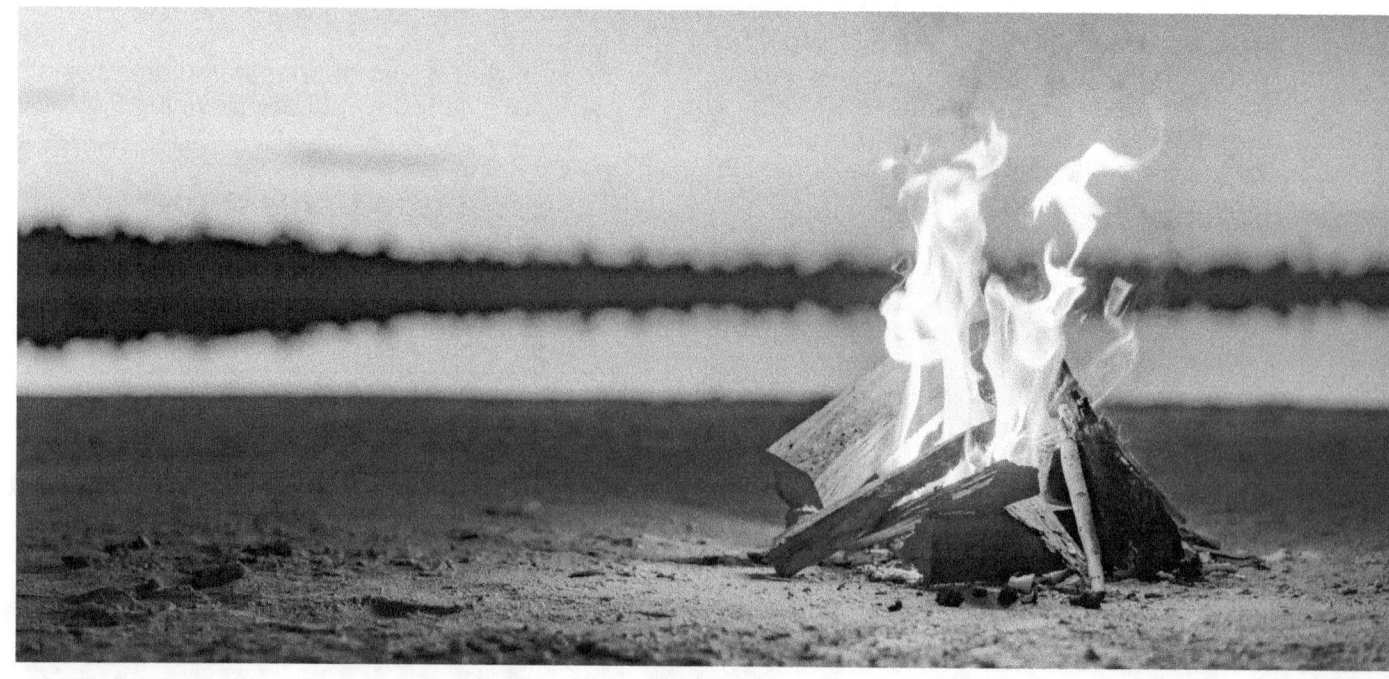

decision such as rice cakes or fat-free coffee cakes. Sometimes the stresses of life just got a hold of us, and food was the only place where we ould escape. We were making bad nutrition choices, while stretch pants allowed us to pretend everything was normal.

The Campfire Effect

The strategies of The Onion Factory are evidence-based. Over fifteen hundred clients have allowed me to teach them the science that will change their lives.

A few years ago, I found myself having to clean up forty pounds of excess fat. That experience honed my skills and forced me to learn the real science to peeling an Onion. After all, there is important science to this. My clients are weighed, measured, and body-comped once a week. Occasionally, I pull them in at mid-week if they are stuck. (When I say "stuck," I do not necessarily mean the scale is stuck at a certain weight, because I really don't care what the number on the scale says. I mean their percentage of fat is not changing.) During my clean-up effort, I checked my body composition daily. As a result, I learned how powerful the science of body metabolism really is!

I learned what to do when your body composition is stuck. I learned how to get unstuck. I learned that this journey is more about sensible eating than non-eating. I also learned I could make a mistake now and then and still get results if I adhered to a few fundamentals.

I learned that my body has to burn fat like a campfire, slow and steady all day long. All I have to do is eat—the right foods at the right times, all through the day—and my body will do the rest.

Imagine you are stranded in the Arctic. Each evening, you need to build a fire so you do not freeze to death. The fire can't go out overnight or you will have to start from scratch the next morning. You need to wake up to a fire that still has a few live embers so all you need to do is add a little wood to get the fire going. This is similar to what you need to do to repair your metabolism. You must ignite and maintain the campfire to burn off your excess fat.

> **If you go past 3 hours without nutrition and you're not hungry, your metabolic campfire has died.**

Dieting deprived your body of essential nutrients in exchange for a number on your bathroom scale. Each time you tried the next diet fad, you actually depleted some muscle. Yes, you lost pounds on the scale, but some of those pounds were the lean mass that sustains your metabolism. You may have accused your thyroid or your age for the lack of long-term results, when the actual problem was at the end of your fork.

Back to the campfire. Building a good campfire takes a lot of preparation. You start with kindling, perhaps a bit of newspaper, then a log or two. Once you start the fire, you may need to add a log occasionally; but if left unattended, the fire will need to be made from scratch again.

Making Changes

Now let's apply this to nutrition. How can you use the campfire effect to melt away your excess fat and reduce the risk to your health? I have found that it takes about 24 hours to wake up your metabolism. You will know it's awake when you begin to feel hungry about 2½ hours after your last nibble. This is also how you'll know when you've allowed your metabolism's campfire to go out. If you go past 3 hours without nutrition and you're not hungry, your campfire is dead. You have entered a catabolic state in which your body puts survival above all else. It preserves your fat as insulation against the cold and burns your lean mass (muscle) to power your normal activity. Not good!

By eating every three hours, your metabolism is safe. Your body can perform the way it was meant to. So don't put your body into survival mode. Don't let your campfire burn out!

54 /// The Fork Is Mightier Than the Gym

Why a campfire? you may be wondering. *I want to burn fat fast, like a furnace!* Remember that your metabolism has to accomplish many things: repairing damaged cells, feeding your lean mass, maintaining hydration, and capturing essential vitamins and minerals. When these processes are functioning normally, your body will be able to consume the excess fat that you have.

You know, babies are smarter than we are. They never skip breakfast, they don't stop eating after 6 PM, and they don't care for the latest food fads. They just want essential nutrition every 3 hours. That's how they become healthy and strong. We can learn a lot from that pattern.

We start and stop. Stop and start. I often wonder: *Why do some Onions go all the way and others go back to their old ways?*

This morning, I completed a weigh-in and measure on a fairly new Onion. After the 8-week camp, many girls stay involved for a month, or two of personal training until they get the bugs out, the light bulb goes on, or they simply need a little extra accountability and support. This Onion is a 68-year-old, and her results have been really impressive. She recently shared some of the trauma she had been working through, and I simply looked up at her and asked, "Why do you think some Onions stop? Why do some girls fall out and never finish? Why do they not go all the way to fixing themselves?"

She shared that she feels three qualities helped her stay on target: First, she has a positive outlook; second, she likes a challenge; and third, she is open to change. In the beginning, she said the formula took a lot of organization, loads of changes, and time to prepare the meals. Eleven weeks into her journey, she says she no longer even has to make a shopping list. She gets it. She no longer misses her old behaviors and patterns.

At first, she used the phrase the food we are "not allowed," and then she restated it as the foods we "are allowed." She says that she just really has a different mindset. She feels that Onions needs to understand why they are doing what they are doing and how to work to reach their goal. She believes there is a good payoff, if you follow the new mindsets to get you where you want to be by learning to change and choosing the tools to help you reach your goals; or even better, not choosing the things that will prevent you from reaching the finish line.

You are developing a new mindset. The choice is up to you. By having a choice, the thoughts of restrictions are eliminated. A person finds a sense of personal power-control! The Onion system all works together to become self-reinforcing. You start seeing positive results, you feel better, and then you are motivated to continue to change and reach for more results.

Body Fat Composition

Throughout this guide, I have referenced the idea that our society is in trouble. We are in trouble because we have lost accountability for our self-care. Obesity, I believe, is a state of losing control of ourselves. Obesity may also be the tool which society utilizes to mask our imperfections. Not just our physical imperfections, but our emotional ones. Has food become not just a source of comfort but maybe even an *addiction*?

I really think a major factor in your completing the journey is to discover your true self, and this will begin with your first dose of accountability. Unfortunately, the old tool of the weight scale will not give you this. Who wants to weigh 120 pounds and still be 40 percent fat and in failing health? Let me share with you a few new ideas that may help you adjust your eating habits and your exercise efforts.

Periodically measuring your body-fat composition will ensure that the only mass you are peeling is the mass with health risk factors, fat. How can we do this?

Hydrostatic measurement

One tool for measuring your body fat percentage is called the hydrostatic method. This is the most accurate and the most respected benchmark of all the methods I will review with you. The downside is the process is a little intimidating. You are submerged in a pod, or chair and must remain underwater without oxygen for a period of time so the machine can determine your fat-to-muscle ratio. The other downside is the cost and

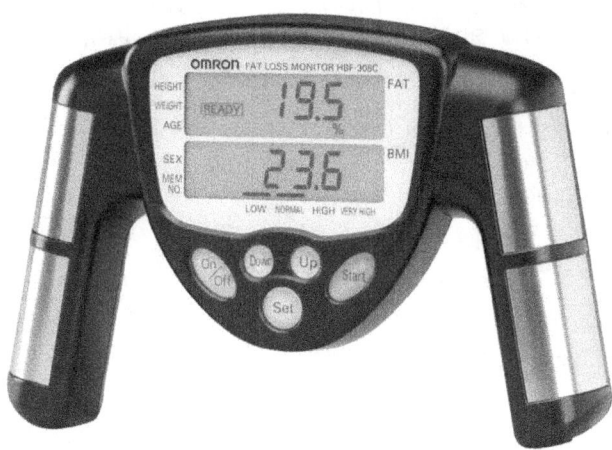

Omron HBF 306-C

lack of locations that offer this method. Hydrostatic testing is normally found in universities or sports medicine facilities and are usually performed by those fit people that we Onions so fear.

Electrical Impedence

Another method of attaining your body fat percentage is through electrical impedance. This process is very much like an EKG. The more expensive type uses gel-like tabs attached to your body so the electrical current can get a reading. In less expensive models, you are able to grip the instrument and sensors will administer a reading. Recently, scales with body-fat-testing capabilities have become available. Whichever method you chose, just remember you are just seeking a beginning benchmark, so you can track where you are today and then weekly information, so you can tweak your nutrition and your exercise intensity.

The high-end electrical impedance machines are amazing, because they will actually give a printout reading and compute your metabolic rate from your lean mass. The printouts are great to work with, however, with the machines costing anywhere from $2,500–$5,000, the cost may be prohibitive for home use. The printout machines are frequently found at hospital wellness centers, or your higher-end fitness facilities. An average cost for the printout is $25–$40.

An entry level body fat machine often can be purchased for under $50 at Ebay. Look for the Omron HBF-306C. The trick to getting optimum use of this machine is not just reading the numbers, but, more importantly, deciphering the information and letting the numbers guide you. Allow me to show you. Let's say you are 303 pounds and the machine tells you that you are 49 percent fat. You take 303 and multiply by 49 percent, which equals 148.4 pounds of fat. That would mean out of the 303 pounds, 148.4 pounds are fat and 154.5 pounds are lean mass.

303 Pounds with 49% body fat

148.4 Fat
+154.5 Lean
303.0 Pounds Total

The good news is that the 154.5 pounds, which is lean mass, has NO health risk factors. This mass includes your bone

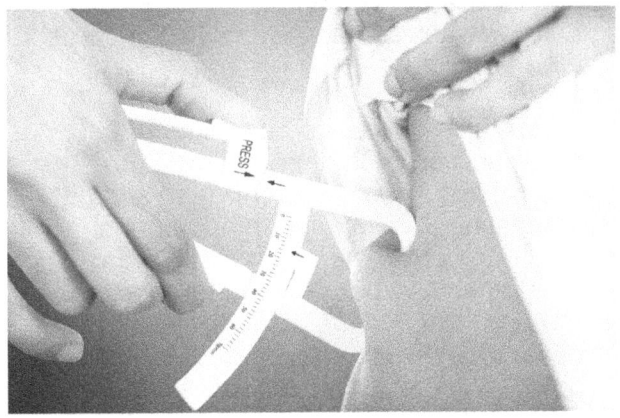

Calipers

density, your organs, your water, and your muscle. The only mass you need to worry about is excess fat. Remember your body needs approximately 25 pounds to protect its skeletal system. In this case, your fat equates to 148.4, you subtract the fat you need for insulation, and you are left with 123.4 pounds that are in your way.

Let's take it one step further. Do you want to learn a really cool way to determine how much you should weigh? You know that height and weight chart created by some insurance company and their bean counters? Well, it never really made any sense. How did you fit the chart if you weighed 305 pounds and had six percent body fat? Guess what? You did not. The

56 /// The Fork Is Mightier Than the Gym

height and weight chart only utilized the weight scale as a guide, and the scale is very misleading! Here is a new benchmark for you:

      154.5 Lean Mass
  +   25.0 Insulating Fat
      179.5 Healthy Weight

Calipers

You might get a chuckle at the next process for checking your body-fat percentage. They are called calipers. They look like something you might find at your OB/GYN's office. Yes, they are very intimidating, and yes, there is a huge margin for human error. You need to understand that in health clubs many trainers are weekend warriors. Many of them are trainers with a certification you can get over a weekend. Very few hold degrees in exercise science, nutrition, or kinesiology. There are some great trainers out there. I am simply saying that calipers have a huge margin for error, even when someone highly trained uses them.

I suppose an inaccurate benchmark is better than none. But imagine this: You take your first step toward better health and call your local heath club, set an appointment with a trainer, and the first thing they do is start pinching your fat. I do not think so. Try to find a facility that uses the electrical impedance method, or even better, the hydrostatic. If your budget allows, purchase the impedence device I mentioned earlier.

I desire for you to be well informed, so let me mention a few more methods that might be utilized in your area.

The *girth method* was utilized in military standards for years. I am not sure if it is still, but the tool of choice is a tape measure.

Body Mass Index (BMI) seems to be gaining popularity, although it is quite misleading. because it does not take into account muscle density. It is very important to understand whether your weight loss or gain comes from muscle or fat. The BMI does not give you a clear indication of this.

In What Mode Am I?

I've come to the conclusion that we fit into certain modes regarding weight loss or gain. I'm sure you will recognize some of these.

Peel Mode

You are in the peel mode when you are actively losing weight. Not any weight but, specifically, fat weight. Taking a diuretic to lose a few pounds is not the type of weight loss I am speaking about. Peel mode is the mode where you are most in control. Peeling is peaceful, once you have gotten temptations out of your way.

How do you avoid temptations? Well, the first step is realizing that sugar makes you crave more sugar. Once you detox your body and eat clean, let's say for a week, you will be surprised how the cravings will start to go away.
The next idea to help you stay in peel mode is: do not go more than three hours without nutrition, specifically, without protein. Protein will keep your blood sugar levels steady and allow you to make good decisions.

Water is also vital. Your body cannot tell the difference between hunger and thirst. When you experience a hunger pang, ask yourself if you are perhaps thirsty instead of hungry. If you put all these ideas together, you will begin to peel away

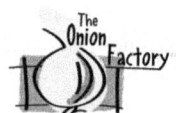

We fit into certain modes regarding weight loss or gain.

Each one calls for a different strategy.

very quickly. It's exciting. When you can pass up the sample lady at your grocery store, you know you are on your best game. You realize, and experience, the terrific feeling of being in control of your appetites.

Gain Mode

Next we have gain mode. Where do I begin? If you find that your weight gain has been creeping up gradually, then a little knowledge and a few new recipes can go a long way to prevent any more gaining. Measure yourself. Add a little cardio with weight training and you are back on track.

Accountability is the key to not allowing the gain mode move into "Oh, my gosh! What happened?" mode.

Clean-Up Mode

Clean-up mode is my least favorite. You know the place, where you feel like you keep peeling the same twenty, thirty, or more pounds over and over again. It is exciting when the weight loss begins to be, what we call in the Factory, "fresh fat." Where we're not just cleaning up the same old amounts, but we're reaching a new level of fitness. Or, you might say, a new level of less fatness. If you can stay in the Peel and Maintain modes, then the lifelong process of weight management will be far easier.

Out-of-Control Mode

What do you do when you are in Out-of-Control mode? How do you recognize it? When can you stop it? How do you find your urgency factor? In seminars, I ask the question: Which client is more difficult to help peel; a client who has gained weight throughout ten years, or one that has suddenly gained excessive pounds? The answer is both scenarios are difficult.

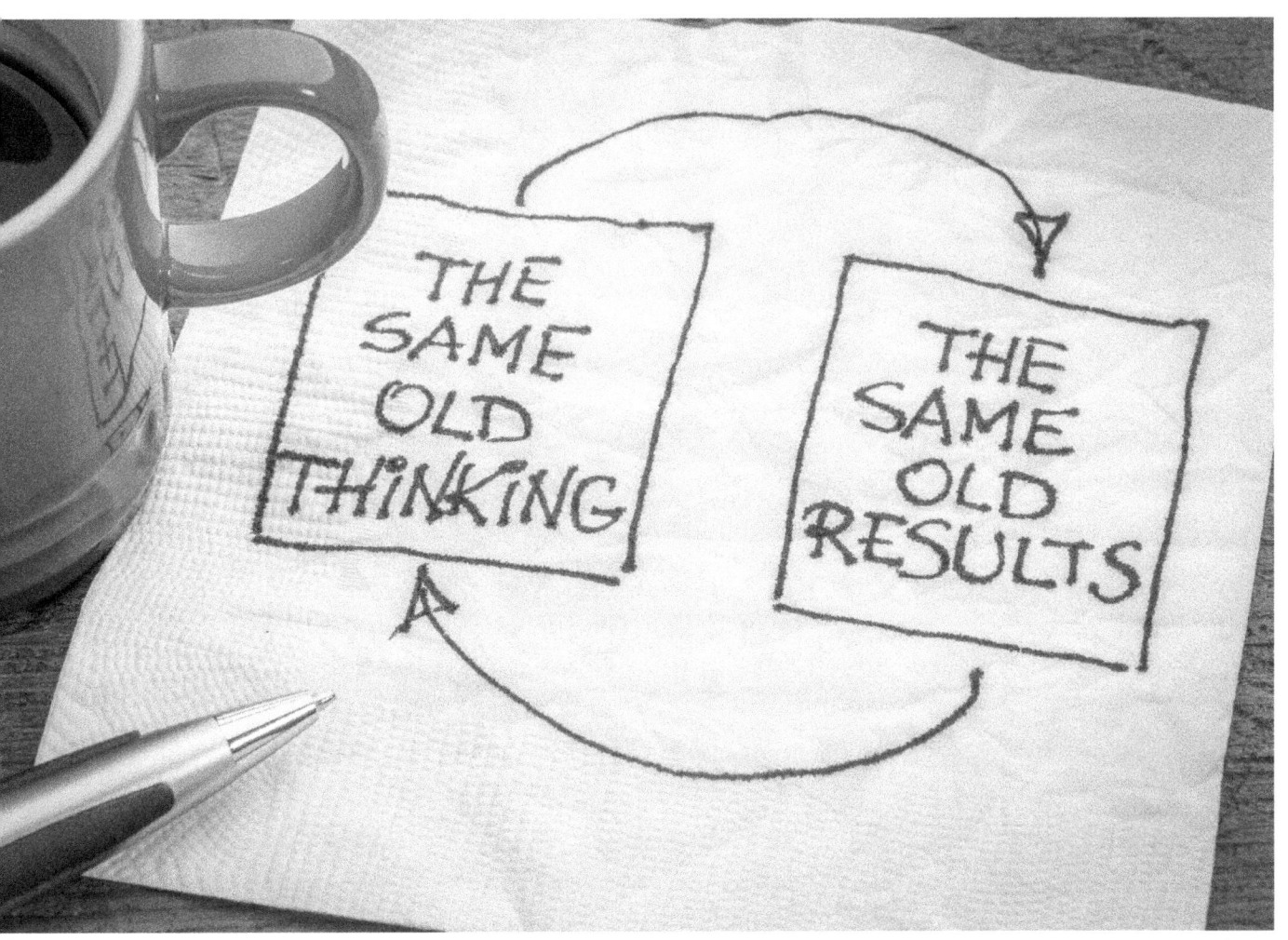

Losing weight takes the mindset of determination. It takes knowledge and discipline, regardless of how fast you found the weight. But if weight gain has been out of control for a long time and is linked to trauma, loss, and/or emotional voids, then the journey will require a lot more than proper exercise and nutrition. The change will involve digging into the voids, doing the work of recognizing them, and fixing the root of the voids.

Maintenance Mode

Maintenance mode is the place where I hope we all land. I hope that all of us can obtain the psychological knowledge we need and then detach the emotions which link us to food. I hope food will become a source of nutrition and not a way to fill a void or a method of escape.

Maintenance is an exciting place to be, once you learn that food is your friend and not your enemy. Normal eating does not have to be boring food or consist of deprivation. There may even be places in time along the way when you allow yourself to be in maintenance mode instead of peel mode. Let's say during the holidays. You might need to understand that just maintaining, despite the temptations, is a victory in itself.

The average American packs on 15 pounds between Thanksgiving and the New Year, just in time for us to refocus, peel it back off and squeeze back into our summer shorts just in time for Spring Break. What a vicious cycle! Maintenance is far more enjoyable than the roller-coaster experience of gaining and losing.

6. Free Seminar

THE JOURNEY YOU ARE ABOUT TO TAKE WILL INCLUDE MORE FOOD THAN YOU HAVE EVER EATEN IN YOUR LIFE.

IMAGINE YOU ARE IN a wood-paneled room. It's fairly large, yet cozy. You are among a group of women who, for the most part, look like you, and they feel like you. This is a one-in-a-million shot to learn how to defeat one of the greatest enemies of your life. Looking around, you begin to feel a spark of hope. You sit down, and the speaker begins:

"Okay, before we begin, allow me ask you a few questions. Has anyone had any weight loss or gain in the past 6 months? How many of you have ever been on a diet? More than one? More than three? How many of you are on a diet now? How many of you are tired?

"First, let me say that I believe you would not have come this morning unless, at some point, as you were getting ready in the morning, you looked at yourself butt naked, and realized you had become over fat. Or have you come to that place that you no longer look? If you don't look, you never really needed to address the issue of obesity.

"I believe the worst thing that ever happened to women were extra support pantyhose and stretch pants; because, these two inventions allowed us to lose track of accountability. At least with the good old Levis, if we had overindulged, the accountability factor was when we had to lay on the bed to zip them up. Moving to the next size would have been sheer defeat. Forget defeat, it would have meant we were bigger; every women's worst fear."

That is the first rant I deliver at all of the Onion Factory's Free Seminars. Now you will be able to read the same information I share with those who attend my seminars.

There are four concepts you will need to embrace to change your life. These concepts do not include a surgery, a pill, or starving yourself. In fact, the journey you are about to take will include more food than you have ever eaten in your life.

We know that starving your body does not work. Now let's peel away those layers.

1. Achieve Target Heart Rate (THR)

The American College of Sports Medicine suggests we need to be in our target heart rate every day of our life. Remember, THR is a tool of accountability to keep us at a level of cardiovascular training, which enables our bodies to burn fat. If you perform cardiovascular activities below this rate, you are just burning time. If you perform above this rate, you may be burning your lean mass, the "engine" which steers your metabolic rate.

The THR formula is great because, let's face it; as Onions, we are eaters, cheaters, and over-indulgers. Most of us would admit that we do not enjoy exercising. The minute we break a sweat is the point at which we wish to stop. The THR formula allows us to be objective about what we're doing, and that assures our intended outcome.

As I was on my first peeling journey, I noticed the same people walking at the park over and over again. They were not changing. Sure, they may have been relieving stress. Sure, they were improving their endurance. But I did not notice their levels of fat changing, or their sizes. If these walkers represented the client base that really does not enjoy working out, how soon do you think they would stop because they saw no results?

If we really do not want to do something to begin with, but we make the effort and do not see results, most of us would give up. Results inspire us to continue.

Earlier, I mentioned that the American College of Sports Medicine (ACSM) recommends that we reach our THR every day of our lives. Allow me to clarify that statement. *Every day of your life means seven days per week.* In fact, it means 20–30 minutes per day. The only variables would be the current level of your health or the results you'd like. What are your medical limitations? What are your personal goals? The desired THR range is 70–85 percent of your maximum heart rate. If you train at the high end of that range, then you can do it for a shorter amount of time. You can also train at the upper end of the range to obtain greater results. The goal in the Onion system is to burn 400 calories per day from cardio-vascular training (see chart on page 37).

It's a silly question, but do you brush your teeth daily? Of course! If not, plaque will build up, you will get cavities, and then it's a trip to the dentist. Remember that cardiovascular training is a tool to prevent plaque build-up in your heart, so practice it daily!

2. Build Muscle

You had better be sitting for step two, because for the past two decades the next concept has been difficult for us to understand. We want to peel our fat layers. If I tell you that in order to peel, you must build muscle; you might think it's an oxymoron like *jumbo shrimp*.

Do you know what atrophy is? *Atrophy* is the deterioration of lean mass. Too bad fat cells do not atrophy! The thought of deterioration is often associated with aging. We Americans hate the thought of aging. We spend a gazillion dollars per year on anti-aging creams and treatments, trying to erase the lines and wrinkles. The best strategy on the war against aging is to prevent atrophy. And the way in which you slow down the process of aging is to build and sustain lean muscle mass.

Muscle works for you even when you can't. Your cardiovascular training burns calories only during the time you are participating in that activity. The great thing about lean mass, specifically muscle mass, is you will utilize stored energy on the day you are breaking down the muscle fiber. Then on your off day, your muscle will consume more stored energy, calories, and stored fat in order to rebuild and repair itself. Muscle is that great mass that takes up less space, burns 50–100 calories per day, and is solid not mushy or flabby.

3. Eat, Don't Starve

Two of the most frequent complaints I receive from Onion Campers are (1) they cannot eat all the food we give them, and (2) they are peeling out of their clothes so quickly. Luckily for most Onions, we have a wide variety of sizes in our closets waiting for our arrival. You know when you get to that point you have made it through the Onion journey. You've made modifications to your behaviors and learned how to feed your engine versus starve it. I believe the moment you come close to that size you dream of; you are ready, willing, and able to set free the larger sizes in your closet. It is both a moment of empowerment and a commitment that you will not return to your former self.

Frequently, I joke with Campers and say, "I was always that girl who colored outside the lines." I have spent a long time learning to stay and play inside the lines. The first step in that growth was when I learned how to peel my onion.

So here we go. The American Dietary Association suggests we daily feed our bodies something like this: 55–60 percent carbohydrates, 12–15 percent protein, and 25–30 percent fat. By now, you are familiar with the concept of metabolic rate. If not, the short version is *fuel in, fuel out*.

Imagine your body is a vehicle that has a fuel tank. If you asked your car to perform on empty, you would be out of luck; none of the engine parts would work. If you asked your body to perform on empty, it still will, but at what price? It will slip into survival (catabolic) mode and burn muscle mass instead of fat.
Let me share an easy way for you to learn how to fuel your engine so that doesn't happen.

If we begin with a 1,500-calorie metabolic rate and plug in the American Dietary Association (ADA) recommendations, it would look like this:

ADA Recommendations Per 1,500 Calories (Female)

	Calories	Grams
Carbs	900	225
Protein	300	75
Fat	300	30

(It doesn't matter which measurement you utilize, but I have found it easier to add up grams.)

You may be thinking, *This is complicated. I cannot do this.* Let me reassure you with a couple of thoughts.

First, you will not have to do this forever. The problem is no one ever taught us how to eat the right way. Learning to feed your engine may take a little work, some preparation, and a bit of patience on your part. But remember, you will not have to calculate your daily food intake forever, just until the formula makes sense.

If you are searching for a long-term solution for the long roller coaster ride of fat loss and gain you have been on, then you will need to give yourself some time to learn.

Second, if you try this and conclude that you are still not ready yet, it's okay. Keep reading. You will be ready when you are ready.

Carbohydrates

Let's start with carbohydrates. I say in my seminars that if you don't comprehend all of the following concepts, please grasp this one. It can make a huge difference in how you see your food in the future.

The purpose of eating carbohydrates is to supply energy for your body. And if you are an Onion, you became one because you have an extra supply of stored energy (fat). Besides eating for the nutritional value of the vitamins and minerals, why in the world are you consuming food that will just be stored? Isn't your storage compartment full?

Way back when I was in the calorie counting mindset, I thought, *If I restrict myself to 1,000 calories, or 800, or maybe even 500, I should be able to lose weight.* I figured I could use those calories to continue indulging in my favorite non-nutritional foods.

Once a cheater always a cheater. I didn't care about learning how to eat better, or how to feed my metabolic engine. I just want to be thinner, so I starved it. I thought my body would move from a metabolic state into an anabolic state. Instead, it moved to the catabolic state, which is sleep-and-store mode. This state of rest was a natural adjustment for the dramatic shock I had inflicted upon myself. My body would no longer release the fat. Yes, I may lose a few pounds on the scale, but those were not not fat pounds. Likely, I lost water, or even worse, my lean mass; muscle. And the roller coaster continued.

The first group in carbohydrates is sugars. In my experience, your body can digest about 10 percent of your daily nutrition from sugar. In this case, it's approximately 24 grams. If you consume more, the excess will be stored as fat, unless your activity level is intense enough to use up the extra sugar.

Starchy carbohydrates form the second group. These are the comfort foods. They include breads, pasta, rice, and potatoes. I have concluded that most things that are white, such as white sugar and white flour have very little value.

The third group is what I call "grass of the lands." These are the natural vegetables and fruits God gave us to eat. In peeling, you will eat from the low glycemic group such as broccoli, cauliflower, lettuce, green beans, strawberries, blueberries, and more.

It's frustrating to think that we were led to follow a food pyramid that suggested we need to consume 9 to 11 servings of grains per day for proper nutrition. That is the first level; the base. The next level up includes fruits and vegetables. The third level is protein. The last and smallest level is fat. Sugars can be found on any level.

A diabetic quickly learns that consuming more than fourteen grapes will raise their blood sugar level. The first level of understanding food is that all carbohydrates are not processed the same. As of late, the buzzwords associated with this process are *glycemic index*. Allow me to explain carbohydrates in a more user-friendly manner. All carbohydrates are processed as sugar. Sugar stimulates your appetite and you cannot make good decisions when you are starving, or should I say craving. We are Onions, so we are not really starving!

Let's take those 225 carbohydrate grams and make sense of them. To make it easy, let's look at carbohydrates in three groups. The simple carbohydrates are first. Also known as refined sugar, each teaspoon you use has four grams. A lot of items have sugar in them that you may have not even realized. Milk has 12 grams of sugar. Foods such as pasta sauce can also vary dramatically. The amount per serving could be as low as six grams, or as many as 12 grams. Loads of products add sugar.

I ask my Onions to limit sugars and eliminate starchy fillers from their nutrition, because

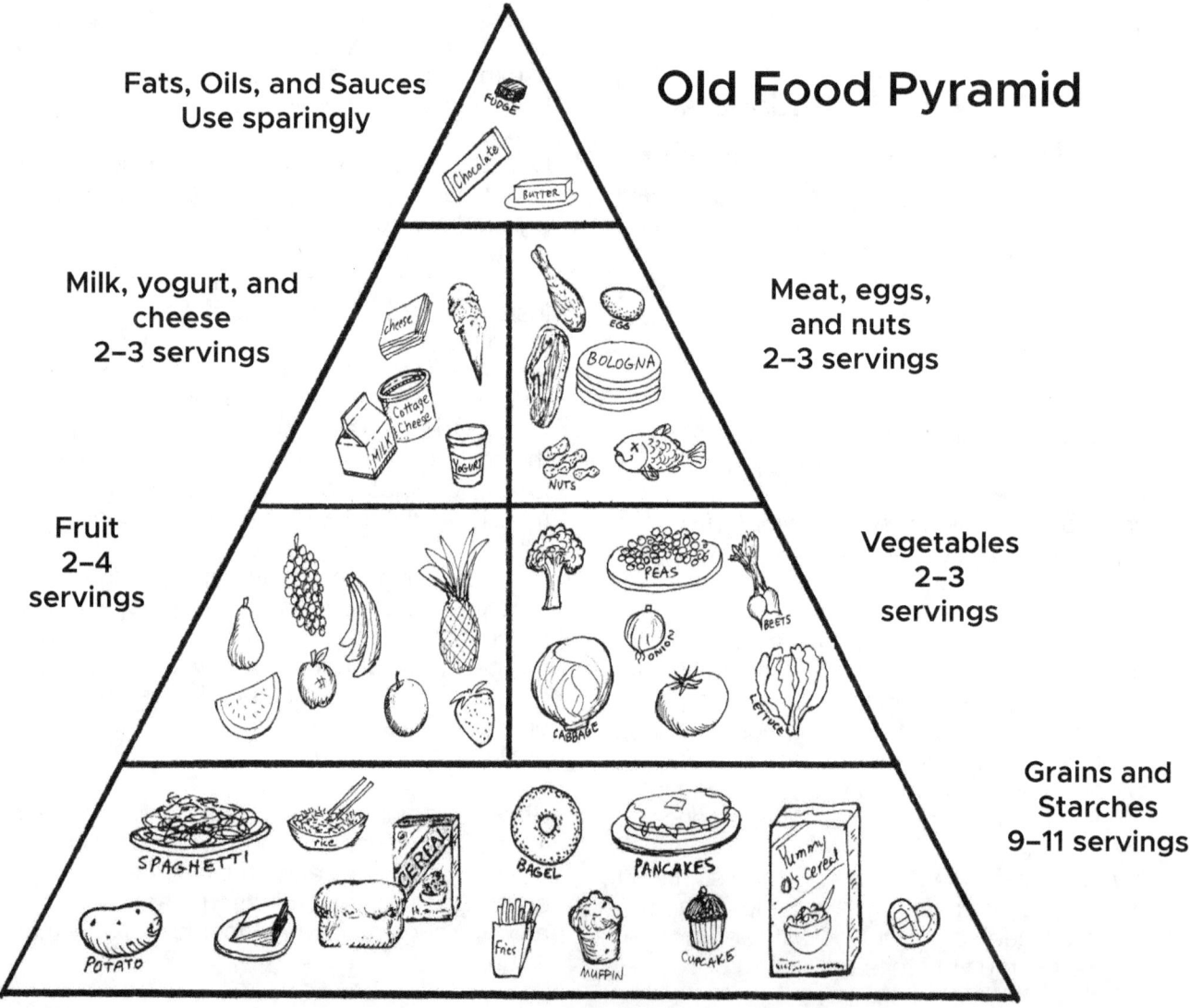

their bodies' storage tank is already full. I assure them that when their body fat is in a safe range, a maintenance range, they will be ready to learn how to bring these carbs back into their nutrition plan. Onions, while they are in peel mode, do not need to stimulate their cravings.

We Need a New Food Pyramid!

During one of my camps, I came across a study by Dr. Oz that validated the principles I'd been practicing with our Onions in Anderson. Dr. Oz quoted a study comparing grass-raised cows to cows raised on grains. The cows raised on grains were fattened for slaughter in 18 months, much faster then the cows that were fed grass. Frequently, when I shared this information in my seminars, someone would blurt out, "That's me, ready for slaughter!"

It's time we go back to eating what God gave us to work with in the beginning. Add lean and clean protein, accent it with some savory fats, dress it up with sugars, and be careful with your fillers. Better yet, use this chart to pick fruits and vegetables you enjoy, then add carbs to total 225 grams for the day.

Again, I don't show people what they cannot eat or teach them portion control. I teach them that if they eat food with real nutritional value it will give them a sense of fullness. In fact, you probably are going to have a tough time eating that much food. Just look at one meal!

Our society has turned tomatoes into catsup for French fries, pizza sauce for pizza, and pasta sauce for spaghetti. These items are poured over starchy carbohydrates, which make you tired and are stored quickly on your

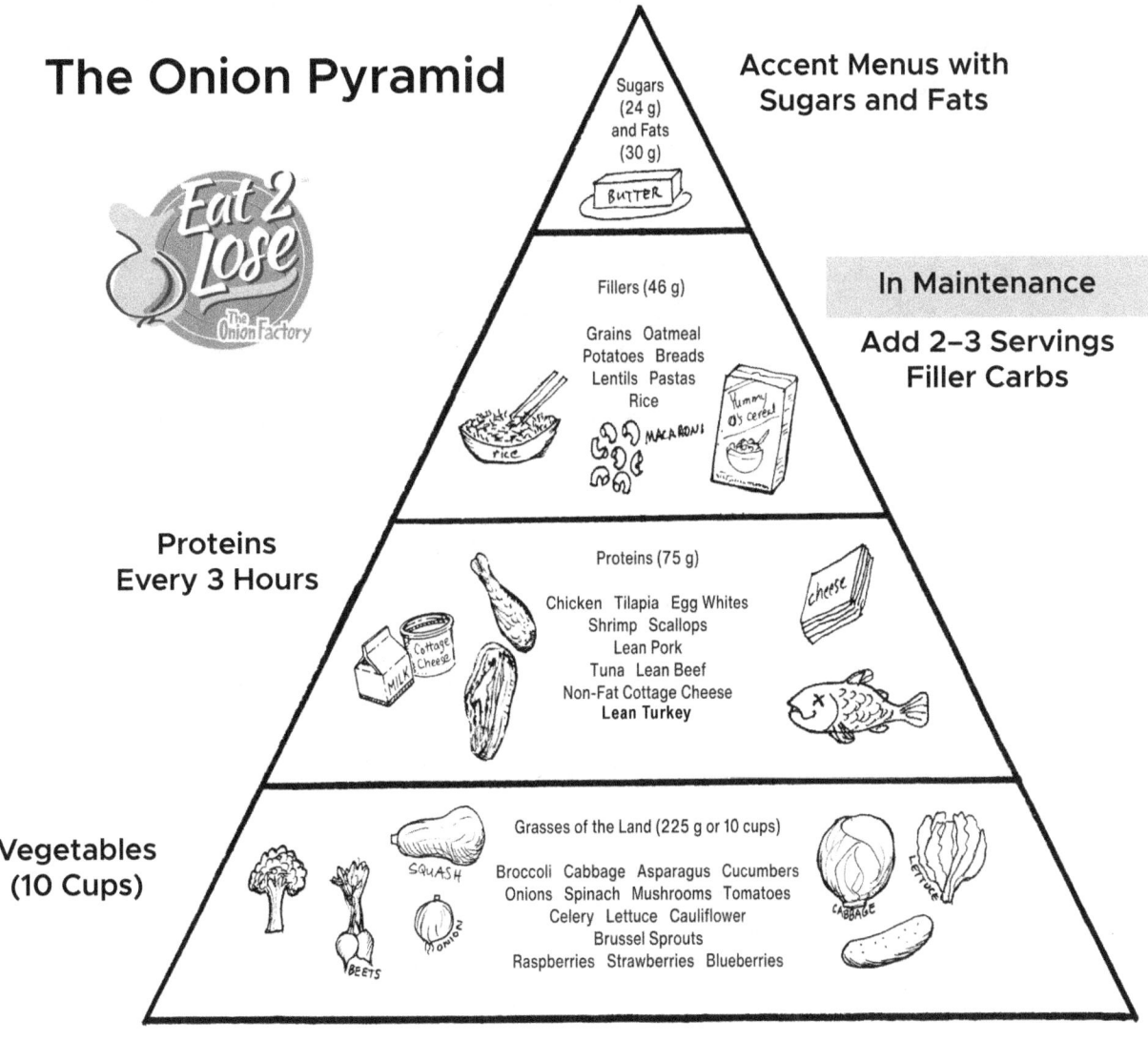

Copyright © The Onion Factory

buttocks. Our recipe section (beginning on page 141) takes macronutrients (i.e., complex carbohydrates or "grass of the lands") and turns them into tasty dishes that will not make you tired, are nutritionally sound, and will not go straight to your fanny pack.

Look at nutrition this way. You would think nothing of eating a steak dinner at a nice restaurant and finishing the meal off with a piece of cheesecake, which might have 80 grams of fat. It's a small reward, right?

You've disciplined yourself throughout the day, so a few bites of that yummy dessert will cause no harm, right? Wrong. This logic would make sense if your body processed all calories in the same way, but it doesn't. It uses protein and complex carbohydrates to maintain your muscles, so that's where the steak and broccoli go. But it stores sugar and starch in your fat cells, so that's where the cheesecake goes.

It's especially difficult for women to adopt this new way of thinking. Women are not accustomed to

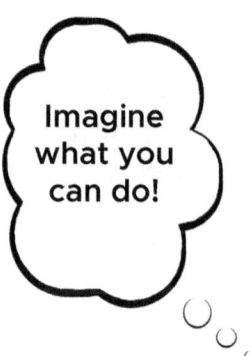

Imagine what you can do!

Vegetables	Carbohydrate Grams	Protein Grams
Romaine Lettuce—1 cup	1.5	.58
Mushrooms—1 cup	3.0	2.0
Zucchini—1 cup	4.0	1.5
Cauliflower—1 cup raw	5.0	2.0
Cabbage—1 cup	7.0	2.0
Green Pepper—1 medium	7.0	1.0
Raspberries—½ cup	7.5	0.5
Broccoli—1 stalk raw	8.0	5.0
Green Beans—1 cup	8.0	2.0
Strawberries—1 cup	10.0	1.0
Blueberries— ½ cup	10.0	0.5
Brussel Sprouts—1 cup	13.0	5.0
Grapefruit half	16.0	1.0
Tomatoes, raw—1 cup	17.0	3.0
Orange—1 medium	21.0	2.0
Apple—1 medium	22.0	0
Mixed vegetables, frozen —1 cup	23.0	5.2

Complex Carbohydrates

- 1 can of green beans   15 grams
- 1 bag frozen veggies   30 grams
- 1 cup fresh berries   10 grams

feeding their lean mass (muscle). Girls do not crave protein as much as we we crave sweets and starches. The body chemistry behind it is very simple: Protein feeds our muscles, which atrophy if we starve them, while fat, sugars, and starch feed our fat cells, which are always ready for storage. So why do we keep eating food that is feeding the very mass we hate to see when we look in the mirror? It does not seem fair that fat cells multiply and muscle deteriorates. Couldn't it have been the other way around? I wish!

Along my journey, I bumped into a writer for *SA* (San Antonio) *Fit* magazine who also owned and operated a successful personal training business in Texas. He and I spent hours chatting—well, really arguing—about our clients. At one point, I said, "You don't get it. I work with obese individuals, not bodybuilders."

He replied that I did not get it, and he would show me how our clients were very much alike. He worked with competitive bodybuilders. He insisted that keeping their nutrition in line was as difficult, if not more difficult, than peeling Onions.

Protein

As I look back on those conversations now, I think I get it. In essence, we are both training people to be body builders. At my friend's fitness gym, his clients built bulging muscles. At The Onion Factory℠, we rebuild our metabolic engines! My friend and I compared notes for one season. During that time, he taught me how to think like a "fit girl" instead of a "fat girl." He shared with me several tools that allowed Onions to shut down muscle loss during their peeling process.

Your body's "engine" needs adequate protein to sustain itself. If you are inactive, you need less protein. As you become active, you need a little more. As you pick up cardiovascular and weight training, you need even more protein. Egg whites, broccoli, chicken, and other lean meat are all good sources of protein. (We offer several great chicken recipes in the recipe chapter.)

When I first began guiding Onions, I saw them work harder and eat more than they ever had; but, I also saw them losing lean mass. As I implemented the bodybuilding technique of adding extra protein, I saw immensely improved results. I've found it a heck of a lot easier to ask Onions to throw down a chocolate protein shake on top of their nutrition than to ask them to add a second or third piece of chicken. After awhile, some of the girls feel like they are beginning to cluck.

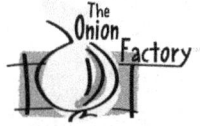

At The Onion Factory,

we rebuild our

metabolic engines!

Your body's engine

needs adequate protein

to sustain itself.

If you are inactive,

you need less protein.

As you become active,

you need a little more.

As you pick up

cardiovascular and weight training,

you need even more protein.

Fat

Fat has gotten a really bad rap! There are two extremely important purposes for fat.

First, vitamins A, D, E, and K are fat soluble, and without the right amount of fat in your digestive track, your body will not absorb these vital nutrients. Nutrients give us great hair, great skin, great mental attitude, and more. As a matter of fact, if you tried one of those fat-free programs in the 90's, you may have experienced some of the side effects from the lack of these vitamins such as your hair falling out, no energy, and feeling weak.

Second, fat insulates our skeletal system. Without fat, we might just be skin and bones flopping around. The issue is really this.

We need about 25 pounds of fat to protect our skeletal system. Anymore and we start contributing to the risk factors. So, once you learn how many pounds over 25 you are, you can start peeling away those layers.

Choose your use of fats carefully. You want to enhance your foods and satiate your palate, but use no more than 30 grams per day.

Start Your Engines!

Along the way, you may get stuck while on your weight-loss journey. During a weigh-and-measure meeting, some girls will say, "I have been so good this week!" But maybe they did not see any results. I see the frustration in their eyes. We talk about their week and look for the holes in their choices.

I will share with you what I share with them. You need to look at the weight-loss equation like this: Your car has an engine and sparkplugs. If one of those sparkplugs is misfiring, your engine will not run as efficiently as it can.

Your body's sparkplugs, in the weight-loss equation, are proper hydration, adequate protein, loads of fresh veggies, cardio everyday, and strength training to prevent atrophy. Atrophy is also known as flabby arms, saggy butts, and muffin tops. It's a puzzle. Put all the pieces together, and the results will come. Skip a piece, and you will get stuck.

I am amazed how the body peels. Until a few years ago, I never really thought about losing weight like peeling an onion. But it is the perfect metaphor. I see the inches lost to be very consistent like peeling the layers of an onion. If a client loses two inches off of the chest area, he/she will usually peel right down the line with two inches off the waist, two inches off the abdominal area, and two inches off the hips. As I review client's weight and measurement information, it is truly amazing to see just how the body does indeed peel. You can decide how many layers you want to peel.

The Scale

Earlier, I mentioned the scale. The short version is stay off of it! It tells you nothing. In fact, the scale can sabotage you. Allow me to explain. The scale is a benchmark of accountability; therefore, the scale is a needed tool in your weight-loss efforts; however, it is not the only tool. If you utilize that scale number to plug into a body-composition machine, you can determine if you are losing water, fat, or muscle. Obviously, we are looking for fat loss, something a scale cannot tell you.

This is the problem with the scale. You get on it, and let's say you lost five pounds. Yeah. You're excited. You celebrate. Maybe even with food? Psychologically, what if you lost five pounds, and your celebration choices were not exactly perfect? You might think you can get the same results next week, even if you are not on your best game. Remember, your five-pound loss was just the scale's results. You are not really sure what fat mass your body set free.

Let's say you had your best week. You made all the right choices. You get on the scale, and the number does not move from your previous weight. You are destroyed. Your emotions take over, and you go comfort yourself. Maybe with food? But what if you put on five pounds of lean and took off 5 pounds of fat? You have no idea by just looking at the scale numbers.

You must put the entire puzzle together. Look at inches you've lost. Check your percentage of fat. Look into the mirror; see how you look. Pay attention to how much better you feel, and allow all those great choices to rack up at the end of the week. You are creating a better you. If you stay on your game, you will win. It's a journey, and I know you have heard that phrase before.

You need to keep in mind four truths: One, you must realize that **you are taking good care of your body**; Two, **be aware of your body type:**

bean, pear, apple, and hourglass and remember that each one peels a little differently; Three, **be patient**, and the results will come if the work is done; Four, **stay focused**.

Measurements

Accountability is a key factor to why these results are typical. Measurements are a weekly

Adjustments = Results

These are the spark plugs of your "engine."

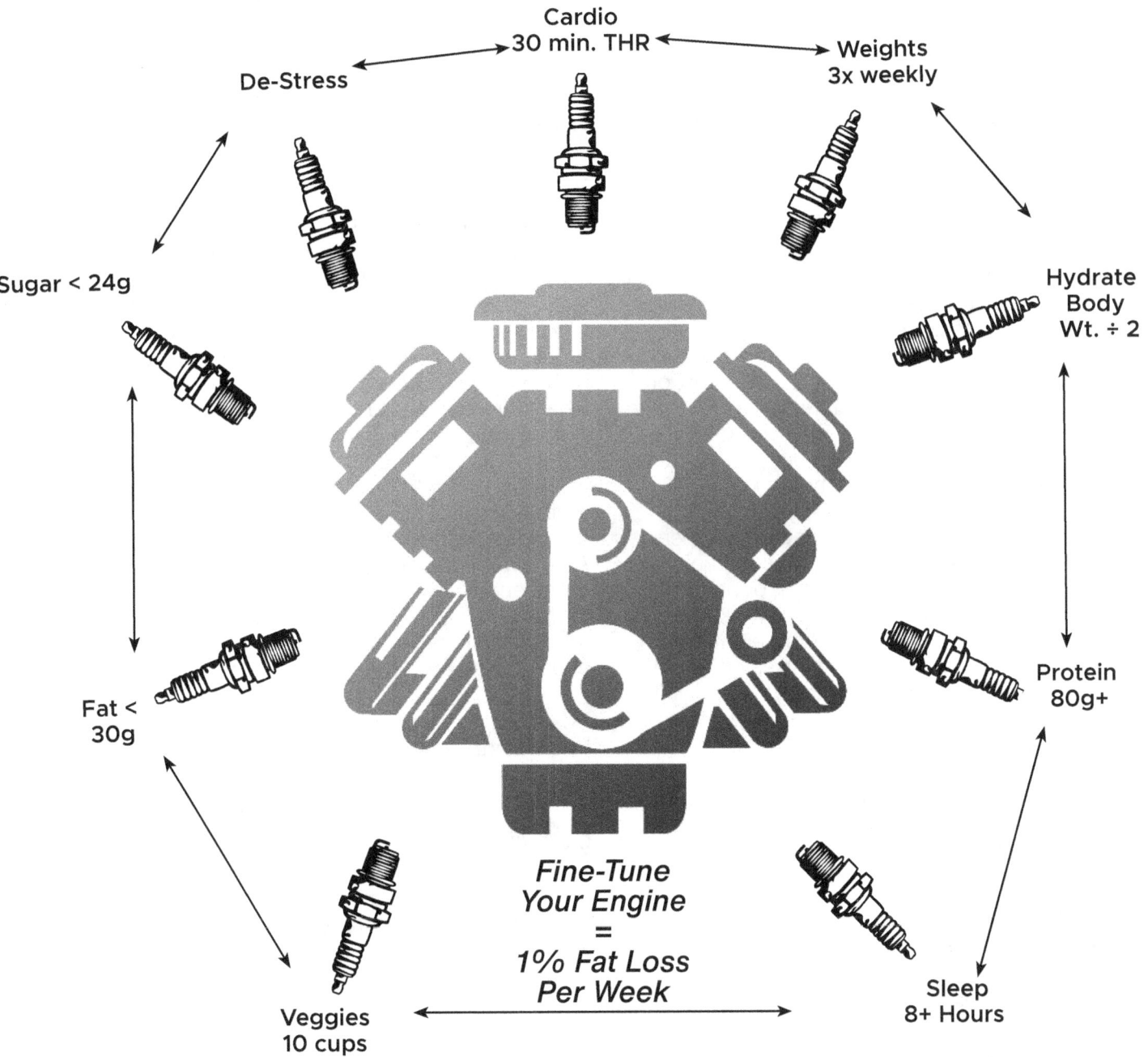

urgency factor. During an 8-week camp in the factory, we perform a weekly weighs and measures. Measures will reveal how your exercise efforts are working for you.

I share this thought with each new camper.: "I am only going to measure you in six places; because, I want to spend my time with you teaching and training, not measuring you." I assume if the left side loses inches, so will the right. I hit the major concerns for a woman: arms, chest, waist, abs, hips, and thighs. For men: chest, shoulders, biceps and waist. In the past, you may have experienced programs that measured every inch of you. Let's face it, if we did not see immediate and consistent results, we'd have a tendency to give up rather than take the leap of faith, make the correct choices, and change completely.

While the scale does not lead you in the right direction, measurements show you how your exercise efforts are coming along. Measurements are not an exact science. You will also need to feel how your clothes are fitting and how you look in the mirror to help you along the way. Weight loss can feel very much like deflating. You will find the décolletage, or cleavage area, to immediately shrink. Your face will become less bloated. But I need to share an idea about measurement to help you, so you do not get discouraged along the way.

You could go out to eat and have a bad meal. Let's say a gazillion calories, but that choice may not show up in your clothes, or on the scale, immediately. It may take a week of bad choices before you notice. With weight loss, I find that a person makes one week of good choices, and they get frustrated if they did not fix the past year of bad choices. It's as if we were good, ate properly for a minute, we should be fixed already. Just like overindulging one week-end did not necessarily show up in your clothes, one week of your best game does not mean you will have your best week in inches and pounds lost.

Victoria's Secret®

When I was running health clubs, I put together a little tool. This tool allowed me to visualize where I wanted to be. Losing 100 pounds in nine months is not really that big of a deal. I have had clients who completed the task faster than I did, five months in fact. The Onion formula is about losing 3 to 5 pounds per week and 3 to 5 inches per week, giving a little wiggle room for set points in the body and plateaus. One hundred pounds in nine months is only 11 pounds per month and only 2½ pounds per week. The trick to the long haul is a head thing. You must keep your head on and stay focused. You must visualize the end result desired. The Victoria's Secret® chart was a tool that helped me stay focused and also has helped other clients.

I looked at the back of a Victoria's Secret® catalog and looked at the size chart. It was my dream, as a big girl, to purchase a normal size bra and normal size, sexy panties. The chart was my benchmark of where I would need to be; it was a form of accountability. It was similar to the chart on the next page..

On March 8, 2008, I completed an Onion's weigh-in and measure. Rose had lost 29 pounds in about eight weeks. It was time for me to take the tape measure and show Rose how much she'd lost. Five inches, when you are looking down at a tape measure, is motivating to want to go after another 5 inches. I used the tape measure results and asked her to imagine, if she stayed focused for another eight weeks, what 10 inches would look like!
Rose's reaction made such an impact on me that I wanted to share it with you. She looked at me and said, "I knew I was big, but I did not realize I was that big. When you showed me how many inches I had lost, it was a shocker." As we went on to chat about her journey and the changes she made, she opened up more to me. She said, "Now, I can look down and see my bathroom scale. My seat belt is no longer choking me. Booth seats are no longer tight."

Rose and all my other Onions realized their true weight-loss from the tape measure and percentage of fat reductions, not the scale.

Detoxification

If you have been on the weight-loss rollercoaster ride before, you know the first week will normally produce a large weight-loss number as shown by the scale. Depending on which diet you had selected in the past, the first week usually represented water-loss. To really change your current level of health, this needs to be a journey about fat-loss, not water. The best examples I can share come from my clients. I've lived it. They've lived it. We made the mistakes, so you do not have to.

Kristy had a background of bulimia. She even questioned if I would accept her in a camp because of her past history and her relationship with food. Ironically, she was the second girl to approach me on the subject of bulimia. Working with the first client gave me confidence that I could successfully support Kristy's weight-loss effort.

One day, Kristy said something so profound that I asked her to write the thought down. She said, "I was not prepared for how bad I would feel from eating so well: headaches, stomach troubles, and not feeling like eating. I kept thinking, how many foods, chemicals, and artificial crap was I unknowingly addicted to? What had I been putting into my body for so long, and more importantly, how long was it going to take to get it out?"

The cleansing process takes about a week. The headaches are horrible, the mood swings may be frustrating to your loved ones, but directly after, you will experience a sense of cleansing and a new burst of energy!

4. Understand the Psychology of Change

The first three concepts I've share are probably not foreign to you. You may have heard bits and pieces of these ideas throughout the past three decades. Many of my Onion Campers share that they are impressed, not because this is new information or a closely guarded secret, but because we package it in a way that makes all the information a little more user-friendly. But most fitness trainers avoid talking about the fourth concept because it's so painful. That's why I've left it until last.

I truly thought at the beginning of my professional journey that a free seminar and a book of knowledge would change the course of obesity. I thought a guide providing practical weight-loss tools would be enough. The book would say, "If you do A plus B and C, you'll receive X results."

But that wasn't true. I discovered that becoming an Onion was about more than sharing knowledge, because our overeating had far more to do with our emotional voids. As Onions, we have tried to hide our voids beneath layers and layers of fat. We don't want other people to see our emotional pain and hunger. We think if we conceal our pain from other people, we can also conceal it from ourselves. Yet neither is true. The pain is always there. Thus, we keep eating, trying to quash the pain and fill in the emotional voids.

We do not want to be fat, never did. And when we got there, we did not know how to change. Most of the fixes available to us were just Band-Aids. Perhaps, if we're truthful, what we really wanted was an emotional Band-Aid or a fairy godmother to wave her magic wand and make us miraculously change. We kept reaching for the quick fixes like diet pills, starving, and purging. But did we ever look inside and search for healing and self-control? Did we try to reform or redesign this life we have been given?

We get one opportunity to live the best life we can. Being an Onion impedes so many basic tasks. It breaks my heart every time an Onion shares that she had to ask for a seatbelt extension to fly, and one of the first benchmarks, the first taste, of success was when they no longer have to request that extension.

Those moments of success that will need to keep you inspired as you put this puzzle together. In less than nine months an image of you, which has been dying to come out, will blossom. However, you will need to find out why you got to this point! This book gives you

	XS	S	M	L	XL
Size	0–4	6–8	10–12	14–16	18–20
Bust	31.5–33.5"	34.5–35.5"	36.5–38"	39.5–41"	43–45"
Waist	23.5–25.5"	25.6–27.5"	28.5–30"	31.5–33"	33–37"
Hips	34–36"	37–38"	39–40.5"	42–43.5"	45.5–47.5"

the tools to change, but it will take a different mindset, a focused will, and an unshakeable determination to change and peel.

Stay Fat

I have this piece of paper in front of me. It must be from a moment when I had an inspiration and felt the thought was worthy of writing down. The thought says, "STAY FAT." I am not sure if the thought is "stay fat?" Or "stay fat!" Or "stay fat." So, let's examine all three ideas. First I need to tell you that I hate the word *fat*. The word is harsh and intimidating. We need to show grace with respect to the shape our society has grown into. All we need is a little knowledge, passion, and motivation to change. "Stay fat," is a general idea, but when you say, "Stay fat!" the exclamation reveals so much about the thought of being overweight. There is anger, there is frustration, and there is judgment. We are not fat because we cannot change. We have become overweight because we were misinformed. "Stay fat!" says that you cannot change. I assure you that you can when you are ready. The choice to change is in your court.

7. Advanced Tools and Tips

IF YOU FEED YOUR BODY RIGHT,

YOU WILL FEEL AND LOOK GREAT,

HAVE MORE ENERGY, AND REDUCE THE RISK OF DISEASE

BY NOW, YOU MAY be thinking: how much more can she possibly say? Well, I am quite a talker. Plus, I love to communicate the information I've learned that can help other Onions travel through their journeys. This section may repeat some of the things you have learned earlier in this guide, but it will also offer more tips and stories.

"I've Just Got to Go on a Diet!"

You've come to a point in your life you are ready, or your doctor has told you, to go on a diet. I'm sure you've already heard that the first three letters spell die. That is because most diets are based on starvation and deprivation, and not on how to feed your mind, body, and soul.

If diets worked after twenty-five years of sugar-free, fat-free, and carbohydrate-free, why are we as a society fatter than we've ever been? As a matter of fact, one of the resources we've followed for many years is the food pyramid. But the pyramid is confusing. For example, look at the grain section. For nutritional value, were they referring to bleached white flour, or whole wheat? Is sugar white, or brown? What is the nutritional value of bleached flour, or white sugar? Flour is a filler, and sugar makes food taste better. Both are empty calories. Use the Onion Pyramid (p. 63)!

Remember, your body is an engine. Feed it with junk and you will look and feel like junk. Feed your body with the proper amounts of vitamins, proteins, carbohydrates, and fats, and you will feel and look great, have more energy than you know what to do with, and reduce the risk factors of heart disease, diabetes, and cancer. Sounds like a pretty easy prescription to me as opposed to increased health-care costs and medications, both of which exhaust our spending opportunities.

So you get up one day and everything is fitting a little tight. Or you go to your doctor, get on the scale, and get a reality check; you have put on a few extra pounds. Even better, you look at your driver's license and realize you have not been at that weight for years, just like Kathy.

Kathy's Story

Kathy says, "I started going to the Onion Factory because the only thing I wanted in life, and did not have, was the ability to control my weight. I also wanted to do all I could to avoid any future health problems that could be caused by excess weight.

"I have always known that I lack whatever it is that tells thin people when they are full and can stop eating. It seems like all of my life has been spent on a diet, sometimes succeeding, but most of the time failing. I really did not think, at age 56, I could succeed at yet another 'diet.' But I decided to give it one more try.

"The Onion Factory sounded like a way to eat the foods I liked but still lose weight.

"Now, after losing over fifty pounds, I have successfully changed my relationship with food without killing my love of food. For me, this has been a process of self-discovery that I am thankful I have made. I feel a tremendous sense of empowerment over food. I now control my life; my life doesn't control me.

"I am almost the ME I was meant to BE!"

Notice how much Kathy's appearance has changed, even though she hasn't lost a hundred pounds. Keep in mind throughout your Onion journey that what the scales read is really unimportant. What matters is the type of mass, lean or fat, you are carrying.

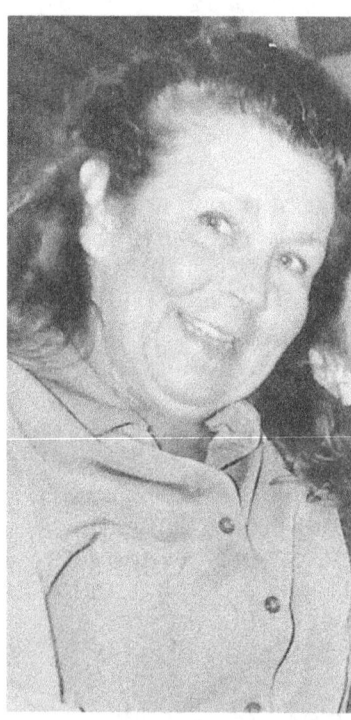

Kathy BEFORE

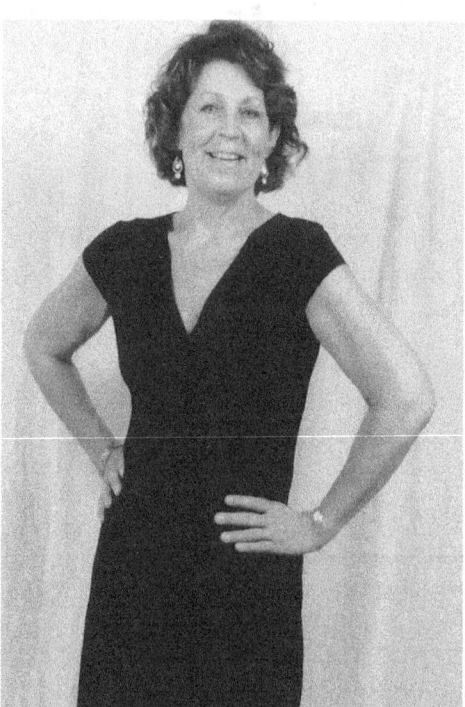

Kathy AFTER

DATE	7/11/07	9/10/07	8/20/08	FINAL
R. ARM	13"	11.5"	10.5"	-7"
BUST	43.25"	39"	35"	-8.25"
WAIST	36.5"	32"	28"	-8.5"
ABS	45"	38.5"	37"	-8"
HIP	45"	41"	38"	-7"
THIGH	26.5"	22.5"	20.5"	-12"
WEIGHT	210	184	156	-54
FAT MASS	92	71	51.4	
LEAN MASS	118	113	104.5	
FAT TO GO	67	46	26.4	
			Lbs. Lost	54
			Inches Lost	50.7
			% Lost	11

Kathy's RESULTS

"I really did not think, at age 56,

I could succeed at yet another diet.

But I decided to give it one more try."

Denver Bronco Player's Mass

My ex-husband played professional football with the Denver Broncos. Years ago, when he went to his first football camp, he was 6'3" tall and weighed around three hundred pounds.

If you looked up his statistics on a height and weight chart, he would have fallen in the overweight category, but he had only 12 percent body fat. He was a lean, mean machine; a defensive guy who could run a 40 yards in six seconds flat. That is fast for a bulky defensive player.

At 12 percent fat, his ratios looked like this:

300 lbs. with 12% Fat Mass

255 lbs.	Lean
45 lbs.	Fat
25 lbs.	Insulating Fat
20 lbs.	Skeletal, etc.

You can see he has a strong metabolic base. And if you are beginning to understand that your skeletal system needs about 25 pounds of fat to insulate itself and the rest are risk factors, well, you can see that he was very lean. However, on the Health Insurance height and weight chart, he would have had a difficult time qualifying for many health insurance programs. Take a look at the chart below.

As you can see, at 300 pounds he was off the chart for weight, yet he was very lean. Another man could weight 202 pounds and be 50 percent fat. You cannot trust these charts to be an accurate measure of health!

As I was in the final stages of completing this guide, I made several calls to talk to him about his numbers and the chart. We even chatted about where he was today. At 48-years old, he weighs 265 pounds and has 18 percent fat.

He shared my frustration with the benchmark of the height and weight chart. I think his words went something like this. "Insurance companies manufactured the chart, and it is an inaccurate measure of the level of one's health and fitness—in this case, the level of fatness. And health risk factors begin with a person's fat mass."

That's it. He said it so perfectly. We have been guided with inaccurate measures and inaccurate tools in this quest for fitness and good health. In fact, that mindset might be where this entire obesity mess began. We have had inaccurate measures for what is okay, what is normal, and what is acceptable. For women, we are never thin enough, and for men, well, I guess they are never buff enough.

When is enough, enough? How about this idea? Let's embrace a new measure of accountability that is based on general health and risk factors. Let's concentrate on risk factors, which are contributing to premature death and impeding the quality of our lives.

We, as a society and as a fitness industry, have come a long way in understanding body compositions and body mass index (BMI) benchmarks. Currently, the most common challenge with the (BMI) benchmark is it is still a benchmark based on girth. Not on fat to lean mass ratios. Clearly, at 300 pounds my ex was in great shape. His lean-to-fat ratios were on task. Even at 48 he still has great lean to fat ratios. Throughout the twenty some years I've spent in the fitness industry, the majority of my clients fell between 30-50 percent fat, or greater. I imagine if you take a look around your community, you will see the same.

Healthy Height and Weight for Men
(A Standard Insurance Chart)

Height	Small Frame	Medium Frame	Large Frame
5'8"	140–148	145–157	152–172
5'9"	142–151	148–160	155–176
5'10"	144–154	151–163	158–180
5'11	147–157	155–166	161–184
6'0"	149–160	157–170	164–188
6'1"	152–164	160–174	168–192
6'2"	155–168	164–178	172–197
6'3"	158–172	167–182	176–202
6'4"	162–176	171–187	181–207

wow!

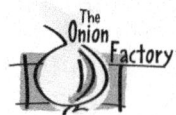

Fit girls take the time to eat.

Fluffy girls do not.

As I've already mentioned, the AMA recommends that to be safe from the risk factors for heart disease, our body fat should be under 26 percent. Fitness gurus are even more stringent; they teach that for a woman to be lean, she must have a fat mass between 16 to 20 percent. Perhaps that is why I never really fit into the fitness industry; I have devoted my life to the well-being of women who are in the 30 to 50 percent range. I have desperately yearned for the industry to understand the needs of this group of women. Perhaps my working in the industry was preparation for writing this guide, so I could share with you what I've learned!

Back to the point, an accurate measurement of your body composition will reveal your body's lean mass (organs, muscles, water, and bone density), as well as your-not-so-lean mass—fat! You need about 25 pounds of fat to insulate your skeletal system. Any more fat becomes a health risk.

You can use your lean mass to compute your metabolic rate. This is the amount of calories your body utilizes per day without activity. The American Dietary Association considers 1,200 calories as the minimum for obtaining the proper vitamins and minerals. Throughout this guide, I am going to work with the figure of 1,500 calories per day as a normative value. However, I've found that most of the Onions I've worked with had a metabolic rate that required an amount closer to 2,000 calories. My personal benchmark was 1,996 calories.

Seriously, think about the workout I was getting as I carried around an extra 100 pounds every day. This took extra muscle, which gave me a higher metabolism. I will explain this more as we go along. Just know this: The higher your metabolic rate, the faster you will lose weight. And contrary to popular belief, your metabolic rate is not determined by genetics! Your level of activity and your food consumption determine the amount of lean mass your body has. So why haven't diets worked for you? Consider this common scenario:

You discover you've been putting on a few pounds, so you gravitate to the latest popular diet fad, searching once again for answers. You choose program x, y, or z, all of which are based on starvation or deprivation. You do lose weight at first; however, the diet is not based on the factors of long-term success, so it's not a plan you can do for the rest of your life. It calls for smaller portions of bad food, or very low caloric consumption. So you do lose fat, but you also sacrifice lean mass—muscle specifically. If you do not feed your engine the basic nutritional requirements, it has no choice but to draw from your lean mass.

Have you ever thought about the meat we eat from a cow, a pig, or chicken? It's their muscles.

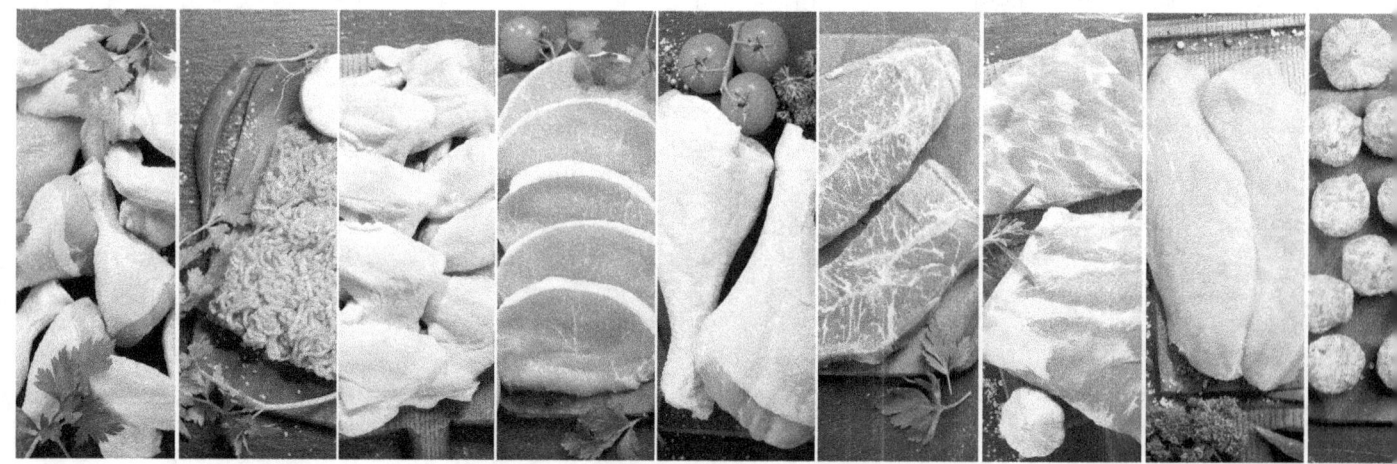

So when you deprive your body of that basic need, you sacrifice your own muscle.

Remember the million-dollar question? *Which weighs more, five pounds of fat, or five pounds of muscle?* Hmmm. They both weigh five pounds. But the five pounds of muscle is like a pot roast, and the five pounds of fat is like a pillowcase full of feathers. And you prefer which one? When you lose the only mass that comes with risk factors, fat, you will melt away the layers and see incredibly fast results in your body image.

In the past, when you based your "diet plan" on starvation and deprivation, you lowered your metabolic rate. If you cannot maintain your weight loss while eating 1,500 calories per day, how will you do it when you go off of the diet, at a lower calorie amount than when you began? You may be told to work out to burn more calories, or just to walk. Well, walk at what pace? Burn how many calories?

In the fitness industry, our demographic group is referred to as the unfit, de-conditioned, and uncommitted. But in my experience, we are the most committed group of all. We've just kept buying into the latest fads, and each time we added on more weight as a result. We have kept trying short-term fixes for a long-term issue.

The first part of your new journey is to learn how to feed yourself then you will spend stored energy, fat, via physical activity, along with a plan to increase your muscle mass, which gives you a higher metabolic rate. That is how I lost 100 pounds in nine months. Once you get to a 26 percent body fat composition and well along your peeling journey, you will find you need to feed your body all the time.

Advanced Protein Theories

Remember this basic protein nutrition formula:

Daily Protein Breakdown

- 12 to 15% of your calories from protein
- Approximately 75 grams or more, daily

A few years into peeling Onions, I discovered that many of my clients were still losing lean mass. Thank goodness for my bodybuilding friends who taught me this advanced formula for protein intake:

Bodybuilders' Advanced Protein Formula

0.5 grams protein per pound of body weighfor an inactive day

0.7 grams protein per pound of body weight for an active day (30 minutes of activity)

0.9 grams protein per pound of body weight for an athletic day (1 hour of activity)

An "inactive" day would be one in which you did no cardio and no weight lifting. An "active" day would be one in which you do one type of activity or the other for at least 30 minutes. An "athletic" day would be one in which you performed both.

With this advanced formula, we were able to slow down the loss of lean muscle for most of my clients; however, not in every case. I realize that we must be careful of too much protein. When high-protein programs became popular in the past the medical community was concerned with too much lipid protein in the urine. I did not desire to teach anything that was not medically approved, yet I still had clients losing lean mass. This was especially true as I increased the intensity in the workout, I would find it to be counter productive to the overall percentage of fat loss.

Members of the team would lose weight, but they lost equal amounts of fat and lean. The percentage of fat was not budging, even though the scale was.

I knew that the overall benefit would be lost if I did not find a way to shut down the lean mass loss. The only result we desired was to achieve a healthy percentage of fat in a safe zone. When all the elements are in line, it can be a percentage lost each week with an occasional set point or plateau.

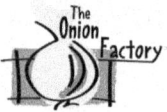

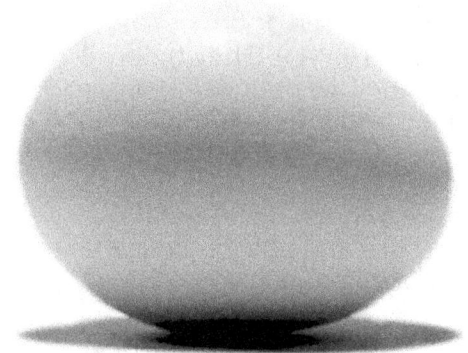

One egg white per hour equals 84g of protein for the day.

In the fall of 2008, I attended Club Industry, a fitness-club trade show in Chicago. I was on two missions. One was to add a few additional ellipticals to the back studio, because the goal for 2009 was to begin specialty camps for teen obesity and a place to work with smaller male camps. (I did not desire to change the culture of the Factory. Women see the Factory studio as a safe place to change.)

The second mission was to learn how to save lean mass and get better results. I had heard of liquid egg whites. Many of our recipes utilize eggs whites. I remember Rocky Balboa putting eggs in his drink during his training in the "Rocky" movies. The sight of him slurping down raw eggs is one we all remember. I did not see myself doing that. What about the risk of salmonella?

The egg white booth at Club Industry taught me a few important things. Their protein recommendation went something like this: Take your lean mass times 1–3 grams of protein per pound of lean mass, depending upon your level of training. Let's review all three based on an average 150-pound woman. First, here are the ADA standards:

ADA Protein Recommendation

For a 150-lb. woman consuming 1,500 calories/day:

12–15% protein=56 protein grams

This number is questionable because it's based on the assumption that an average woman weighs 150 pounds. As I said earlier, I'm confident that the average iwoman n the Midwest weighs more than 150 pounds. Let's take a look at a 200-pound person and base our calculation on that person's level of activity. (Refer to the "Bodybuilders' Advance Protein Formula" on the previous page.) Here's how the real world looks:

Daily Protein Need By Activity

(Based on 200 lb. Person)

0.5 protein grams/lb.=100g for an inactive day

0.7 protein grams/lb.=140g for an active day (30 min. cardio)

0.9 protein grams/lb.=180g for an athletic day (1 hr. cardio)

So far, so good. Yet what could I do when I had a client still losing lean mass with the above formula? I would need a different tool for this.

Robin was a client with an athletic background who was still losing mass. I asked her if we could try the athletic theory of protein intake I had learned at the trade show. We bumped her up to one and a half grams of protein per

Trade Show Formula For Protein Consumption

(Based on 200 lb. Person)

1g Protein/lb. Body Weight = 200g

2g Protein/lb. Body Weight = 400g

3g Protein/lb. of Body Weight = 600g

Fat Content Of Breakfast Meats

2 slices pork bacon = 15g fat

2 slices turkey bacon = 7g fat

2 patties turkey sausage = 7g fat

4 slices Canadian bacon = 1.5g fat

pound of her body weight. The proof was in the pudding. She had a successful week of fat loss with no lean mass sacrificed.

Using this new protein formula has proven successful for many clients since Robin. Onions complain about all the meats and protein drinks they take in. But why wouldn't you want to lose the most amount of fat as possible? You must get in all your protein grams each day.

I've found these new formulas to be helpful for my clients. Yes, I specialize in working with beginners, but as beginners start to see results, they want more results. The three formulas give me a tool to insure we are providing adequate lean protein and feeding our muscle in order to reduce the percentage of fat. Then we can change the course of obesity.

The irony is this. I'm often asked, "Isn't that a lot of protein?" Well, weren't we eating a lot of fat and not blinking an eye? I would rather teach someone to feed their muscle than teach them to feed their fat. (My guess is that all of us already know how to feed our fat cells.)

Bet You Didn't Know This

Breakfast is a great time to get started consuming your protein grams. However, not all breakfast meats are created equal. Allow me to explain.

When we moved from regular bacon to turkey bacon, that was a good move; however, many of us began eating four slices of turkey bacon instead of two. Partly because our brains told us it was okay, it was low-fat turkey. Partly because we were not satiated with the leaner choice of the turkey bacon.

But do you know what is really cool? Four slices of Canadian bacon are more satisfying with just a fraction of the fat content. So get creative and chop it up, add some veggies, egg whites, and make a great omelet. The following chart shows how the fat grams shake out with breakfast meats.

My position on fat consumption goes like this: In my nutritional layout, I budgeted 10 grams of fat for each meal. For me, I prefer to save my fat for a little later in the day. Fat keeps you satiated. I seem to struggle with cravings and temptations later on in the day rather than first thing in the morning.

Now that we have breakfast figured out, let's look at lunch and dinner meats. Notice the difference in fat content of some commonly used meats (chart below). In essence, you could consume 30 servings of chicken before you would consume the amount of fat in that one ¼-pound burger.

Fat Content Of Dinner Meats

(Each has 20g protein)

¼ lb. hamburger=30g fat

¼ lb. turkey hamburger=10g fat

¼ lb. chicken=1g fat

1 piece (20g) talapia=1g fat

If you find it difficult to consume enough protein for your daily nutrition, try RTD (ready to drink) protein supplements. It's a lot easier to supplement your meals with drinks instead of trying to eat enough protein in the form of chicken or fish!

Protein Supplement Drinks		
Product	Protein Per Serving	Fat Per Serving
EAS	20g	3g
MML	20g	2.5g
Matrix	20g	1g
Nectar Supreme®	20g	0g

The pros to using these products are that they are easy, already made in cartons, and you can buy them at most grocery stores. The cons are that you cannot add three, or four, without too many fats, and they are expensive. Matrix chocolate and Nectar Supreme® Fuzzy Navel are my favorites. Everyone needs a chocolate fix, and breakfast isn't the same without OJ.

Fat Recap

Earlier I explained two benefits of fat, one as an insulator, the second to help your body to absorb vital vitamins and minerals. But with all of the dieticians' talk about good fat, bad fat, and saturated fat, the information becomes very confusing. Here is the short version.

Remember that the good fats still add up. Fats have more than double the calories per gram than protein or carbohydrate. This is probably where we got the term "empty calories."

The sooner you realize that fat is not the big deal, the sooner you will be able to begin to change your life. I joke and say that I have gained and lost over 1,000 pounds in my lifetime. Seriously, I became fat like many other individuals who did it due to starvation—depriving themselves of the nutrition their bodies need while eating foods that supply nutrients of which they were already full.

Imagine filling up your car at a gas station. The nozzle clicks off, telling you that the tank is full. But you keep filling and filling. Fat is just stored energy; it is your reserve tank that is waiting to be used! One pound of fat equates to 3,500 calories of stored energy in your tank. You simply need to learn how to spend them and start eating!

We've said that fat serves two purposes. First, fat insulates your body. Without it, your organs, skeletal system, and skin would be unprotected from the elements. To be healthy, your body needs approximately 25 pounds of fat. Any more and you begin to collect risk factors for serious health issues.

Second, fat plays a crucial role in the absorption of some vitamins. Vitamins A, D, E, and K are all fat-soluble. They require fat in your digestive system in order for your body to use them. If you eliminate fat from your nutrition plan (you know, we all bought in to the rice-cake and pretzel fads of the late 80's), you will begin to feel sluggish, lose hair, and just not feel as healthy as you would if your body was absorbing those nutrients. Although you want to lose weight, the only mass you need to lose is fat mass. I would bet that if you've ever been on a starvation or

The Skinny on Fats

Good Fat:	nuts, canola oil, avocados
Bad Fat:	fried foods, butter, cheese
Saturated:	animal fat, palm oil, coconut oil
Polyunsaturated:	salmon, tuna, tofu, walnuts, mackerel

deprivation program, you lost some fat but you also sacrificed lean mass.

Lean mass consists of your organs, water, bone density, and muscle, all of which contribute to the good level of your health. The most important muscle/organ is the heart, where the greatest risk resides. Did you know fifty-eight percent of our dying population is dying from heart disease? If not fed properly, your body will consume muscle mass. And what is the most important muscle you have? Your heart! Hmmm, you don't want to lose that. Muscle is the "fountain of youth." We all know that we would love to maintain a youthful appearance. By the way, why is it that when a man gets older, he seems to get better looking; but as we women age, we just get older? Maybe it has something to do with men's percentage of muscle mass being higher than women's.

Understanding how the body processes fat can be overwhelming, especially when we were brainwashed to believe that "fat-free" was the way to become thin. Little did we know that by eating "fat-free" we lacked the ability to absorb vital vitamins and minerals. In addition, when we saw "fat-free," we assumed "free" meant its quantity could be "unlimited." Therefore, we kept filling, feeding, and gaining. We didn't realize (or ignored) the fact that when food is processed to become fat-free, sugar is added to help replace the taste that had been removed. While our fats may have been on target with a "fat-free" regimen, our sugar intakes were not.

Even as a health professional, I found it confusing to decipher the difference between good fat, bad fat, saturated fat, and trans-fats. The comparison between olive oil and butter was the best visual I had.

Let's look at fats in French nutrition versus Italian nutrition. A study to compare the consumption of fat in different cultures' cuisine found that Italians use less fat with their bread and olive oil than the French do with their bread and butter. Specifically, the Italians consume one tablespoon of oil to the French's two tablespoons of butter. So what's the difference? The first difference is in the amount of fat grams it takes to satisfy their tastes.

The French require double the amount of fat on their bread. The second difference is that Italians use olive oil, which is heart healthy while the French use butter, whose cholesterol clogs arteries. At least so far as fats are concerned, the Italian cuisine is much healthier than the French.

Fiber: Are Beans Okay?

When you eat efficiently, your body utilizes all the wonderful components of nutrition. Hence, there is little waste. However, our bodies do require a certain amount of fiber to function properly. So what are the proper amounts of fiber and where do we get them?

I can assure you that If you consume 10 cups of green veggies and fruits from "the grass of the lands," you will obtain more than enough fiber for your body to regulate itself. Howerver, here are some good "rules of thumb" for fiber consumption:

Stay away from fiber additives or fiber bars because you will also get carbohydrate fillers in them. And you are already full of carbs. Here are better dietary sources:

Fiber Sources

Broccoli	¾ cup—7g
Spinach	½ cup—7g
Kale	½ cup—4g
Turnip Greens	½ cup—4g
Cabbage	¾ cup—3.5g
Brussel Sprouts	¾ cup—3g
Blackberries	½ cup—4.4g
Raspberries	½ cup—4.6g
Celery	¼ cup—2g
Green Peppers	½ cup—1.2g
Cauliflower	¾ cup—2g
Mushrooms	½ cup—2g

Often, I get asked this question. "Are beans okay?" Yes, I know beans are high in fiber. Green beans, black beans, chili beans, and garbanzo beans, all healthy, right? Of course. But not all beans are weight-loss worthy, and not all beans are going to get you the quickest results you desire.

You need to consider that what is taught in fitness magazines is for fit people who are already under 26 percent fat. The choices we Onions need to make are far different. If you find yourself to at 30, 40, or even 50 percent fat, you will need this bean knowledge to help you find your way. Once you reach a safe percentage of body fat, then the abovementioned beans are definitely part of a balanced nutrition plan.

For the moment, you need to focus on your fat reserve tank. You will enjoy the affirmation of quick results, which will mentally charge you and give you the motivation to continue to make modifications in your behavior.

Green beans such as Italian, French cut, or just regular green beans are unlimited. Eat away!

Black beans are often promoted as a good protein source. I evaluated the nutrition label of a typical can. One-fourth cup of black beans indeed has 9 grams of protein. However, you will need to factor in the 23 grams of carbohydrates that come with it. Refer back to our carb chart on page 39 and guess which column these carbs are coming from. No, not sugar. They are not green and leafy, so they are not coming from the "grass of the lands" column. They are coming right down the middle column—fillers. And you are already over full!

Fiber Requirements

Women under 50	25g
Men under 50	38g
Women over 50	21g
Men over 50	30g

When you are in your maintenance mode, maintaining your weight and not gaining, you will have 46 grams to carbs to work with. If you desire at that point to utilize a helping of black beans as part of the equation, go ahead. Just be aware that while you are still in weight-loss mode, 23 grams from the middle column (the starches) will not get you the same results as 23 grams of broccoli, which is from the "grass of the lands" (complex carbs).

Mom's Sugar Vice

My mom's vice is sugar. It always has been Specifically, chocolate. When she would get a box of chocolates for Valentines Day, or any holiday, she would take a bite out of various pieces until she

What Fiber Does

- Adds bulk, increasing satiety and helping in weight management.
- Lowers cholesterol.
- Attracts water and turns to gel during digestion, trapping carbohydrates and slowing the absorption of glucose.
- Decreases risk of heart disease and Type II diabetes.
- Speeds the passage of foods through the digestive system, facilitating regularity.
- Maintains gastrointestinal system health.

found the piece she wanted. Sooner or later, all the chocolates were gone.

Gradually, she moved to fruit. Fruit is healthy, right? The questions would go like this. "Are cherries okay to eat? Is pineapple? Certainly bananas are good!"

But fruits are not created equal. Fruits are carbohydrates, and all carbohydrates are processed as sugar. Sugar stimulates cravings and makes you hungry. You cannot make good decisions when you are hungry. It's not really about what you can or cannot eat; it is an awareness of how your body will process your choices. In addition, if you have excess weight you are trying to lose, you do not want to slow down the process by selecting a piece of fruit to eat that will be difficult to burn off as well as stimulating to your cravings. It will make only make things harder on you.

When you understand how your metabolism works, you'll realize that peeling is much easier when you to select from better, unlimited choices that are lower on the glycemic scale. Fats, sugars, and starches feed fat cells. Protein feeds your muscle. Most women do not crave protein, men do. When you feed the craving, you often desire more. Not the case with protein. If you feed your engine consistently with lean protein, you may find you are more satisfied and you will shut down the other cravings. You can make good decisions when you are not hungry.

Once you are at a safe body fat percentage, then you will be able to enjoy fruit occasionally.

Stay with the berries above during your peel time. They are great in fiber, antioxidants, and they are less likely to get in the way of your goals.
This guide is not a magic pill; the Onion journey is a process of change, knowledge, and understanding. Once you see success from clean eating and peel a few layers, you will be ready to bring fruits like cherries, pineapples, and grapes back into your daily nutrition. We have spent decades satisfying our cravings and feeding our fat cells. This is your opportunity to learn how to feed your muscle with protein.

I did an experiment with my mom. She had come to visit while I was getting the new Factory ready. Mom is great at painting, cleaning, and jumping in to help whenever needed. After a long day of work, we came home to the boxes of food left for us by the food division. I think we had chicken, a vegetable, and broccoli salad. I watched my mom eat almost everything, but as usual she asked for a small portion of meat. Why some women do not like meat is beyond me; however, I see this frequently.

Being the dutiful daughter that I am, I harassed her about finishing her chicken. I went into my normal rant about feeding the muscle instead of feeding the fat. I am sure she knew it was coming. Then, in a split-second inspiration I said, "Mom, you have to try my new Caramel Crepe recipe.

Love Those Berries!

Fruit Lowest in Sugar

- blackberries
- raspberries
- strawberries
- blueberries
- lemons
- limes

Fruit Moderate in Sugar

- grapefruit
- apricots
- apples
- honeydew melons
- cantaloupes
- nectarines

Fruit Highest in Sugar

- tangerines
- mangos
- figs
- bananas
- plums
- kiwi fruit
- pineapple

I think I will become famous just for this recipe."

"Okay," she replied.

Our Caramel Crepes create such a great presentation. I sprinkle the plate and the crepe with cinnamon, top it with a dollop of caramel sauce, and finish it off with of smidge of light, or fat-free aerosol whipped topping. Keep in mind, this crepe is 100 percent protein (28 grams) made from egg whites, fat free, sugar free, and this treat would compete with any five-star restaurant crepe.

I proudly placed my masterpiece in front of her. Guess what? She ate every bite. I looked at her and said, "I thought you weren't hungry?" At least I now know how to help my mom eat her protein. If I can accomplish this, protein will shut down her cravings for more sugar.

Artificial Sweeteners

For the past few years, I have been researching how artificial sweeteners play into the weight-loss process. One day, I had just completed a consultation with a stuck client. She had lost 68 pounds to date and had not been able to get back on her game to reach her goal of 150 pounds. We looked at the possible kinks: lack of hydration, training too hard, not eating enough macronutrients, not eating enough protein, and her use of sweeteners. I asked her to take one week and clean up everything we'd discussed. I was attempting to help her reconnect to her weight-loss goals.

At times, the process of losing 100 to 150 pounds can seem overwhelming. A client might need a minute to refocus and go back to the basics. In some way, they need to clean up their act.

We finished our consult with a refreshed focus. The following Monday, she came in chuckling and said, "Did you see what was on the news today?"

I said, "No."

She went on to tell me about a big Purdue University study that revealed how artificial sweeteners could be preventing weight loss. She also shared that she had gone home after our consult and thought about how many sweeteners she had been consuming and was amazed. She decided if her body was trying to process all the chemical sweetener junk, perhaps it couldn't eliminate fat effectively.

I asked another client if she would look online for the article and forward it to me. When I arrived home later that day, she had sent me the study. Below is a condensed version of what I read.

Artificial Sweeteners Tied to Weight Gain

If you're watching your weight, those no-calorie sweeteners could be doing more harm than good. A Purdue University study found that artificial sweeteners might actually foster weight gain by confusing the body in a way that makes it harder to burn calories.

In the study, one group of rats were fed yogurt sweetened with glucose, a simple sugar with the same calories as table sugar. Another group received yogurt with saccharin. The saccharin group went on to consume more calories, gain more weight and put on more body fat.

"The research might explain why other studies about the effects of artificial sweeteners on weight have largely been inconclusive," Swithers said. It might also explain in part why obesity has risen in parallel with use of such sweeteners.

APA Feb. "Behavioral Neuroscience" 2008 AOL LLC All Rights Reserved.

Allow me to expand your horizon just a tad more. At the beginning of an Onion Boot Camp, clients frequently ask, "Can I have Diet Coke?" I usually take a deep breath before I attempt to answer this question.

Can you lose weight drinking diet soda? Yes, I have seen it. But is diet pop healthy? No,

I answered, even before I read the Purdue report..

Consider this:

Our society eats too much white flour and white sugar, over-processed, prepackaged, and low-nutritional items. A person could be as far to the other extreme, using no preservatives, consuming nothing with a face, or a mom, and no pesticides—a strictly organic approach. My goal with this guide is to teach you how to get to the middle of the road.

As you begin to obtain a safe body-fat percentage and feel incredibly better, you might find yourself seeking more pesticide-free, organically grown foods. You will find that free-range meat tastes dramatically different from the meat we typically purchase in the grocery store.

Yes, a few of our recipes do use products containing artificial sweeteners. And yes, occasionally, we need to use those sweeteners. But the goal is to eat as pure as you can.

This means eating lean protein, loads of veggies, not too much fat, and a dash of sugar or a tiny bit of artificial sweetener.

Why You Should Drink More Water

- About 75% of Americans are chronically dehydrated.

- In 37% of Americans, the thirst mechanism is weak it is often mistaken for hunger.

- Mild dehydration will slow one's metabolism as much as 3%.

- One glass of water shut down midnight hunger pangs for almost 100% of the dieters in a University of Washington study.

- Preliminary research indicates that 8—10 glasses of water a day eases back and joint pain for up to 80% of sufferers.

Please, just drink water!

8. A Side Order of Psychology

TO ACCOMPLISH THIS CHANGE in your way of life, you must also work on your psyche. The mind is a powerful weapon. You will need to learn how to utilize the mind to help you make changes and get rid of your risk factors, so you can begin living your life.

A few months ago, my guardian angel, Chris, came to me and shared that we had a guest speaker and author coming to church. "I really want you to meet him," she said, "So, don't miss church on this Sunday." She is very much like my second Mom. Chris was convinced that this speaker's path and the Onion path should cross, connect, or at least mingle. Chris is one of the best cheerleaders The Onion Factory℠ has. She has lived it, learned it, and she has changed her life. We have so many of these cheerleaders now!

I am not sure if the author and I will ever cross paths. I am thankful for Chris' belief in me and in the system I've created. I made it to church that Sunday, and what I did pick up from the guest speaker's sermon was the psychology of ourselves. *Hmmm,* I thought, *a tool to help peel Onions?*

It's often said that *insanity* is doing the same thing over and over again and expecting different results. I'll admit that I had a certain kind of insanity for the twenty years I spent starving myself to lose weight. So do the women who meet with me on a weekly basis. A client can spend an entire week doing all the right steps and then, in a blink of an eye, an emotion overcomes her and she makes a decision that sabotages or derails the path she is on. Isn't that a little insane?

One definition of *psychology* ("the study of going nuts over a brownie") made me giggle, but this is serious business. While the process of peeling an Onion is truly easy, the mental part can be tough. It will take something to make you want the results of this process more than you want the temptation directly in front of you. (Note to self: *If I could discover what this "something" is, I will tell all of my clients.*) Each person is wired differently, and I have not yet figured out how to describe the mental attitude that is the essential "something" of weight loss. This book is a first step in that direction.

I knew in the beginning the Onion concept worked. It does not feel good to say I am on a diet. Especially if it is the fourth, fifth, or what seems like a lifetime spent saying you were on a diet. I found out, way back at the first camp, that being an Onion was, in part, an acceptance of the current mode a person was in. Attending the seminar was the first step to understanding and realizing that a change of thinking must occur or you will stay on your diet rollercoaster process forever.

This is one of the main reasons the "diet" concept does not work, because "diets" are about temporary change. Obviously, if you go back to your old behaviors, you will grow back into the old you. Becoming an Onion is an awakening. Team members know they are on a new journey, a true journey, yet some of them do not tell anyone they are on it, because they are afraid of failing.

One of the funniest girls I ever worked with told her family she was going to an anger management meeting rather than a weight-loss camp. She flipped over the cover of her workbook to hide the name of of it and she attended Boot Camp only twice a week. Even so, I liked to think she indeed went home with a new attitude, because her endorphin and serotonin levels would have kicked in after her workouts.

Does Anorexia Have a Mirror Disorder?

Over the past three decades, we have been exposed to more and more information regarding better health. Yet as a society, we have continued to get larger and larger. If fat-free, sugar-free, and carb-free was the answer, why are we fatter as a society then we have ever been. We have been desensitized. The acceptable size has grown. Oh how we, Onions, just relish the idea of not having to walk into the large section of the clothing store.

A few years back, I caught an interview with the singer Nancy Wilson. I was always a huge Heart fan. She shared the pressure she was under by the record labels to be thinner because fat doesn't sell records. In fact, I remember her saying that at one point in her career even though she was the lead vocalist of Heart, the PR team started placing Ann the guitarist in the front of the photo shoot. I remember her sharing how cool she and Ann were about the entire thing, but how difficult the pressure on her to lose her weight felt.

For whatever reason, I really connected with Nancy during this interview. You see, she did not really see how big she had gotten. Nor did I. I did not dress like a fat woman. I did not buy mu-mus. I did not wear clothes that were big and baggy. In fact, looking back I probably wore things a little tighter than they should have been.

So if an anorexic looks in the mirror and sees this fat person when in reality they are skin and bones, do you think there could be a disorder that is opposite? Like Nancy Wilson and I looking into the mirror and seeing slimmer images than we actually were.

Star Jones and Anna Nicole Smith were both, at one time, large women who were beautiful and sexy. They did not dress like the majority of larger women do. The big and beautiful Delta Burke created a line of clothing that did not look like a sack and allowed women to still be fashionable in their larger versions.

Perhaps we should take this reverse disorder seriously. Instead of seeing an inaccurate image of our bodies in the mirror, we might have our picture taken. Somehow a picture seems to reveal our true size. In fact, I challenge you right now to put the book down and have a family member, or friend, take that first step with you. Take a picture, tape it to the fridge, and start your journey of accepting where you are and where you want to go.

Instead of covering up our layers and trying to hide our imperfections, let's face them. We need to find the real woman who's been hiding behind all this stuff. It's not for vanity sake, although fitting into a size 8 feels pretty good; but it is more for the sake of living, for the sake of being the best you that you can be, for the sake of having more energy, better heath, and being in control, as opposed to being out of control.

Signs

In the original Onion Factory℠ studio, there was a sign that read, "Nothing tastes as good as thin feels." I probably got more feedback from that one sign than most of the snippets I have hanging around the Factory. Is that feeling we desire control? Self-control? Or is that feeling a body with loads of energy, or perhaps a body that does not need to suck in its stomach, or does not have a muffin top?

You do know what a muffin top is, don't you? It's that bulging layer hanging over the top of your outfit that should probably go to the next size, but moving to the next size might mean we had gotten bigger. So, we stay in the current size as long as we can, take it until we are busting at the seams, or we finally give in and purchase the next size up. We just can't take it anymore.

You know what else Onions do? When we find an outfit that fits, or we feel good in, or one that hides our imperfections, we buy it in every color. What in the world is that all about?

The first thing Onions do as we start to peel is tucking in our clothes again. Did we think big and sloppy and/or ugly and baggy clothes were really hiding anything? I think not!

That original sign which caught new Campers' attention all goes back to this matter of control. It is control that completes our psychological health. It is lack of control that has encouraged the majority of our society to find an emotional escape in food. We'd better change, because obesity is literally killing our nation!

The "It" Girl

I walked into the Factory recently and encountered an Onion I had worked with the previous day, who was getting ready to begin the "Beast" (a workout on the largest elliptical machine we have). All Onions are special to me, but I had clicked immediately with this one in our Onion Camp over the holidays. However, Kelsey admitted that the week before this morning conversation had been a tough one for her.

A bit of explanation: During Camp, we learn how to train the body's various muscle groups. My first goal is to teach team members, who normally hate exercising and have spent a lifetime dieting their way in and out of their clothes, to learn how to take care of their muscles.

The first week of Camp is spent teaching clients how to clean out their pantry and relearn how to eat. Then I ask them to start building their cardiovascular endurance (THR training). By week three, they are very comfortable lifting free weights. (You know, the ones that you can buy at any Wal-Mart®, Kmart®, or Target®.) I love that we work with free weights, because it forces a person to utilize their entire body, learn good form, and you can always have a set handy. It is exciting to see Onions lifting free weights and learning proper weight-lifting form.) By week four, the Onions' fitness foundation is built.

Dear Lisa,

After my weigh and measure today. I was very down and defeated. I wanted to break, or at least reach my goal of 30 #'s lost. I was even ready to accept my loser goal of 25 #'s lost. When I saw it was only 22 #'s, I felt like a failure. I did not even want to go to graduation knowing that I had only conquered 3 #'s in the second half of camp.

Then I thought... How many people would've loved to lose 22 #'s in the last 8 weeks?

One of my co-workers told me that she was jealous of my progress. Then, I thought about how selfish I sounded. I am thankful for each pound and inch I have lost, and I am thankful for you and your patience and knowledge. I just hope that this summer when I am 100 #'s down, you pull this out, and we can chuckle about my desperation at graduation.

I have every intention to complete this journey. Hopefully, most of my trials in this area are in the past. I plan to work hard, and see where it gets me. Thanks for not giving up on me, or any of the rest of us Onions!

A lighter & still sassy,
Kelsey

In the second half of the eight-week Camp, we are ready to turn up the intensity and peel Onions. A camper usually takes off 25-40 pounds during the eight-week Camp. Kelsey was one of my "big hitters," she took off 19 pounds and 21 inches in the first four weeks. I was certain she could could break the record of 43 pounds in eight weeks.

But then the holiday month of December hit her. A significant life change hit her, so negative emotions hit her, and the last four weeks of Onion Camp were not kind to her. Here is the card she gave me at graduation:

Kelsey started advanced training with a new attitude (actually, her old sassy one had returned). She told her husband she was starting the Factory food plan, she was training full force, and she was reinventing herself. That is the key. When life hits us with unexpected events, hurts, joys—all kinds of emotions—we can allow ourselves to feel them, but then we have to get back in the box of our new healthy lifestyle.

Day one of Kelsey's advanced training concentrated on her chest and triceps. Body-part training was a whole new world for her. It is muscle specific, rather than a major muscle routine where you work an entire muscle group. We exercise one or two muscles repeatedly and increase the intensity.
(The advanced training studio is in the back of the Onion Factory, and Camp graduates frequently tell new Campers, "Don't let her take you back there.") The back room is very much like that place in fitness centers where fit people train. It has very intimidating machines and looks like a torture chamber instead of a fitness room. By contrast, the Factory is non-intimidating and has color-coded free weights. The Factory looks like fun and is fun.

After Kelsey's first day in the advanced room, I received a text message saying, "I am sore." Bear in mind, this is a love/hate relationship. The clients who are invited to train in the advanced studio are ready, or I would not invite them to do so. Advanced training is tough, but the results are amazing. You begin to see body parts that you did not even know were there because they were hiding behind layers of fat.

Day two includes the back, biceps, and shoulders. The following day, I received a text from Kelsey that said, "I hurt," with a smiley face. Remember, this is the type of hurt that results from lactic acid build-up in the muscles. In this level of training, muscle fibers are broken down and rebuilt. In your
mind, you know muscle will utilize stored fat as an energy source for rebuilding as you reinvent your body. So this is soreness for a good purpose. Its another expression of that love-hate relationship. You hate the place you are in, but you love the results.
Day three concentrates on the legs, your largest muscle group. I decided to egg Kelsey on, so I texted her, "Ready for legs?"

She replied, "If I say yes, will you take it a little easy on me?"

Of course, by now you must realize I could not. So on Friday, we did legs. Saturday morning she looked at me and with an odd expression and said, "I am not that sore today." She was reconditioning her body.

I smiled and she said, "I brought that picture you asked me to bring." The prior week I had asked her to bring in a past photo of herself in which she looked fat.
This was Kelsey's opportunity to show me that even as a thinner version of herself, she still had "cankles." I asked what she meant.

She lifted a leg and said, "You know how most people have a transition between the calf and the ankle?"

I said, "Yes."

"Look, I don't. My calf goes right into my ankle. Hence, I have a cankle."

I looked at Kelsey's yearbook cheerleading picture and thought, *WOW. She had been the girl I wanted to be. I bet she was even Prom Queen.* I said, "May I share a story that might offend you?"

She said, "Yes."

"In high school, I was never that 'it' girl," I explained. I was taller than all the boys, bigger than all the girls, and desperately wanted to

Failures of the past may be so deeply imprinted on your psyche that you are not aware of their connection with food.

be 5'2" and size two, but I was not made that way. To top it off, I spent 20 years dieting myself into a 300-pound girl, when I did not even like myself at 180 pounds."

I told Kelsey that she represented everything that I wished I had been back in high school. However, we both ended up in the same world of obesity. Now she had to do the hard work of conquering it, too.

Class Reunions

As big girls, one of the ways we resolve our self-esteem issues is through just-look-at-me-now moments at our class reunions. At least this is how I wanted to resolve mine. I always heard the stories about class reunions where the "it" girls were no longer "it." They ended up getting married and growing fat. At the same time, girls who were rarely noticed and never dated usually went on to do great things, find Prince Charming, and walk into the class reunion without anyone knowing them, because they had blossomed and found themselves after high school.
Years ago, I thought to myself, *I will go back to my class reunion and show what I've achieved. Everyone will see what was hiding behind THIS fluffy girl.*

Guess what? Last year was my twenty-fifth class reunion and I did not attend. I was busy completing my Factory and writing this guide, and going back to describe the journey was not really that important anymore. How liberating. I was free of my past and enjoying the here and now.

The Root of the Problem

Let's go way back to the root of our obesity problem. I am not going back to the cradle, but to gym class. You see, as I help clients find themselves and change, one question often tells me a lot about that individual: *How did you feel about gym class?*

In gym class, when they selected players for kickball or another team sport, were you chosen first, last, or somewhere in the middle? Can you remember the first time you had to undress in the locker room and let other high-school kids see you take a shower? How mortifying was that? No matter what shape, size, or body type you were, I think it was still mortifying.

Curly-haired girls always desired to have straight hair, tall girls wanted to be shorter, and brunettes wanted to be blondes. The imprints and expectations from our past never end. Were you the girl, like me, getting an excuse slip to avoid going to gym class? I think gym teachers make a mistake when they give most of their attention to the athletic students, instead of embracing those of us who are chosen in the middle or last. We just get lost. When we cannot do a sit-up, they teach us a crunch. When normal push-ups are too tough, they teach us the "girlie version."

I can honestly tell you that in my 40's I can run a faster mile, perform more real sit-ups, and do more real push-ups than I could ever do in high school. With a little patience and persistence, you can do anything you want. But failures of the past may be so deeply imprinted in your psyche that you are not aware of their connection with food.

I want you to think about the psychological roots of your problem. Ponder these questions:

- ❏ Do thoughts about food occupy much of your time?
- ❏ Do you binge and feel guilty afterward?
- ❏ Do you hide food to eat in secret?
- ❏ Do you consider food your friend or comforter?

- ❏ Do you eat specific foods when you are upset, sad, angry, afraid, anxious, or lonely?
- ❏ Have you tried to diet, repeatedly, only to sabotage your own weight loss?
- ❏ Do you overeat to the point of discomfort?
- ❏ Have you ordered too much food from a fast food restaurant and gotten two drinks to cover up the size of your order?
- ❏ Do you sneak food after others have left the room?
- ❏ Do you get up in the middle of the night to eat?
- ❏ Do you feel afraid to give up any particular food that is not good for you?
- ❏ Do you get upset if you cannot have the exact food you desire?
- ❏ Do you escape from stress by eating?
- ❏ Would you consider the idea that you might be addicted to food?

As you continue to read through *The Fork Is Mightier Than the Gym*, allow yourself to go to your truths and acknowledge the real source of your problem. Then determine to learn how you can change.

Change Is Good

Changing your old habits and changing what you have believed for decades will be tough. You might even be frustrated no one took the time to teach you these basics early in life. You will need to want the results more than the brownie sitting in front of you. You will need to focus on the big picture and not the temptations. Remember, you already know what that brownie tastes like, and later down the road when you are at that safe body-fat percentage, you will learn how to enjoy a bite (not the entire pan) of brownie again. Let me remind you, "Nothing tastes as good as thin feels."

Here's an even better thought: Nothing tastes as good as loads of energy, feeling good, and relief from pain.

The great thing about change is you do not need to be perfect, you just need to make better choices. This journey of reaching a healthy weight is not a race against anyone but yourself. The change does not need to be dramatic. Remember the example of "what if" you lost one pound in January, two in February, and so on? By the end of the year, you are 78 pounds lighter. Your journey must be a consistent process of change with better choices.

The first step to changing is to gather the ideas and collect the knowledge you will need. The next step is making a reasonable plan to change. You will need to dig deep in your soul to find the will to change. You must find the right mindset to take care of you. For me, I can accomplish anything if I get mad enough. When I have had enough, change is bound to happen. I want to ask you: Can you get motivated to change? What emotion do you require in order to motivate change?

What trips your own trigger to start, or stop, a life change? Is it a season? I find that some clients are motivated to change by a change of seasons. Usually, it's the reality that last season's clothes no longer fit. That's a huge wake-up call.

Perhaps you have a class reunion coming up, and the reality of seeing all your old schoolmates horrifies you. Guess what? They are probably in the same shape you are in, or worse. But if the thought of a class reunion gets you started, great! Just keep in mind what are you going to do *after* the class reunion. Go back to your unhealthy habits? I hope not. I hope you find that this new energy level and new health level are motivating enough to keep you on task.

Could a medical concern bring you to this fork in the road? Prevention is such a wonderful tool. Why is it that a marriage or divorce can become an instant weight-loss program? I love it when clients change because they wish to have more fun with their grandkids. I cannot imagine a better motivation than quality time with children.

Life triggers such as these are very important in the process of change. We need to get rid of our old habits because they obviously are not working. We need to find new habits that support the new lifestyles. we want If you find that food is filling voids in your life, or you have compulsive behaviors with pans of brownies, then you will really need some motivating force, an urgency, to help you change.

A few paragraphs back, I mentioned eating a brownie; let's revisit that. Are you a person who nibbles until the entire pan is gone? Can you eat just one potato chip? Do you mindlessly eat? Or here's my favorite: Do you nibble and sip as you cook for your family and then sit down to have a meal with them? I did. The mistake of this behavior is that we cannot make good decisions when we are hungry, so we wind up eating two meals' worth of food!

Are You Hungry? Angry? Lonely? Tired?

One of the best things I've learned along the way is the acronym H.A.L.T. The psychology link was a missing component in the Onion world until now. We needed more tools to help clients keep their focus, and H.A.L.T. is one of them.

H.A.L.T. is not a new idea. The term is used with people who have various addictions, and I've found that it works for Onions like us. Simply never allow yourself to get too *hungry*, too *angry*, too *lonely* or *tired*. In these moments it is very difficult to make the proper choices.

Recently, I was working with another health professional, and she shared with me that a smoker attempting to quit will work through the physical addictions within three days; however, it's not until the ninth day that a smoker deals with the psychological withdrawal from the smoking addiction. So consider this as you change your behaviors. If you keep going back to your old habits, you are probably stuck in the third- and ninth-day syndrome.

The first step to overcoming an addiction is to reach the point where you really desire to change. The next step is to make sure you have the proper information with which to change. And the final step is to find the self-discipline to make the change happen.

Addictions are tough, whether we are addicted to food, alcohol, drugs, sex, or something else. Detaching yourself from any of these weaknesses is a process. Be patient but relentless and you will break out of the prison of addiction.

Food and Discipline

If you have an addiction to food, one piece of pizza rather than the entire pizza may be a problem for you. If you have taken off 25, 50, 75, or even 100 pounds, you have been retraining yourself on a whole new lifestyle. And at the end of the day, that is truly the only weight-loss solution out there. When we eat clean, we have loads of energy. When we bring back the high-fat selections or the grab-and-go nutrition that is processed and full of fillers, we begin to feel sluggish again. Addiction means you must change the mental or psychological element of your relationship with food.

If food has been your escape, your comfort, or your pacifier, then you have to replace that behavior with other behaviors that make you healthier and make you feel better.

This is a journey, as I said in the beginning. It is a new beginning, a rediscovery, and a regaining of your true identity. You will need to manage your results with your new knowledge of food and a new understanding of your habits—the good ones and the ones that you must continually work on.

A Fit or Fat Mindset

I am thankful that I've spent more than two decades on the front lines of the fitness industry. I would hate to think that someone would attempt to write a guide on how to change your life after reading research papers alone. I am the most thankful for the past few years, because I had the opportunity to conquer my own obesity. I learned what works and what does not, as well as some of the issues behind a society that is crippled by this disease. If obesity could have been cured through a pill, changed with a Nordic-track, or conquered by some other fad, our nation would not be in this condition.

However, as with many things in life, there is a point at which more is not better. If you are a trainer working with clients, you may

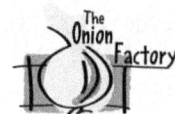

Two bad weeks did not get you out of your skinny jeans, neither will two good weeks get you back into them.

see them give you more and more, without immediate results. What went wrong? Was it a medication? Were they eating outside of the box? Perhaps you inspired them to over-train; or perhaps you push them too hard, convincing them that working a few extra minutes may get the results they want. This may work, or not.

Often, I have felt that I wanted results for my clients more than they did. I did not realize that, although I had taught them the necessary information, I had not gotten under the layers of denial deep in their souls to the root of the problem. Again, I thought the correct knowledge and formulas would be enough. They weren't.

You must go back to the hurtful places in your life, or go to the situations that caused an eating binge. Identify what you are hiding from, and realize that you no longer need to be afraid to reveal the real you. No matter what you've heard in the past, you are worthy to be seen and acknowledged. You are worth the effort it takes to lose the layers you've be hiding behind.

I believe taking body composition readings, weights, and measures at weekly meetings are the tools by which we can make adjustments—not just the scientific ones, but also the mental ones. Did we need more hydration? Did we need more protein? Was our cardiovascular training at the correct intensity? Did we fatigue the muscle? If any of these strategies are not in proportion, your body may decide to hold on to its fat for a while longer. Did something happen to upset you? Did you lose focus because of an emotion?

If you are an Onion, you became fat because you trained your body to be lazy. Now you will be re-training it, learning how to get the most out of your engine. The past few years have taught and re-taught me that fat loss can be a five-pound-per-week journey. But faster weight loss is not likely, no matter how much harder you try. So don't go that route and risk becoming discouraged. Remember even one pound lost will encourage you, so that you begin thinking and believing you are becoming fit!

Weight Loss Versus Weight Gain

The psychology of weight loss and weight gain intrigues me. The psychology of change was one of the most difficult parts of this program to learn. Finding examples that make sense and speaks to others took many years. As a coach, I see patterns. These patterns and stories give you the opportunity to take a look in the mirror and see if the examples are speaking to you.

One factor that works in the Onion world—more specifically, the Onion eight-week course—is our weekly weigh-ins and measurements. These validate the choices Onions made during the previous week. Weight and measurement stats inform a client if they need to make adjustments for water, protein, complex carbs, and/or workout intensity. Weekly accountability aligns the psyche for yet another week as you continue to learn, grow, and modify your behaviors. There is a psychological component of the weigh-and-measure session that I need to explain to you. It's about how your brain can get the best of you.

Have you ever had a bad week or two of eating wrong, yet your jeans still fit? The scale does not seem to be changing. Then, all of the sudden, Week Three hits and you can no longer zip up your jeans.

Frequently, what happens in the emotional center of our brain is this: If Weeks One and Two do not give us the validation we are looking for, then we are tempted to sabotage the new choices and go back to our old ways.

Call this a moment of transition, a plateau, a set point, or whatever you like. You need to realize that two bad weeks did not get you out of your skinny jeans, neither will two good weeks get you back into them.

Meltdown Fix: Candy

Sometimes, life is so difficult and so messy that only some chocolate will help. Old psychological imprints and our taste buds' memory can take over our wills to convince us of reasoning like this.

While standing in the line at the grocery store, I picked up a package of mint patties. I turned over the bag and began my review. I wanted to check the nutritional chart to see whether we Onions might be able to squeeze in a patty or two.

(Let's be frank, if we are going to manage our weight for a lifetime, then we need some back-up plans for the days when nothing but a piece of chocolate will make us feel better.)

This particular bag markets its diet value as only one point. I have never been on the point system, but have many friends on it who have done well. What I do know about the point system is that the program provides good nutritional knowledge, and knowledge is where change begins. Of course, what you do with the knowledge makes ll the difference.

What if you utilize all your points for something that has very little nutritional value? Counting points may help you lose pounds on a scale, but you may not reduce your overall percentage of fat, improve your blood sugar level, lower your cholesterol, gain more energy, and feel better. You may still, after all that effort, be a smaller version of a fat you.

I asked my current campers, as I showed them the bag, "How many of you would have eaten just one serving? Because the front of the bag reads 'one point,' how many of you would have thought, *These little patties are okay*? And once you opened the bag to satisfy your craving, it was all over. Before you realized it, you had finished most of the bag. Then guilt set in. And you tried to regroup and figure out what you would not eat for the rest of the day to make up for the over-abundance of mint patties and wasted points. Sound familiar?"

I felt I needed to inform my Campers of a few facts as we learned together how to feed our metabolic engines:

1.) This little bag of mint patties contains two and a half servings, so be very careful.

2.) One point is for *one piece*, not one serving. If you eat a serving, you must count *three points*. If you have a meltdown and eat the entire bag, you need to count *seven points*.

3.) One serving looked like this:

Nutrition Facts

Serving Size 27.00 g
Servings Per Container

Amount Per Serving

	% Daily Values*
Total Fat 2g	2%
Saturated Fat 1.0g	6.0%
Trans Fat 0.0g	
Cholesterol 0.0mg	0.0%
Sodium 10.0mg	0.0%
Total Carbohydrates 22g	8%
Dietary Fiber <1.0g	2.00%
Sugars 18.0g	
Protein <1.0g	
Calcium 0.0% Iron	4.0%

*Percent Daily Values are based on a 2,000 calorie diet. Your daily values may be higher or lower depending on your calorie needs.

I have a few questions for you. If you subtract 18 grams of sugar from the total carbohydrates (22 grams), where are the remaining 4 grams of carbohydrates coming from; a fruit, a vegetable, or a filler? Will this candy aid your weight loss? Or will this "fix" make you crave more sugar?

The same day I reviewed the package of mint patties, I met with an Onion who is working extra hard at her weight loss, so she can gain it all back with a pregnancy. For several weeks, she has been stuck with small losses. Minor

Hershey's® Bar (43g)	210 Calories	13g fat	26g carbs	24g sugar
Kit Kat® Bar (42g)	218 Calories	11.1g fat	26.9g carbs	20g sugar
Snickers® Bar (57g)	271 Calories	13.6g fat	34.5g carbs	28.8g sugar
M&M's® (48g)	236 Calories	10.1g fat	34.2g carbs	36g sugar

mistakes on the weekends were getting in her way. She needed a good week for her psyche. You know how it goes: A little success fuels more good choices and more drive to stay on your game. It encourages you to do the little extras that help weight loss. But once you forget a meal or a workout, it seems like a slippery slope back to old habits.

Bravo! She got her validation this week. She had a five-pound loss in her weigh and measure. When this happens, you can see a client's eyes light up. This feeling empowers a person to want more and go for more results.

During this Onion's workout, she stops, looks at me, and says, "I need to confess something. I had a meltdown Friday night and had to have a candy bar." (I love this part of the story.) However, she took the time to flip every label, because she wanted to make the best "bad" choice she could.

Her thought process reminds me of the question, Which is less harmful, too much sugar or too much fat? Which chocolate fix could she work into the equation? To get where you want to be, you need to remember that your body will burn about 24 grams of sugar per day, and fruit contains fructose, which is sugar. Any more than 24 grams, and it's going back to your reserve tank.

On a meltdown, she decided to use a few grams of sugar for a little chocolate in order to get over the temptation and move on.

After the fact, as she works out she says, "Darn, if I would not have eaten that candy, maybe I would have lost six pounds." She is getting it. She is realizing she is in control of her change.

Every step toward a new you begins with the choices you make. Just for fun, let's look at a few of those candy bars we all love and see how they add up (see chart below). Then consider this alternative:

Chocolate Fudge Bar (66 g):

- 110 calories
- 4 fat gm.
- 16 carb gm.
- 13 sugar gm.

Which bar would give you the best nutrition? I want you to learn how to read nutrition labels on prepared foods and ask some perceptive questions when you do. For example, when you subtract the sugar grams from the total carb grams, where are the remaining carbs coming from, a filler or "grass of the lands"?

Of course, a cleaner option than any of these candy bars would be a chocolate protein drink. The drinks will help curb your cravings while feeding your lean mass.

Feeding the cravings may indeed make you want more sugar, or it might satisfy you enough that you can work your way through another week of better choices. My goal is to bring you critical knowledge about how your body works. Then this game of a "new you" is in your ballpark!

The Cheating Psche

Oh, those weekly weigh-ins! We love them; we hate them. We forget to bring our logbooks when we know they will not look good. We call for an early weigh-in if we suspect it will be great. Then the weigh-in is when you get validation for your choices of the past week. (Be honest, you know when you are on game.) Regardless of what I teach you, I understand that you may still have a love affair with the bathroom scale. If I have not talked you out of the scale, then at least make sure it can give you all the information you need to make educated changes. Get one that reveals both pounds and percentages of fat.

This journey requires mental focus. The tools are just the tools. But the mind is an entirely different ballpark. Let's talk about cheating. At first, we look at the obvious desserts. If you gave up the desserts that you desired so badly, then you deserve a number on the scale that makes it okay, you know, worthwhile. We all know that number on the scale is so accurate. NOT!

Let's talk about cheating with an entirely new perspective. Keep in mind that when you are on your game, there will be countless examples of how the body can, and will, change one percent per week if you will do the work. Therefore, anything outside of not doing the work is cheating! RIGHT?

The Question

I caught wind of a conversation from an Onion Camp that included repeater Onions as well as new Onions. This made for an interesting mix. A new Camper asked a returning camper, "Can I cheat?" When the question was shared with me behind the scenes, I just shook my head.

Imagine investing in an eight-week course to change your life. You want to know how to change but still ask where the shortcuts are. In essence, someone is asking for results without doing the work. I am not sure anything in life works that way. I wondered why someone would want to know if there were any shortcuts, as if they were looking for Cliff Notes in weight loss. Guess what? There are none. We fluffy people have been looking for the Cliff Notes for decades, and look what happened to us.

Physical change is not about cheating. It is about learning how to eat rather than starve. It is about learning how to eat and not cheat. And change is about learning how to eat nutritious food, so you can obtain the essential vitamins and minerals every day, enabling you to feel better. It is that simple. You are learning how to eat in order to feed and protect your metabolism and metabolic rate. You are not going to cheat yourself any longer by feeding your fat cells. I won't let you!

Let's review the purpose of food. Food is for obtaining essential vitamins and minerals. Food is for energy. And food is for prevention of what ails us. Food is not to fill our social needs. Yes, go out be social; however, do not sabotage your goals for a moment with food. Enjoy the company you are with. If you need to change the setting or the menu to avoid making poor choices, then do so. Food is not there to fill the emotional voids in your life.

A pizza is not meant to be your Saturday night date. Try a walk in the park or a bubble bath and a book. Heck, buy a romance novel if you need to, but stay away from the bon bons.

Last, but not least, food is not simply something to satisfy your cravings. It has an emotional dimension, too. Remember, we celebrate with food. We stress with food. We comfort with food. We sabotage with food. If you start understanding the self-destructive relationships we may have with food, then you can begin to make positive changes in your food habits.

"Starving"?

Let's face it. Most of us really do not know what true hunger feels like. We know cravings and we know temptations to eat, but when we say we're "starving," what do we really mean? After all, when we look in the mirror, we know we really *aren't* starving.

We have already established the fact that it's difficult to make a good decision when you feel hungry. For me, cooking dinner on an empty stomach was one of my recurring mistakes. I was so hungry I would nibble while cooking, and then I would eat dinner with the family. One might call this an example of mindless eating.

Whatever you call it, cooking on an empty

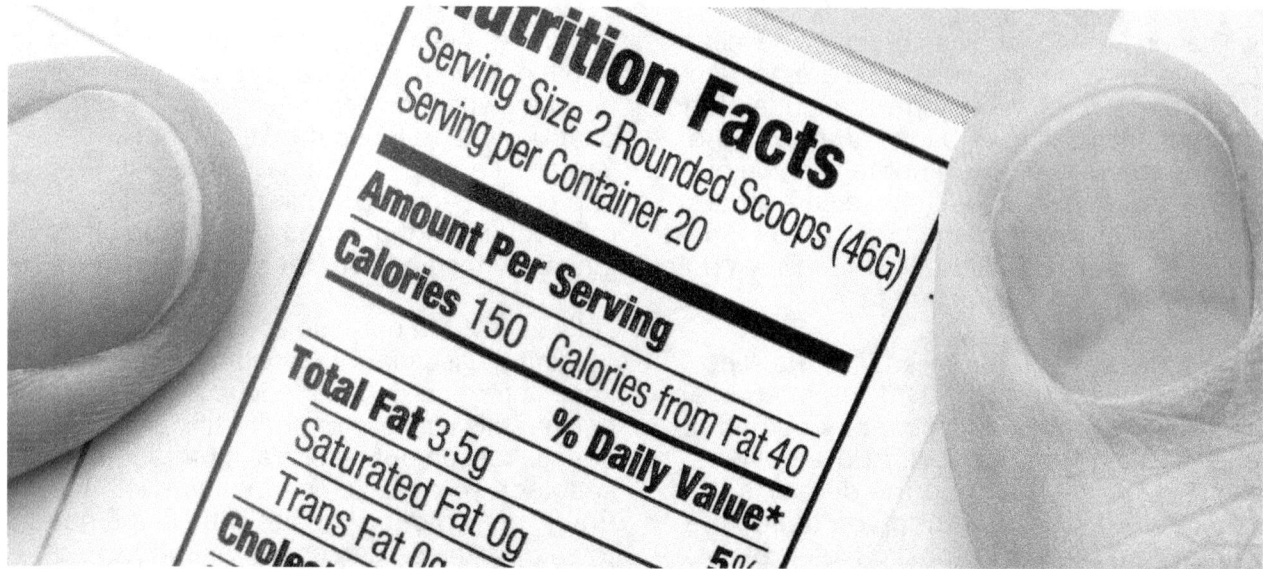

stomach or buying groceries that way both prove how difficult it is to eat properly when you are not well-prepared to make objective decisions.

Psychology in Advertising

How about this one: *Limited time only.* What happens to your thought process when you see this tag line? Guess what? It is a marketing tool (an urgency factor) to stimulate you, the consumer, to buy this product.

You have heard of the tag line: *Part of a reduced-calorie diet.* Have you ever wondered what that really means? What type of calories? We see *reduced-calorie* and again, as consumers, we think this food is okay. The mind can play so many tricks on us.

We have been exposed to all of the *free* stuff for a very long time: *fat-free, sugar-free, carb-free.* The manufacturers kept producing these products, we kept buying, and look what we bought into: We got away from the basics of nutrition. Change can be as simple as returning to basic nutrition.

The nutrition labels tell us a lot. What does a food producer mean when a yogurt's label reads, *only 100 calories?* Let's take a look. Maybe Yoplait® has a bigger marketing budget, but Kroger has a better yogurt for weight loss. Examine the labels below and answer these questions:

1. How many grams of sugar are in each?

2. How many grams of protein?

4. Sugar feeds your _____ cells.

5. Which yogurt better feeds your lean mass?

General Mills Yoplait® Yogurt

Serving Size: 6 ounces

Calories: 100

Fat: 0

Carbohydrates: 19g

Sugars: 14g

Protein: 5g

Kroger Carbmaster® Yogurt

Serving Size: 6 ounces

Calories: 80

Fat: 1.5g

Carbohydrates: 4g

Sugars: 3g

Protein: 12g

9. Food, Food, Food

YES, CHANGE IS MENTAL.

BUT FITNESS RESULTS ALL BEGIN

WITH FOOD.

I WILL NEVER TEACH you to eat smaller portions of valueless foods. Those foods only stimulate your desire for food that tastes good, but has little nutritional value. My goal is to teach you (and give you recipes for) foods that are nutritionally sound, that serve the purpose of feeding your muscles, and that supply vitamins and minerals. Why would we continue to create and consume smaller portions of trigger foods? It goes back to the internal/external understanding of your motivation.

How You Are Going to Eat

A tough part of peeling Onions, changing the course of obesity, is to change individuals' mindsets about the consumption of grains, milk, and bananas. Remember, what you will eat when you are in a safe body composition and what you will eat when you are trying to peel away layers of fat are two different menus. While you have a reserve tank of stored fat, you do not need to eat fillers, or starchy carbohydrates, for energy. You want your body to pull from your reserve tank.

In the following pages, you will learn many things that are contrary to what you have learned about food over the past few decades. Everyone still finds eating to lose weight very difficult. So you must ingrain the thought process of which foods are healthy and promote weight loss. Surround yourself with these food selections. I am going to share with you information I've learned during my journey of losing weight. If you keep these examples in mind, they will help you during your journey.

Healthy?

In front of me, I have two cans of soup. They caught my eye at the grocery store because their labels boldly say, **Healthy**. I am always reading food labels, searching for new ideas and tools to create recipes. The can of soup in my right hand is tomato, and the one in my left hand is cream of chicken. If you were on a mission to make better choices, which one do you think would be the better choice? Most clients would say the tomato soup. Certainly, we have been trained to believe that a cream soup could not possibly be better than tomato. The tomato soup has 1.5 fat grams per serving, which is less than the 2.5 fat grams for the cream of chicken. But did you realize that a can represents two and a half servings? So the can of tomato soup has a total of 3.75 grams of fat while the cream of chicken can has 6.75 fat grams. At this point, it would appear the tomato soup is the best choice because it contains less fat. Let's look closer, though.

The next amount to look at is protein. Each soup has the same amount of protein with two grams per serving. If you ate the whole can (by the way, many people do), you'd have fed your body five grams of protein, which is a far stretch from the minimal 75 grams per day your body requires.

When I was in my former life, eating out of control, one of my favorite comfort foods was a big bowl of tomato soup made with milk and loaded with crackers. While my stomach was full and I felt comforted, I had not given my lean mass enough protein from this meal to sustain its needs. I had fed it only five grams of protein (plus seven from the milk), which falls far short of the body's requirement of 75 grams or more per day. But let's keep going.

This piece of the puzzle might blow your mind. To see if these soups were worthy to create a recipe, I checked their sugar content. Can you imagine this? The tomato soup has 10 grams of sugar and the cream of chicken has zero. Make this innocent can of tomato soup with milk and you get more than the 24 grams of sugar that your body can digest in a day.

As I shared this trip to the grocery store with Onion Camp 15, I told them that I would rather use the cream of chicken soup. I would grab a pound of chicken breast and a bag of frozen broccoli. I'd season the chicken and grill it on my George Foreman grill. Then I'd throw the broccoli on top of the chicken, pour the soup (diluted with water) over the top of that, and bake it for 20 minutes at 350 degrees. Now I have a recipe with ingredients that will feed my muscle protein (the chicken), give my body macronutrient vitamins and minerals (the broccoli), and utilize the fat and flavor from the soup to create a meal with real food value.

Dressings and Sauces

It was Thanksgiving Day. Mom, my oldest son Jake, and I were at Starbucks when I informed them that I needed to stop at the local grocery store to complete some recipe research. Because of my obsessive dedication to this kind of work, even on Thanksgiving, Jake blurted out, "Mom, I am going to get you a poster from the movie, 'The Blues Brothers.'" I looked at him confused, so he said, "The poster says: 'We're on a mission from God.'"

We all chuckled. I imagine he still feels this way, because I want to do all I can to give you the best information about healthy eating habits, even on Thanksgiving. I want this book to empower you with knowledge that will help you create a new you.

We Onions have been led astray for a long time. Simply desiring to be thinner, we have jumped on lots of bandwagons, so I'm trying to break that cycle.

Frequently, people at my Onion Camps ask, "Can't you just write down what you eat?" Not really. While I can certainly explain the basics of the nutritional formula, I am not a dietician, so I cannot write you a comprehensive food plan. Besides, the diet concept has not worked. Even if I could clear those hurdles, we do not like all of the same things. But if I teach you how to feed your metabolic engine, you can make your own decisions about what specific foods to eat.

The first step is knowledge, so here we go.

One of the biggest mistakes Onions have made over the past few years was eating too many fat grams. Fats add up very quickly. Although fats are satisfying, they are empty calories, which is both good and bad. If fats leave you satisfied so that you do not eat the foods you need to sustain your lean mass, they will sabatoge your goals. However, if a small portion of fat embellishes your base food with a tasty flair so that you feel satisfied until your next meal, then it is good. Dressings and sauces fill this role.

Salad Dressings

Recently, while I was at my younger son's basketball game, I sat with an Onion who was currently in our Camp. She, like most of us working women, was behind the eight ball of a tight schedule and had to grab her dinner on the fly. Basketball-game food is not known

> ### Cream of Chicken
> *with Broccoli*
> ### Smashed Cauliflower
>
> ☐ 8 grilled chicken breasts
> ☐ 2 16-oz bags chopped broccoli
> ☐ 1 8-oz can fat-free cream of chicken soup
> ☐ 1 soup can of water
> ☐ 4 cups smashed cauliflower*
> ☐ sprinkle of 2% cheddar cheese
> ☐ sprinkle of Durkee® fried onions
> ☐ sprinkle of Mrs. Dash® seasoning
>
> *Directions:*
> - Grill chicken, season with Mrs. Dash®
> - Whisk soup and water in measuring cup, pour over chicken
> - Top with broccoli and cream of chicken soup
> - Cover and bake at 325° approx. 1 hour
> - Garnish with cheese and fried onions.
> - Plate cauliflower, baked chicken, and gravy.
>
> *See p.189 for Smashed Cauliflower recipe. Make more if you like!.

to be help people lose weight. Those breadsticks and nachos go straight to our tushies. So this Onion had a great idea. She stopped at a local restaurant and grabbed a grilled chicken salad. Great choice. She also grabbed two packets of dressing. Ouch, there were 30 grams of fat in each packet. Ironically, she was on her cardiovascular game and was weight training at full capacity, but she was stuck on her way toward losing weight. I soon figured out why: Too many fat grams!

So I flipped over the dressing packet and began to guide her. Who would have thought a grilled chicken salad with dressing could add up to 60 grams of fat?

Later, on my Turkey Day at the grocery, I decided to spend some time in the salad dressing aisle. Dressing is usually the first place we make our mistakes. The two biggest mistakes we make will be in our consumption of too many fat grams and too many sugars. Salad dressings, if you are not careful, can be loaded with both.

I started my store research with ranch dressing, which is most people's favorite. (Kind of like chocolate ice cream!) I have learned that if someone is not a ranch person, then they are more likely to go after the high-fat and high-sugar dressings like poppy seed or honey mustard. At least with ranch, blue cheese, oil and vinegar, or Caesar dressing, you just need to pay attention to the fat content, not the sugar. These dressings are naturally low in sugar or sugar-free.

If you watch your portions and carefully select the *light* version of a dressing, the following are good choices:

☐ Blue cheese
☐ Caesar
☐ Ranch
☐ Oil & Vinegar

Unlimited Portion Selections

We at The Onion Factory℠ have discovered a tasty brand of salad dressings that are both fat-free and sugar-free. These are the Walden Farms dressings This company offers a wide selection, including these:

☐ Ranch
☐ Bleu cheese
☐ Thousand Island
☐ Raspberry Vinaigrette

Portion-Control Selections

I want you to consider something. Do you truly use only two tablespoons of salad dressing? Before I understood the entire picture, I was a dump-and-go girl with my salad dressings. Pay attention to portions. Toss your lettuce with the tablespoon you use to measure your dressing; it'll go a long way.

100 /// The Fork Is Mightier Than the Gym

- ❑ Trader Joe's Champagne Pear Vinaigarette
- ❑ Ken's Light Vidalia Onion
- ❑ Ken's Light Caesar

Do-Not-Touch Selections

You will risk using all your day's allotment of sugars and fats in one helping of salad with an out-of-bounds salad dressing. When in doubt, read the label on your dressing bottle.

- ❑ Poppy Seed
- ❑ Honey Mustard
- ❑ Creamy Ranch
- ❑ Creamy Bleu Cheese

Secret Weapons

Allow me to share two secret weapons in the fight against obesity. I have to brag about Walden Farms® again. They have a line of condiments for diabetics that is one of the rare fat-free, sugar-free, carb-free lines out there. It is very difficult to find all of those "free" ingredients in one item. Thank you to my bodybuilding friends who taught me this secret! Aside from their salad dressings, here are the Walden Farms® products that we at The Onion Factory℠ love:

Walden Farms® Favorites

- Chocolate syrup
- Pancake syrup
- Caramel dip
- Chocolate dip

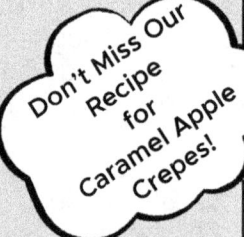

Don't Miss Our Recipe for Caramel Apple Crepes!

I'm going to be honest with you. I've tried all this stuff, and there are a few products you may not want to invest with your grocery budget. Avoid Walden Farms® peanut butter; it's not worth it. Try Better 'N Peanut Butter®, available at Trader Joe's®, but take a shot at analyzing the label and figure out how it works into the equation. It's not unlimited, but it's good. Instead of 17 grams of fat from off-the-shelf peanut butter, Better 'N Peanut Butter® only has 2. But watch out for the filler carbs. Use sparingly.

My vice is not sugar. I love breads, pasta, rice, potatoes—you know, all that warm comfort food! When I began writing recipes, all of my Onions voiced that they needed more desserts. Not a sugar-holic, I never got it, but I started creating them. Walden Farms® products made it very easy. Check out the famous Blueberry Cobbler using Walden's Blueberry syrup (recipe on page 208). If your vice is sugar, this indulgence will delight you.

The second secret weapon is from Susan, a.k.a. 911, because she is a dispatcher. And she is truly amazing! I really considered putting her picture on the cover of the book, not mine. She lost 91 pounds in a little over six months. She started at 46 percent body fat, and last week she was 29 percent. I tease her every day that when she hits 26 percent she will be kicked out of the program. Maybe that is why she agreed to help train newcomers to the Factory.

We were all working in the kitchen recently and she shared her favorite salad dressing. This Kraft® dressing is not marketed as fat-free or sugar-free, but check this out: Two tablespoons of Kraft® Red Roasted Pepper Italian with Parmesan has only two fat grams, four carb grams, and three sugar grams. Susan peels and slices cucumbers and marinates them in this dressing. It's incredible! One last word about sugar. As I began creating recipes to help Onions stay in the nutritional box, I was extremely concerned about opening the sugar demon. Once you consume a little sugar, you desire more.

A protein works the opposite way. Protein levels out your blood sugar, and then you are satisfied. Most of the sweet treats in this guide are protein-based and enhanced with a variety of Walden Farms® items. The sugars and fats are strategically placed to enhance the taste of the protein.

I've found that adding Fat-Free Cool Whip® to protein powders or topping off a protein drink with it fills the sweet-tooth craving. Our Food Division team has to analyze various options while creating new treats, and they found that Cool Whip® can bring a light, sweet taste without a lot of sugar.

Cool Whip® Nutritional Values

	Fat Grams	Sugar Grams	Carb Grams	Protein Grams
Regular	1.5	1	2	0
Lite	1	1	3	0
Free	0	1	3	0

Warning: Dipping into the Cool Whip® container too frequently will get you in trouble. Remember that two teaspoons, not the entire container, equals a serving. If you find yourself eating the entire container in a day or two, put it away. You are not ready. Go find a protein drink or some fresh berries.

Here is the breakdown of Cool Whip®. The serving size is 2 teaspoons, so there are 25 servings in a container.

Remember that Cool Whip® really has no nutritional value. If you find you are feeding a craving, but neglecting the rest of your nutrition, you may decide to leave Cool Whip® alone.

I've had plenty of Onions come to the realization they were not ready for Cool Whip® or peanut butter. Sometimes it may be better to keep those two doors closed until you are able to peel a few layers.

Sauces

Now let's look at ingredients in some of the most common sauces.

Tomatoes are a huge part of our society's food. Pizza sauce, pasta sauce, and catsup are three American staples. Unfortunately, in these processed foods tomatoes have been used on top of filler carbohydrates. Too many fillers and too much comfort food might be part of the reason why Type 2 diabetes has grown to epidemic proportions. Carbohydrates composed a large portion of the food that I so loved to consume. I am sure the majority of my carbohydrates came from breads. If you really look at the average American's eating habits, you will probably find that more than 225 grams of a day's carbohydrates are coming from starches.

A large portion of the recipes in this book use tomatoes and pasta sauce. When we

Pasta Sauce Nutritional Values

	Fat Grams	Carb Grams	Sugar Grams	Protein Grams
Newman's Sockarooni®	2	12	11	2
Ragu®	4	12	9	2
Bertolli®	2	13	9	2
Classico®	1	11	6	2
Barilla® Sweet Pepper	2	10	4	2

started the Food Division, I quickly learned that not all pasta sauces are created equal. I wanted this book to be full of sauces you could use in unlimited amounts. I wanted you to learn how to eat, not starve. I did not want this journey to be about portion control. I wanted to find food that would fill a plate. Remember, I am an eater. I love food. If you are an Onion, I assume you feel the same way.

Not all sauces are created equal. Why waste sugar grams on a sauce with loads of extra sugar? Save the sugar for something else you might enjoy more. All of the sauces compared below are based on a one-half cup serving. The sauce with the highest sugar content will lead the list, and the others follow in descending order.

As you can see, all the fat grams are about the same. However, the amount of sugar varies. You can save 7 grams of sugar and have the same serving amount just by selecting the Barilla.

We have analyzed fat and sugar; now, let's play around with protein. Cottage cheese is a wonderful low-fat, quick, and easy source for your protein needs. Cottage cheese is not as clean a protein as egg whites or chicken breast; however, it can make recipes taste richer. Cottage cheese is a great breakfast choice if you are on the fly. It is also an easy snack item.

Low-fat, no-fat, and regular-fat proteins can be confusing. I see so many items that are advertised as good protein sources; however, they are full of high-fat and high-filler carbohydrates. I hope to teach you how to select proteins that feed your muscles, from low-fat, no-filler selections. Let's break down a serving of small curd cottage cheese (chart below). As you start learning how to make better choices by reading labels, you will often find that when fat is taken out, sugar is added. Buyers, beware.

Remember I mentioned that I could not indulge in any food that tastes fake or flavorless. I struggle with the cottage cheese options. I have found cooking with the fat-free cottage cheese works great. You cannot tell the difference; however, if I were going to choose one for a snack, I would probably select the low-fat. Did you notice that the fat-free cottage cheese has more sugar? Did you ever analyze the difference between regular milk and fat-free? I am going to have you do that comparison on your own. Then, go to the cream aisle and plug that information into your new understanding of food. The crazy part is when an item has more fat we tend to use less. This entire food journey and all its selections can be overwhelming.

Apologies to Ralph Nader

I used to tell my Onion Campers that I did not wish to be the Ralph Nader of food. Well, I take it back. I DO want to be the Ralph Nader of food, because I DO want to impact society with knowledge and insight as he did. And I can only hope to accomplish as much as he has. (If you're reading this book and don't have any idea of who Ralph Nader is, bravo! You're a much younger person than most of us.) If you are seeking knowledge and solutions as relentlessly as he did, you have found the real deal.

Allow me a Ralph Nader rant. In our town, there is a huge billboard on which a brewing company declares how wonderful their beer is for all of

Cottage Cheese Nutritional Values

	Fat Grams	Sugar Grams	Protein Grams
Regular (4%)	5	4	13
Low-Fat (1%)	1.5	4	13
Fat-Free (0%)	0	5	13

the runners out there. The billboard proclaims that this product has only 95 calories and 2.6 grams of carbs per can. It assures all would-be marathon runners that this beer is a perfect complement to our fitness goals.

Let's do the math together. That's 95 calories from what? Beer doesn't have any calories from fat, so we can eliminate that column. Protein? Nope. Beer has NO protein. So all 95 calories must come from carbohydrates. Normally, carbohydrates have 4 calories per gram, but alcohol carbs have 7 calories per gram. So let's do the math in two ways:

1. If we said all of these 95 calories came from alcohol, we would divide by 7, which tells us that the can's 95 calories equal 13 grams of alcohol.

2. If we use the usual divisor of 4 calories per gram of carbohydrate, then the beer has 23.7 grams of carbs.

Although the billboard says you are only consuming 2.6 grams of carbs, you are really consuming between 13 and 23 grams, depending on which formula we use. A slice of bread has 15–20 grams of carbohydrates, so drinking one of these "low carb" beers is really like eating an extra slice of bread.

No wonder beer drinkers get such big bellies!

The Keto Effect

The one rule I have about dieting is this: If the plan is not one you can follow for the rest of your life, then don't start it. The reason is simple. When you go back to your old way of eating, your old results will come back. Nutrition is about balanced eating. There are no secrets, no shortcuts, and no magic new idea. Perhaps this is the best way I can illustrate it:

For your car to perform at 100% efficiency, you have to give it gas, change the oil, rotate the tires, etc. If you neglect one of those maintenance items, don't be surprised if your automobile poops out on you.

There's a lot of buzz about the Keto diet right now, and medical experts say that the Keto diet will produce weight loss for a short period of time. However, it is not meant to be a lifelong way of eating. Can the Keto diet give you results? Of course! Most diets can give you results on a bathroom scale. However, we are looking for more than a change in numbers on a scale. We want to sustain a healthy metabolism so that we look healthy, have plenty of energy, and prevent disease and premature death.

The Keto program is a favorite of people who prefer to eat more fat. Fat keeps them satisfied. But the long-term health consequences can be disastrous.

This is why I am not trying to persuade you to begin yet another diet program. Instead, I want you to learn balanced nutrition. It's not sexy and not likely to be endorsed on television by the latest spokes-model. But the results are real.

I like to think our work is like balancing your checkbook. That little chore is important. If you don't balance your checkbook, the consequences could be overdraft fees and unwanted penalties.

Good nutrition requires you to find your balance. Learn to enjoy what great food feels like when you reduce the pain in your joints, walk without gasping for air, and fit your favorite clothes again. The journey may be challenging at times, but the health benefits are totally worth it.

Am I Going to Get Sick of Chicken?

Do you get sick of hamburger? Probably not. We've learned how to get inventive with hamburger. We make burgers, chili, lasagna, meatloaf, and more. A serving of hamburger has as much as 30 grams of fat for 20 grams of protein. If you look closely at this protein selection, the bulk of what you are eating is fat. Artery-clogging fat at that. We are lucky that we have leaner choices of hamburger available, but you need to pay attention to the label to realize the fat percentage you are purchasing and how to plug the fat grams into your daily allowance.

That same size portion of chicken has 20 grams of protein and only one gram of fat. In essence, you could eat 30 chicken breasts in place of that one hamburger. The journey is a whole lot easier if you do not have to worry about portion control, or being out of control, as you are re-training yourself

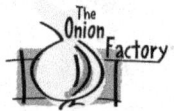

We want to sustain a healthy metabolism so that we look healthy, have plenty of energy, and prevent disease and premature death.

on weigh-loss worthy options. Focus on what you can eat without having to pay close attention to the portion quantity. For example, look at some of the wonderful dishes you can make with chicken:

- Chicken broccoli Alfredo*
- Verde omelet*
- Friday's chicken
- BBQ chicken
- White chicken chili
- Chicken taco salad
- Chicken cauliflower Cheddar soup*
- Chicken broccoli mushroom soup

Which Is the Lesser Evil?

As I review these case studies, I've come to realize that Onions sometimes do step out of their boxes. I would love to think a person could grasp the good-eating formula and find enough discipline to complete the peeling journey within nine months. In reality, I have learned that, although staying on your game for that long a period does happen, just as frequently, it does not.

Continually, I tell our Onions it does not matter how long it takes you to get in your safe range, just make sure you get there. I love working with a client who can stay in the box and finish sooner versus later. However, I have learned more from those who occasionally come out of the box—i.e., those who depart from the Onion Camp plan.

I do not want to teach you how to cheat, but I do want you to understand the pros and cons of off-plan foods, so you can make the best decision possible when you are tempted to cheat.

*Recipes in the recipe section of this book. Others are coming soon in a new cookbook!

When you face such a decision, ask yourself this simple question: Which is the lesser evil, consuming too many fat grams or too many sugar grams? Choose wisely!

If you decide to indulge in too many fats, remember that a fat gram contains more than double the amount of calories found in a sugar gram—9 calories per gram (fat) versus 4 (sugar). If you equate the calories to how much extra time you will have to spend on the elliptical machine, then you can clearly see you would have to do double duty to make up for your fat indulgence. The good thing about fat? Fat satiates you, so you feel satisfied. That's the bad thing about it, too. If you indulge in a high-fat item, you will find you aren't hungry, so you'll have no appetite for high-nutrition foods such as broccoli, asparagus, spinach, and lean protein. Your brain will tell you that you are already full because you have satisfied yourself with fat. Nutritious food sounds appealing when you are hungry, but not so great when you are full.

Earlier, I mentioned there are good and bad fats. Non-saturated fats, which are good for your heart, are found in foods such as avocados, nuts, and olive oil. Saturated fats that clog your arteries are found in dairy products and red meat. Usually, if Onions choose to step out of the box, we do it with extra fat. We revert to old behaviors by choosing foods like French fries, pizza, and cheeseburgers. All of these are filled with heart-threatening saturated fats. Plus, because these foods fill us up, we'll probably neglect to eat the foods containing important vitamins, minerals, and overall nutrition. High-value foods enable you to feel good, look good, and enjoy loads of energy.

(Continued on page 108).

Connie's Story

Connie was the first, and perhaps the only, Onion who put on weight her first week of Onion Boot Camp. She came in for her initial weigh and measure anticipating a great week. She thought she had grasped the information provided in the free informational seminar, she'd made her choices, and now was seeking validation for her efforts. As Connie stepped off the scale, her eyes welled up with tears.

Connie is also extremely hard on herself. The closer we get to her goals, the harder she becomes on herself. About halfway into her weight loss journey, I was in the middle of a training session with her. While reviewing her week's results, Connie looked up at me with her big blue eyes and said, "Occasionally, you need to dip your finger in the frosting." I looked at her and just starting laughing. I understood exactly what she was saying.

Eating in the box the first month is exciting. As you reach your second month, you begin to think surely one cracker could not hurt. And by month six, you may congratulate yourself for all the great choices you made during the week with a weekend pizza fix or a finger full of frosting.

While this is not a competition, every time you go back to your old behaviors you risk the chance of getting back your old results. This journey is much easier if you focus on all the food you can eat now, versus all the food you used to eat. I am not saying that you will never have frosting or pizza again; however,

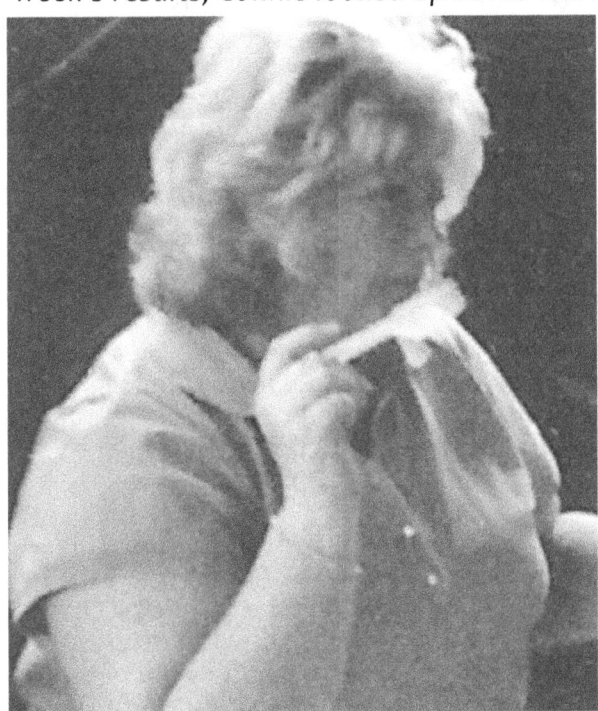

Connie BEFORE

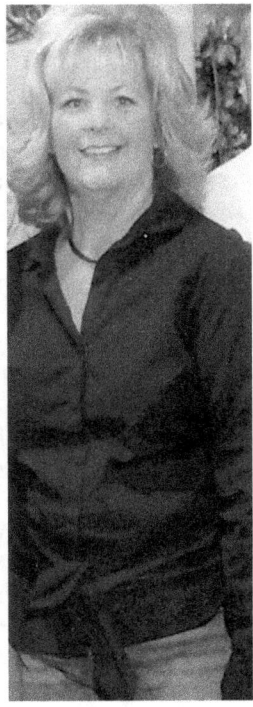

Connie AFTER

DATE	3/11/07	7/24/07	5/22/08	FINAL
R. ARM	15"	13"	12.5"	-5"
BUST	50"	41.5"	38"	-12"
WAIST	45"	36.5"	32"	-13"
ABS	53"	44.5"	41"	-12"
HIP	52"	45"	41"	-11"
THIGH	26"	23.5"	22"	-8"
WEIGHT	240	199	171	-69
FAT MASS	108.7	80.5	60.5	
LEAN MASS	131.3	118.5	110.5	
FAT TO GO	83.7	55.5	35.5	
		Lbs. Lost	69	
		Inches Lost	61	
		% Lost	10	

Connie's RESULTS

Connie said, "I have something to show you."

She pulled out a pair of shorts she had bought the previous summer.

With a huge grin, she said, "I can fit in one leg now!"

if you are still in peeling mode, stay in peeling mode to get fast and efficient results. When you get to maintenance, you will have more wiggle room for an occasional finger dip in the frosting if you still want one.

If you sat down with Connie right now, she would tell you she is stuck. For the past few weeks she has been grabbing her mid-section and asking, "How do I get rid of this?" There is no way to spot-reduce, short of liposuction. However, if you do not change your choices for the long haul, you will regain the fat in those fat cells you've emptied. (By the way, I have heard from liposuction clients who have regained their fat weight, and the fat comes back in new places. Yuck!)

Certainly, you can strengthen your abdominal wall. In fact abs are one of the few muscle groups you can work every day. The secret to a flat stomach and great abs goes back to the beginning. It all starts with great nutrition.

After several weeks of the same question from Connie, she came back one day with a new thought. She wondered if she had a stomach tumor. I looked at her puzzled blues eyes and burst out laughing. I said, "You have got to be kidding me!" This time, I grabbed her midsection and said, "This is not a tumor; this is stretched skin and excess fat. Now get back to work."

I'm not sure if my sessions with Connie are really training sessions or counseling sessions. We have spent a year together. Connie started Onion camp as a size 22. Last week, she bought her first size 8 dress. The closer she gets to her goal, the more critical of her body Connie becomes. She is extremely tough on herself. She has invested a year in changing her habits and exercising, something she thought she would never do. As she neared the finish line, I feared I was out of pixie dust to take her through.

In desperation, I said, "I am coming to your house tomorrow night. Come in and get your cardio training, then I will follow you home." I was planning an intervention.

The Intervention

Intervention is not a new idea. In fact, there are several shows on television that are based on the premise of holding an intervention. I am passionate about helping people reach their health goals. I hate it when a client gets stuck! I mentioned I felt like I was all out of tricks with Connie. A fridge and pantry inspection was the last step to see if I could help Connie get the bugs out of her nutrition.

Connie didn't think I was serious, so she hadn't prepared for the inspection. When she arrived to the Factory on Friday, I directed her to begin her exercises. I told her I was going to change and would be ready to leave in thirty minutes. She started giggling a nervous laugh.

On the drive to her house, Connie called her husband. I thought she was warning him to dispose of some evidence in her kitchen. She'd already admitted to me that she had started eating popcorn each night while cooking her clean dinner. (I often find that little, seemingly harmless nibbles are usually the reason Onions get stuck. That's when it is time to get back to basics, and that was one reason for the home inspection. I wanted to see if there were small adjustments I could make to refresh Connie's Onion-peeling nutrition. I also wanted to see if there were any pieces of the nutrition puzzle missing.)

Remember, otherwise healthy food may not be weight-loss worthy. Read your labels. Look at fats, sugars, and carbohydrates, and think about where the carbohydrates are coming from.

When we arrived, I looked in Connie's fridge. I was impressed with the amount of fresh vegetables and fruit. For the most part, her fridge looked clean. But a bowl of bright red strawberries, a container of Cool Whip®, and several sugar-free Jell-Os sat right in front. I knew exactly what had been happening with Connie. In the evenings, Connie was satisfying her cravings with artificial stuff. Remember that if your liver is processing the extra chemicals found in sugar-free, fat-free food, it cannot do its job of processing fat. Also, what begins as a dollop of Cool Whip® to accent fresh berries quickly becomes a tubful of whip as an ice cream replacement.

(One time in the grocery store, I ran into a client who was also stuck and saw three containers of Fat-Free Cool Whip® in her

Little, seeminly harmless nibbles are usually the reason Onions get stuck.

---

shopping cart. I asked, "How long will those last you?" She looked at me innocently and answered, "The week." "Then you'd better put some of them back," I ordered with a giggle.)

While at Connie's house, I also inspected her cupboards to see how much processed stuff she had. When a client is stuck, I wonder if they making major nutritional mistakes such as too much fat, too much sugar, not enough whole foods, or not enough hydration. Perhaps the client is making minor mistakes such as an extra animal cracker here or there, too many artificial sweeteners, too much artificial stuff, which we are not sure how the body processes. Carbohydrates, whether they are simple, starchy, or complex, are still carbohydrates. If the body doesn't use them immediately (i.e., if you're not running a marathon while you're nibbling on that cracker), carbs will be stored as fat. Some companies try to convince you that you count net carbs rather than all the carbs. Well, I count them all as what they are, carbohydrates.

Connie's cabinets looked good. The items I found that were outside of the Onion food box belonged to her husband or her son. I verified this with her husband. Then I divided her good stuff from the items she needed to leave alone. At this point, you may be thinking that an intervention is brutal. However, I had promised Connie to help her ready for her family vacation in June. So the intervention was needed.

I can always tell when Connie knows she is having a good week because, instead of waiting for her normal time slot, she will call me early in the day and say, "Wha'cha doing?"

I'll usually say, "Peeling Onions." But when she did this a few days after our intervention, I replied, "Let me guess, you would like an early weigh and measure?"

This early call means Connie has been on her game and wants validation now! So I squeezed her in between clients and found that the intervention was a success! She'd lost four pounds, reduced four inches, and lost one percent body fat in only six days. Connie was back on track.

However, Connie did not attend our group session on the following Wednesday. That means she would be missing her final body-part workout for the week—legs! When I saw at her training session on Thursday, I said, "Missing a body part this week is not an option. We are too close to your vacation." I suggested that she come for an extra consult on Saturday morning at 8:45, and I would train legs. It would have to be quick and hard, or fast and painful, depending on her condition. I had fifteen minutes to fatigue her legs, which are the largest muscle group.

That Saturday, we had our work cut out for us. We started on the Smith machine and she performed full leg squats. Squats are tough and definitely not for beginners, but remember; I had been working with Connie for more than a year, so I was confident she could handle advanced leg exercises. On the second set of squats she Isaid, "My eyes are going to pop out!" Well, at least we were off of the stomach tumor excuse!

One Saturday morning, I was making a soufflé while a few Onions were hanging out. In walks Connie. She said, "I have something to show you." It was Memorial Day weekend, and she pulled out her shorts from the previous year.

The previous summer, Connie had told her husband she had nothing to wear on the boat, so he suggested she buy some new shorts.. She had. Now she showed us those shorts. With a huge grin on her face, she said, "I can fit in one leg now!"

The Fork Is Mightier Than the Gym

Connie had made a similar demonstration to her family a night or two before. Her son had looked at her and shook his head in disbelief. He said, "Mom, I don't remember you being that big." (My boys said much the same thing to me when I lost so much weight. I guess our children continue to see us as "just mom," regardless of our weight loss.) Now Connie was carrying those famed shorts in her car to show others. She enjoyed her moment in the spotlight when she completed her next 8-week segment and I read her story to the current Boot Camp. And I imagine it gave some of them a wake-up call.

(Continued from Page 104.)

Now let's say you decide to cheat with sugar. I already mentioned that you wll only need to work half as long on the exercise machine to make up for your indulgence than you would with fat. So sugar may seem like a better choice, but let's probe this option a little deeper.

We know that sugar is a simple carbohydrate, so sugars will stimulate your appetite, and you cannot make a good decision when you are hungry. Allow me to clarify that statement: You are *less likely* to make good decisions.

Since you are reading this book, your history would probably reveal that you have not made the best nutritional decisions that you could have. So why make it any harder on yourself? If you step out of the box with sugar, you will crave more sugar. It never ends! If you can avoid the sugar temptation, your journey will be easier.

To repeat: Stay on your best weight-loss game, finish the journey, and learn how to choose your fat and sugar grams at the right time and place.

"But I'm Not Hungry"

In front of me is a popular fitness magazine with a small article that has caught my eye. It claims that chewing gum may reduce your appetite. As I read this article, my blood pressure began to rise because this is the root of our society's problem. We are not eating enough!

How do I know this? Because I have spent several years collecting food diaries of what Onions were eating before attending a Camp, what they ate as they learned the principles of body health, and what they ate when the light bulb of insight came on. These diaries convince me that non-eating did not help any of these people to lose weight. Like them, I tried anything and everything before I figured out what does not work. Then I put a few basic ideas together and came up with this system to feed our bodies instead of starving them. I learned there is no long-term benefit from feeling deprived, which only stimulates our cravings.

The Onion system stresses what you *can* eat rather than what you *cannot*. It teaches you what foods stimulate cravings and make you want to eat more of what will be stored directly on your derrier if you are not active enough.

"But I don't feel hungry," you may say. That is exactly my point. Besides, when did anyone ever need to feel hungry to eat a doughnut? Ask Danny Devito in the movie "Other People's Money." You don't need to feel hungry to indulge in cheesecake, candy bars, or doughnuts. They always sound good. We feed the sugar craving, then we eat sugar and we want more. Sugar is very addictive. When you flush white sugar out of your system, you will be amazed how much easier it is to make good health decisions. You will also be amazed how sweet fresh berries will taste.

Two phrases that I hear every eight weeks as we start a new Boot Camp: "I am not hungry," and "I am not thirsty."

Brace yourself. Here comes another Ralph Nader-like rant.

Imagine your body's need for food and water are like a vehicle's need for gas and oil. Does your car need gas and oil to operate? Of course. So what happens to you when you don't get enough to eat or drink? Let me ask you a few questions that I ask in my free seminar:

- Are you tired?
- Do you feel lousy?
- Are you here because you want to change these conditions?

If you answered yes to these questions, then I hope you will ponder the next paragraph with an open mind.

If you have not been a water drinker, be assured that when you start drinking the proper amounts of water, your brain will trigger you to realize you need more water. Many people are so accustomed to living in a dehydrated state that they do not realize how great it feels to be hydrated. Dehydration slows down your metabolic rate, and Onions need every element on their side to peel away the stored fat. Just think, by drinking the proper amounts of water you can increase your metabolism. Wow, that was easy!

If you say, "I'm not hungry," I would ask this. If you are not hungry, how did you become obese?

I mentioned earlier that the pattern I see in the demographic of people whose body fat falls in the 30–50 percent range, or higher, is they are not eating enough. Typically, they are eating only one or two meals per day.

This stems from the high-fat food they have depended on. When you eat high-fat foods, you stay satisfied longer.

Have you ever been out for Chinese food? You consume what you think is a lot of food, and a few hours later you feel really hungry again. That's because your body worked very hard at processing all that stir fry. Chinese food is loaded with clean protein and more veggies than the standard American cuisine of hamburgers and French fries. Hamburgers and fries are loaded with fats and starches, but few veggies. A McDonalds® Quarter Pounder with regular fries contains 980 calories with 107 grams of carbohydrates and 49 grams of fat. Yet you get very little nutritional value.

You feel full for a long time after eating a Quarter Pounder, while your body stores those surplus carbs and fats as...fat!

How did non-eating take our society to an epidemic of obesity? The answer is simple: We ate too much fat, white sugar, and flour, but we forgot to feed ourselves good nutrition. The food we ate made us feel tired, so we stopped being active. Day after day, we repeated that pattern.

Ray Croc, the founder of McDonalds®, did a great job of capitalizing upon our busyness. His objective was to create a system that would ensure customer satisfaction and repeat business. He made it easy for us to drive thru and grab food to go. I doubt he ever imagined that eating fast food would become a contributing factor in the problem of obesity in our society.

The solution to our obesity epidemic is equally simple. First, we must understand how to feed our bodies well. Then we must stop making the wrong food choices. Drive-thru eating seems easier, but it makes life shorter.
Let's face it. If we're given food that's not in a box, bag, or drive thru, we no longer know what to do with it. My passion, my commitment, is to teach you the basics of what to do.

Read Your Food Labels Carefully

Today, a client brought in a label to see if her new protein drink would be okay. I have a few lines of powdered protein drinks I really love to work with; however, her daughter had some protein product left over from another weight-loss plan. My client felt the leftovers might be a great way to add a drink toward her daily goal of getting enough protein in her nutrition.

When I look at protein drinks, or bars for that matter, I don't look just at the amount of protein. I look at the calories and the grams of fat, protein, sugar, and carbohydrates. How high are the fat grams? Is the protein amount high enough to justify the amount of calories per serving?

For example, if the item has 7 grams of protein but 12 grams of sugar, the item is probably not the best protein source you could select. If the item has 20 grams of protein but 10 grams of fat, it still might not be the best choice. There may be other options that would be cleaner sources of protein. Next, I look at carbohydrates. How many does the product have? Where are they coming from? You can safely assume the carbohydrates are coming from a starch or a sugar rather than "grass of the lands," since there are no green, leafy vegetables in that powder.

You do not want to consume more than 24 grams of sugar carbohydrates while you are trying to lose your storage tank. And for starchy carbohydrates such as breads, pastas, and potatoes you need to leave them alone completely, especially if your percentage of fat is over 30. Eating for weight loss will require you to obtain all 200 grams of each day's required carbohydrates from your complex macronutrients, a.k.a. fruits and vegetables. When you no longer have a storage tank of fat, you can bring the starchy carbohydrates like breads, pasta, grains, and certain fruits and vegetable back into your nutrition. That amount will be approximately 46 grams, or 20 percent of the total amount of carbohydrates required.

As I continued to review my client's protein drink label, I stopped and smiled. To the right side of the label, a short paragraph confirmed a thought process I have been teaching Onions for the past three years. I ask all Onions to forgo their milk during their eight-week Camp. This request usually stirs up questions. "Give up our milk? How are we going to get our calcium?" I will explain why this request is so important in a moment. The reason may surprise you.

The blurb on a protein drink said,: **For Mass Gaining: add higher calorie foods such a** peanut butter, 1-2% milk, and fruit juice. Hmm. Let's take that thought one step further. We grow up believing milk, fruit, and peanut butter are good for us. Milk and fruit are healthy. Peanut butter has been the staple of brown-bag lunches for a long time. Now in front of me is a nutrition label stating that these foods are needed to put on mass.

I spent thirty years trying to manage my weight, and now a little label explains what I should have known a long time ago. So this protein drink was not designed for weight loss, but for weight gain. It should be used only by bodybuilders who need extra calories for the many hours they spend lifting huge weights, trying to bulk up. Most definitely, it was not a good choice for Onions.

"Gotta Have Milk and Bananas"

The Factory's Girl Friday planted a fascinating fact in my head one day. She said, "You know, humans are the only mammals that continue to drink milk after they are weaned."

I looked at her and thought, *Wow. What is the link between milk, digestion, calcium requirements, protein, and weight management?*

We are the only mammals that consume another mammal's milk, and we think that's good for us? Milk is actually very species specific regarding health benefits. That is why many babies have episodes of colic and many elderly people experience intestinal cramps. We all associate drinking milk with calcium intake, but did you realize that one cup of milk contains 12 grams of sugar?

When we were into the fat-free eating craze and began drinking lower-fat milk, some of us actually started drinking larger servings of milk. We bought a lower-fat content and drank a larger amount because we were not satiated. Have you ever consumed eight ounces of whole milk? Whole milk is very rich. A little goes a long way.

Let's debunk some old beliefs. When I teach an Onion about weight-loss worthy choices versus what we are led to believe is healthy, I am frequently challenged on this idea of not drinking milk. Where in the world are we going to get our calcium if we are not drinking

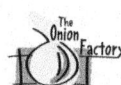 *Did you realize that one cup of milk contains 12 grams of sugar?*

milk? As you learn more about nutrition, you will be amazed with all the calcium options you have.

I see what people have been eating. I have all new Campers write one week's worth of "how they were eating" before they come to a Camp. I want to see if they leaned on sugars, fats, one-meal eating, or some other habit that may lead to obesity. I also pay attention to what they in their grocery carts like processed, prepackaged, and high-calorie selections. So if you are really worried about your calcium intake without milk, consider the following information.

Weight-Loss Worthy Calcium Selections

- Salmon
- Seafood
- Dark green leafy vegetables
- Asparagus
- Broccoli
- Cabbage
- Tofu
- Turnip greens
- Watercress

"I'm Chiquita Banana and I am here to say...." I love bananas. In fact, during one phase of trying to lose weight, I would have yogurt and bananas for breakfast. I think I mentioned earlier I really wanted a Belgium Waffle, but I thought I was making a healthier choice with the banana and yogurt. Healthy? Yes. Weight-loss worthy? Probably not. It is very difficult to find a yogurt with under 20 grams of sugar. I've found one that has 8 sugar grams, so I use a dollop of it to accent items such as berries. I make a container last for eight servings. My latest find is Kroger Carbmaster® Yogurt. It is low fat, low carb, and sugar free!

Now comes the question, "Don't I need to eat bananas to get enough potassium?" Allow me to broaden your nutritional horizon. A banana has 24 grams of starchy carbohydrates. If you are an athlete in sports training or at a safe body composition, a banana is a wonderful way to enhance a protein shake or eat on the fly. However, if you are trying to lose weight, don't be surprised if your efforts get stuck when you are eating bananas. Here are some other high-potassium sources that won't sabotage your weight-loss efforts (see chart).

Be careful with the winter squash, yams, and yogurt. They are higher on the glycemic index and contain a higher amount of sugar.

Grocery Cart

I hope things are beginning to make sense to you, and you are beginning to make changes. I want to reinforce the new way you will look at groceries.

Take a look at what we are putting in our grocery carts. Is there any wonder why we feel depressed, or why we are we are growing fatter? Most items in the cart are processed foods, not whole foods. Remember, everything we need for good nutrition is on the outer rim of the store. Everything we crave, or that looks fun, is in the middle of the store. So what should you look for? I've put together a sample list for you. (See the following page).

Weight-Loss Worthy Potassium Selections

- Fish
- Beef (low-fat)
- Poultry
- Garlic
- Spinach
- Winter squash
- Yams
- Yogurt

Grocery List for a New Onion

Proteins	Veggies	Fruits	Miscellaneous
Cottage Cheese (1% or Fat-Free)	Asparagus	Blackberries	Mexican Shredded Cheese
Ground Turkey Sausage	Broccoli	Blueberries	Light Ranch Dressiong
Ground Turkey (99% Lean)	Brussel Sprouts	Strawberries	Molly McButter®
Chicken Breast	Cauliflower	Raspberries	Pam® or Crisco® Non-Stick Spray
Tilapia	Cucumbers		Taco Bell® Seasoning
StarKist® Sweet & Sour Tuna	Celery		Mrs. Dash® Seasoning
Canned Tuna in Water	Garlic Cloves		Classico® Alfredo Pasta Sauce
Canned Chicken	Green Peppers		Ragu® Traditional Pasta Sauce
Shrimp	Onions		Parmesan Cheese
Hardboiled Eggs (No Yolks)	Shredded Lettuce		
	Caesar Salad in a Bag		
	Tomatoes		
	Frozen Veggies		
	Zucchini		

Grocery Cart No-No's

Bananas (Starch)	Carrots (Sugar)	Ice Cream (Sugar)
Potatoes (Starch)	Lima Beans (Starch)	Peas (Sugar)
Corn (Starch)	Milk (Sugar)	Cereals (Starch)
Breads (Starch)	Waffles (Starch)	Rice (Starch)
Pasta (Starch)	Olives (Fat)	Avocadoes (Fat)
Adult Beverages (Sugar)		

Shortcuts from Trader Joe's®

Frozen Proteins	Frozen Veggies	Frozen Fruit	Miscellaneous
Ahi Tuna	Asparagus	Very Berry Medley	Caesar Salad Dressing
Turkey Meatballs	Broccoli Florets	Strawberries (no sugar added)	Parmesan Ranch Salad Dressing
Chili Lime Chicken Burgers			Pear Champagne Salad Dressing
			Pure Protein Drinks
			Traditional Marinara Sauce
			Trader Joe's® Pizza Sauce
			Trader Joe's® Electrolyte Water
			Trader Joe's® Green Bean Chips

Portion Control

When I was searching for answers about how to lose weight and keep it off, I did not want the issue to be about portion control. It is tough enough to learn how and what to eat. I have always said, "Do not show me what I cannot eat; show me what I can eat." I am an eater. I love food. I do not want a smaller portion of a brownie that has little or no flavor, or a frozen dinner that leaves me unsatisfied. I would much rather indulge in a treat that's rich and decadent and satisfying than eat something that tastes artificial.

Show me what I *can* eat so I do not feel deprived. The moment I feel deprived is the moment I seem to sabotage my efforts. I realized several years ago that I would need to stop the roller-coaster ride of weight loss ups and downs. I had to figure out how to feed my body rather than starve or deprive it.

The crazy thing about portion control is our portions have been so out of control. Way back when, I can remember my mom purchasing whole milk. With whole milk you do not consume very much because it is very rich. At some point, we switched to two-percent milk and, later, skim milk. Many of us began drinking larger portions. We just kept pouring our milk and eating our chocolate-chip cookies.

Seems innocent enough, doesn't it? But take a look at how 16 ounces of skim and two percent compare to an eight-ounce serving of whole milk (chart at bottom of this page).

Our society has a love affair with weight control. From my recollection, Jack Lalane was the first spokesperson for fitness and a healthy lifestyle. Then came Arnold Schwarzenegger, the bodybuilding icon, and Richard Simmons for obesity. If you look back at our grandparents in old family photos, you will soon realize that what we thought was big was nowhere near what big is today. We are indeed super-sized.

If we have a love affair with weight control, then we certainly love the word *free*! Didn't our parents tell us a long time ago that nothing in life is free? First, we were exposed to sugar-free, then fat-free, and then carb-free. If "free" was the answer, why in the world are we fatter then we have ever been? Is the picture starting to make sense yet?

Honestly, I think the first mistake I made in my diet effort was my first diet, because it was all about food deprivation! What I really needed to do was learn how to eat.

The Truth about Healthy Eating

We have grabbed onto so many farfetched diet ideas. Maybe we really wanted someone to tell us that eating a doughnut was okay, even though the doughnut was full of transfats and sugars, and had no nutritional value.

I want you to take a look at how you ate before this journey, how you will eat during the peeling stage, and how you will eat to maintain the new you. The peeling part is far tougher than

Milk by the Numbers

	8 oz. Whole Milk	8 oz. 2% Fat Milk	8 oz. Skim Milk	Double Portion (16 oz.)
Calories	150	130	90	180
Fat Grams	5	3	0	0
Carb Grams	12	13	13	26
Sugar Grams	12	12	12	24
Protein Grams	8	8	8	16

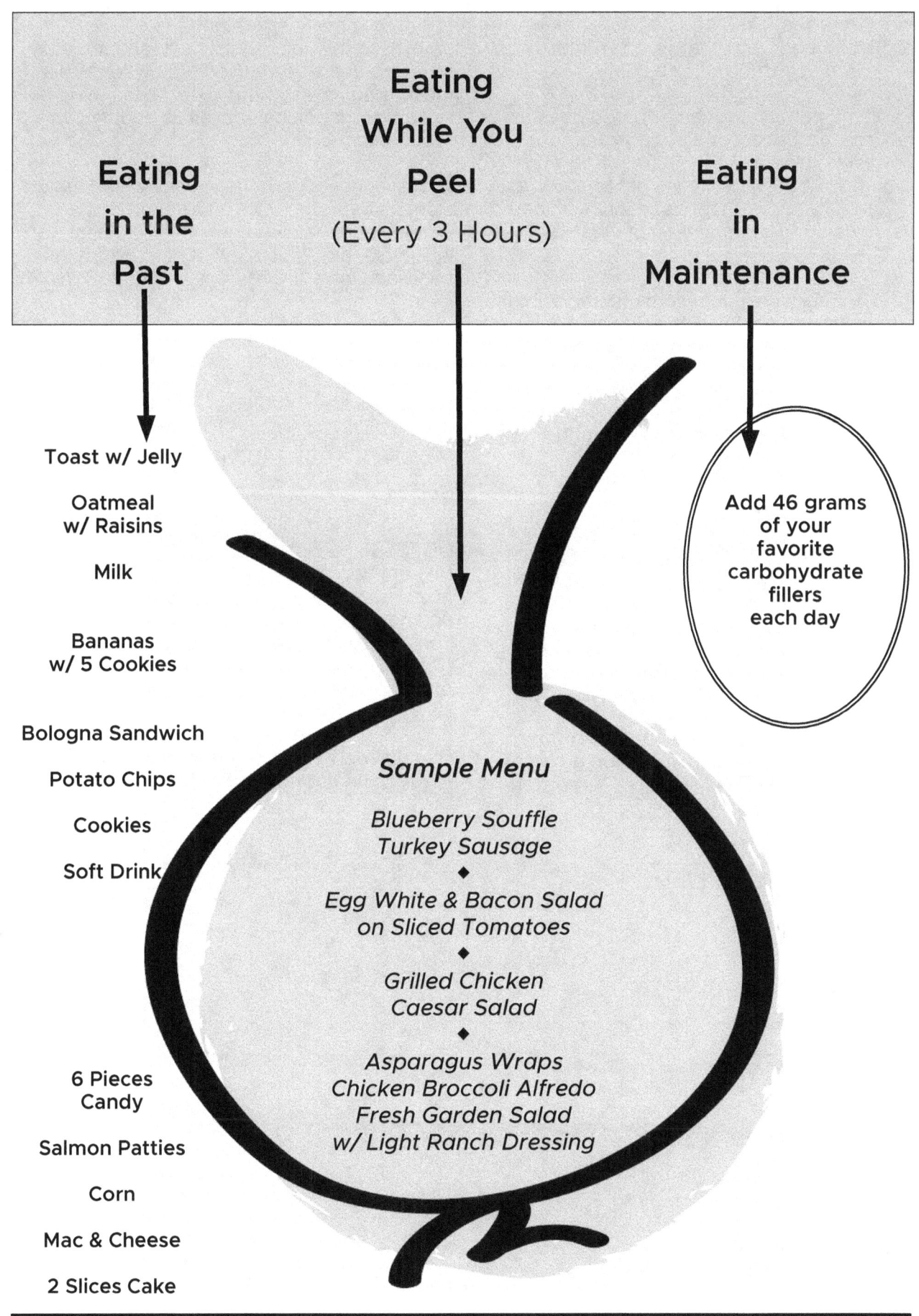

maintenance. Peeling is about making the right choices, and that is often more fun than making the bad ones.

Earlier, I mentioned America's fad diets of fat-free, carb-free, and sugar-free foods; however, I would like to share a few more thoughts about what types of food are really healthy. To answer that question, we need to have a clear understanding of what we mean by "healthy."

First and foremost, a "healthy" person obtains a high level of health without high risk. That means a healthy body weight to begin with; that alone will go a long way toward preventing bad backs, bad knees, bad joints, high blood pressure, and type 2 diabetes. Remember, 26 percent body fat ("fluff") and no more is your goal.

Great nutrition begins with healthy food habits, NOT quick fixes. I know, we all wish there was a shortcut or magic potion that would confer good health upon us, but there isn't. So, in this book, we aim to go back to the fundamentals of good nutrition.

This section of the book grew out of a conversation about low sodium. I usually find that when a client throws at me a catch phrase like "low sodium" or other supposed nutritional "lows," they do not have a proper baseline of what "low" really is. I have even found they may understand the concept of low sodium but are still confused about the how, where, and when of how to build a menu around their nutritional needs while not violating what dieticians tell us about "low" requirements.

I don't want you to be derailed by marketing slogans that urge you to select products that may not help you build a great menu. So let's make a quick review of healthy eating baselines for a 150-lb. female or a 200-lb male:

	Female	Male
Fat	30g	40g
Carbohydrates	225g	300g
	(Ah...but choose wisely, grasshopper!)	
Protein	80g	100g
Sodium	?	?

NOTE: Sodium does NOT inhibit weight loss. Sodium may make your bathroom scale fluctuate, but we know the scale is not an accurate measure of your current level of health. This is a journey about how much good mass you have (bone density, vital organs, water, and muscle) and managing the layers of fluff (fat).

Remember: Feed your lean mass and STOP feeding the fluff!

10. Eating Out

BALANCED EATING TAKES A LITTLE PRACTICE, BUT YOU CAN DO IT, EVEN IN A RESTAURANT. I'M HERE TO COACH YOU.

AS I SIT HERE pecking away at my computer, my girlfriend calls. I tell her I am stuck, not sure what to tell you about how to eat out. She says, "Just tell them, 'Don't eat out—EVER!'"

I know what she means. I also know her well enough to know she is not joking. When she puts her mind on peeling a layer, the process is all or nothing for her. It is not unusual, when she is getting ready for a trip, for her to cook her food, pack it on ice, and carry it on the plane.

You gotta know Abby. We first met when she was my front-desk girl. She had just graduated from high school and I was deep in the trenches, working in the fitness industry. She is incredible. Let me see, she is the former Miss Teen Indiana, funny, intelligent, and beautiful. She is truly my inspiration. And yes, she has had a battle with her weight just like the rest of us. While her battle with weight was not as dramatic as mine (in her 20's she grew to 165 pounds, measured 30 percent fat, and wore a size 15 junior), just look at us now.

Abby gets it. Food is a science. She knows exactly the amount of sugar, fat carbs, and protein she needs to get the results she desires. When you eat out, you really do not know what the kitchen is adding to your food. Even if your selection is perfect, such as a salad (actually a bowl of lettuce—no croutons, no cheese, no extras), grilled fish, or chicken with a side of broccoli. I gasp every time I see Rachael Ray spin her EVOO (olive oil) all over the pan. That move could add 10–30 grams of fat into the equation, even if what you added to the pan was a bunch of weight-loss worthy vegetables.

So when Abby says to tell you, "Don't eat out ...ever!" she's really saying you will lose a little of the control when others, who do not cook or think like Onions, cook for you. When I eat out with her, here is how Abby's drill goes with the server: "I would like a plate of

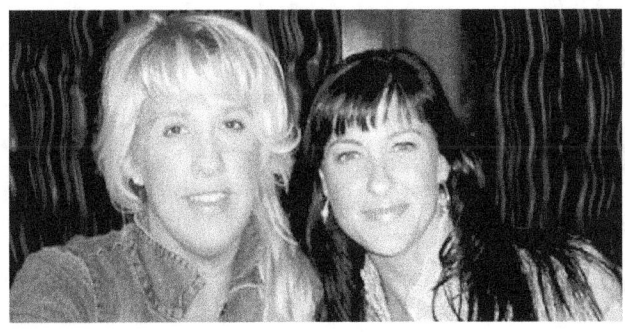

lettuce, chicken grilled with nothing on it, and steamed broccoli with no butter." And if it's not done right, she will send it back to the kitchen because her results are on the line.

Take a tip from Abby: Be specific when you eat out! Especially in the beginning, because those beginning results will motivate you to fight, learn, and yearn for more results. This journey of peeling and creating a new you can become very addictive. The more results you get and the more you discover how the body can repair itself, the more results you will desire.

Once you've learned the formula for feeding your body, you will find eating out is a breeze. I say over and over again the best vacation I have ever taken was a cruise, because as an eater, I had unlimited resources to all the food I could eat.

I think the answer to changing the course of obesity is to change the relationship you have with food. Eat! But eat the stuff that is not going directly to your assets. We became an over-fat society partly because we stopped eating. At frequent intervals, we experienced deprivation for short periods of time, and then went hog-wild with food later.

The tools you need to make a life change are in this guide, but the will to change is within you.

I think that by now you understand I love food. I love culinary art. I believe that presentation is nearly as important as taste. Food is a visual pleasure, so I want to satisfy my visual appetite as well as my taste buds.

Some people escape at the shopping mall, a casino, or indulge in their hobby. Mine is food. Take me to Ruth Chris or the latest bistro and I will melt. How in the world do you think I grew into a 300-pound girl? Now I can still eat out, but my choices are far different.

A Restaurant Plan

Why is it when we go out to eat we are already starving? Talk about stacking the odds against making good choices. You sit down at a restaurant with all your friends, knowing that you want to make good choices, and just about that time the waitress delivers bread

Secrets to Success When You Eat Out

- Have a protein drink before you go out to eat. Remember protein levels out your blood sugars and eases hunger. You cannot make good choices when you are experiencing hunger pangs.

- Ask your server NOT to bring the rolls or chips.

- Select an appetizer that helps you reach your weight-loss goal. Shrimp cocktail, a small salad, or a clear soup are great choices. French onion soup WITHOUT the bread or cheese is another good starter. Ask your server to bring your starter as soon as possible.

rolls or tortilla chips to hold you over while you look at the menu. You cannot make good decisions when you are hungry. At that point of hunger, sheer willpower has to kick in.

I want to share three secrets with you that will set you up for success:

When you go out to eat, you must have a plan. The first step is to understand what your lean protein choices are: grilled chicken, baked fish, or lean pork. The second step is to select two or three whole foods (complex carbohydrates) such as a salad, coleslaw, or fresh veggies. Remember to pass up the bread, pasta, rice (even if it's brown) and potatoes. Fresh berries make a great dessert.

Eating Out: Client Specific

I have come to the conclusion that I have three types of clients at the Onion Factory. That's why this portion of the book has been so difficult to write. There are so many options (and distractions), but bear with me.

This journey all starts with the basic eating formula and continues from there. However, how you continue beyond the basic formula is where it gets a little tricky.

Loves to Cook

Are you the Onion who loves to cook and has the time to do it? Are you someone who can cook, but time gets away from you, so occasionally you eat on the fly? Or are you an Onion who should never be left alone in the kitchen? You see the dilemma these questions pose.

I will start with the Onion who can cook or wants to learn how to cook. This book has 70 weight-loss worthy recipes. We have provided their nutritional values so you can mix and match them. Remember, the magic is not in the recipe. The magic to eating and peeling is consuming the correct amount of fats, sugars, carbohydrates, and proteins so your body will burn off the fat and save the lean muscle mass.

If you find yourself eating on the fly, you will need a few extra suggestions to help you manage your nutrition. The challenge with eating on the fly is you might choose from fast-food places, chain restaurants, and fine dining. I'll give you some pointers about all three.

Believe it or not, once you grasp the basic formula and understand where the mistakes can be made, you will find that you can eat out very successfully, and it's actually simpler (no dishes or grocery shopping). If my budget would allow, I would chose fine dining every night of the week. I've found that the finer restaurants are the easiest for Onions because we can avoid the temptations of high-fat, deep-fried food such as French fries, burgers, etc. But let's start with the fast-food establishments.

Fast Food

Fast-food restaurants are the places where you go through the drive thru and eat in your car, because your life has gotten too busy to get a table inside. Answer this question: Have you ever been eating in your car and glanced over to see someone else eating on the fly? Do you think they were enjoying their meal? More importantly, were they overweight? Like you, they were probably eating so fast they could not enjoy their food. Could that person be an Onion? Maybe the first behavior to change in this scenario is to stop a moment, think about what you are going to feed your body, and (most importantly) take enough time to enjoy your food. Studies suggest that it takes twenty minutes for your brain to realize you are full. A heck of a lot of food (especially high-fat and high-sugar items) can be consumed in twenty minutes. And how many times after you feel full do you keep eating anyway? Why do we do that?

Let's take a look at the everyday stops. Fast food consumption has grown into a multimillion-dollar-per-year industry. We rarely eat at home. We are eating on the fly. We probably aren't going to change eating on the fly. But we can change the choices we're making at the quick and easy eating establishments. As I evaluated all the choices of fast food for this guide, I found it interesting that the original choices like a hamburger or a taco were not too far out of the weight-loss box. However, when the fast-food industry grew creative in attempting to encourage our fat cravings to a greater degree, they made us want to eat more. They super-sized our choices. Singles became doubles or triples. They built the Baconnators (like we weren't getting enough artery-clogging fat already). Now we are simply out of control. Once our fat and starch cravings are satiated at one level, we want more, we crave more of what will be stored on our assets. We didn't increase our vegetable consumption, so perhaps the fast-food industry thought we were getting bored with the basic taco or burger.

What I Would Order

Onions always ask, "What do you eat when you go out?" I think, *I wish I could eat out everyday; it would be so much easier to explain.* They assume I have been studying nutrition and fitness for so long that it will be easy for me to explain fast-food eating in a way that will be easy for Onions to grasp. So in this part of the book, I'll share what I would order at a fast-food restaurant, why, and the nutritional holes I look for.

120 /// The Fork Is Mightier Than the Gym

Let's take the eating-on-the-fly concept and plug in some baseline nutrition, so you will have enough information to eat fast food occasionally and still peel a layer, or two. With drive-thru eating, select grilled over fried. Skip the French fries. Get rid of the bread (fillers), watch sauces with high sugar (catsup) or high fat (special sauce, mayonnaise, and those darn salad dressings).

Let's see what eating on the fly looks like.

Fast Food Favorites: McDonald's®

When fast food was introduced, you could occasionally work in a hamburger and a side of French fries and still maintain your weight. The problem began when "occasionally" turned into "more often than not."

We women were busy working, so fast food offered us an easy alternative—no shopping, no prepping, and no dishes. So McDonald's® became our friend. But look what happened to the nutritional counts as our taste buds and our posteriors grew.

You could plug a burger and fries into the equation occasionally! But then the menu grew to include fried chicken sandwiches, and we grew as well. Who would have thought that a chicken sandwich would have more fat than a McDouble® burger? WOW!

What if you decided to indulge in a chocolate shake? See the "Small Shake" below. At face value, 14 grams of fat looks doable and 13 grams of protein...not bad. But look at the total of 102 grams of carbohydrates. Which kind? Well, 58 of them are from sugar, which leaves 44 from either "grass of the lands" or fillers. Which would you guess they are coming from? If you guessed fillers, you guessed correctly.

Instead, try the Caesar salad and grilled chicken breast from McDonald's®. (See below.) These are satisfying selections and their nutritional values are much better across the board.

Avoid the last two McDonald's® choices AT ALL COST. (Can you believe these burgers?) French fries are usually packaged with them, not to mention a few cookies (You smelled the aroma of a fresh batch when you entered the place!) or even that chocolate shake!

These best-selling McDonald's® items will sabotage your health.

McDonald's®	Serving Size	Calories	Total Fat	Carbs	Protein
Hamburger	3.5 oz (100g)	252	9g	31g	12g
French Fries	Small (74g)	230	11g	29g	3g
McDouble®	151g	390	19g	33g	22g
McChicken®	5 oz (143g)	360	25g	34g	14g
Small Shake	16 oz	580	14g	102g	13g
Caesar Salad	7.5 oz	90	4g	9g	7g
Grilled Chicken Breast	1 piece	120	2g	2g	24g
Dbl ¼ Pounder w/ Cheese	9.9 oz	740	42g	40g	48g
Big Mac®	1 sandwich	590	34g	47g	24g

Wendy's®	Serving Size	Calories	Total Fat	Carbs	Protein
Small Chili	227g	190	8g	19g	14g
Chicken Caesar Salad	1 salad	490	33g	20g	31g
Small Frosty®	12 oz	330	8g	56g	8g
The Baconator®	1 sandwich (276g)	840	51g	38g	56g
Plain Baked Potato	10 oz	270	0g	61g	7g

Wendy's®

Wendy's® is a strong competitor to McDonald's® for several reasons. One reason is this: A smart shopper often can find better food choices here.

For example, if you are out and about but forgot to pack a snack, try Wendy's® small chili. You can work with the chili's 8 grams of fat; you get 30 per day. The protein looks good; enough protein to keep your blood sugars in line. It's quick, it's easy, and very affordable. Remember to take its 8 grams of sugar into account. Subtract those from the overall carbohydrates, and you'll still have 13 grams of carbs for "grass of the lands."

On the other hand, Wendy's® Caesar salad has some unpleasant surprises. Ouch! Just when you think you know what you are doing. Again be careful. I assume the high fat content in this salad is in the cheese and the dressing they use. Who would have thought a salad would be a higher fat choice than a burger?

Oh, how we love Wendy's® Frosty®! But look at that heavy load of carbs. Forty-two of the 56 carbohydrate grams are from SUGAR, a two-day supply. Even worse, you will crave more sugar after you indulge. I am sure you can find a better way to satisfy your cravings than spending 46 grams on just a small cup of soft-serve!

Wendy's ad campaigns make people sound and look cool if they order one of these specialties. Don't believe it!

I think Wendy's® is one of the few fast food locations in which you can order a baked potato. A plain one, even. How can a plain potato be harmful to your nutrition goals? Certainly potatoes are only evil if you turn them into French fries.

My grandmother had a fish & chip shop in England. I thought she made the BEST French fries. In fact, we even made them into French-fry sandwiches with her homemade bread and fresh English butter. Her secret was she would soak the fries overnight to allow the starch to float to the top of the water. Did you catch that? *Starch.* Starch is used to thicken sauces and is processed by the body very slowly.

So if you are struggling with a reserve tank (your weight), a baked potato is just going to slow down your results. For now, you need to see results.

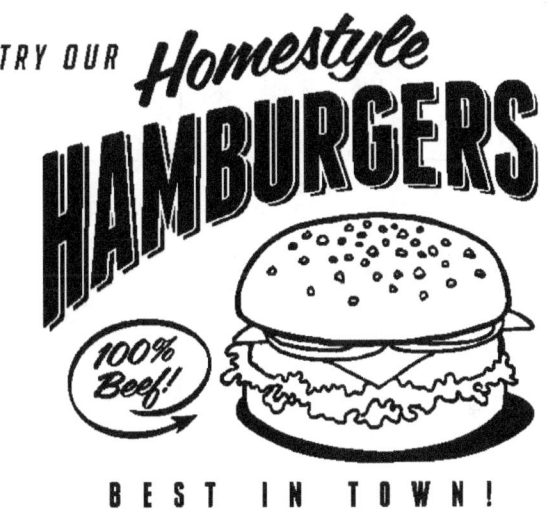

Arby's®

I like the freshness of Arby's® food. The selection is not always perfect, but there is a lot to be said about avoiding artery-clogging (deep fried) fat of alternative drive-thru food options. I really like Arby's® because, if I am going to select a bread option, I prefer the dark breads such as pumpernickel. Arby's® has a few garden-fresh sandwiches that are a nice change. Remember, you can always throw away half of the bread.

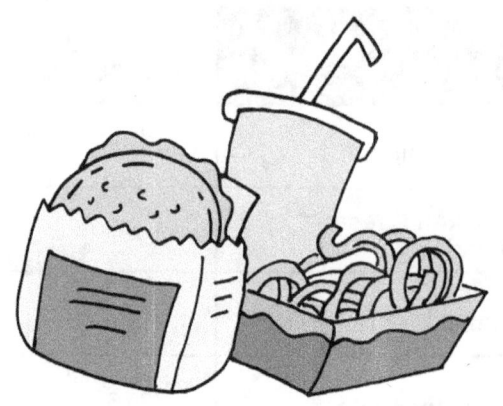

I am more than seven years into managing my behaviors. I am not always in losing mode. Occasionally, I am in clean-up mode from a few bad choices. Those choices are usually around holidays and weekends. The good news is that the more we understand, the better chance we have of not growing back into the old version of us.

Need a sandwich? Try Arby's® Turkey Deluxe sandwich and throw away half the bread. I love to err on the side of protein, and the Turkey Deluxe has 24 grams of it. The protein will help level out blood sugar and shut down the cravings for bread, or sugar. The moment I satisfy those cravings,is exactly the moment that I desire more.

The fat is a little high; however, if you ask for mustard instead of any of their extra sauces, the fat will be reduced. You can eat 30 grams of fat per day. On this particular day, if you select this sandwich, you could just lean up your dinner.

A salad will always be your safest bet as long as you pay attention to the dressing you select. Let's compare several of Arby's® salad selections with this guideline in mind.

You can make the Raspberry Vinaigrette work; however, this selection will give you less wiggle room for fat for the rest of the day.

Arby's® Jalapeño Bites® ALWAYS get me in trouble. How can a jalapeño be bad? Isn't it a "grass of the lands"? Well, when you stuff it with cream cheese, deep fry it, and add a high-sugar

Arby's®	Serving Size	Calories	Total Fat	Carbs	Protein
Turkey Deluxe Sandwich	1 sandwich (7 oz)	375	17g	33g	24g
Grilled Chicken Salad	284g	229	11g	9g	20g
Lt Vinaigarette Dressing	1 packet	110	6g	13g	0g
Raspberry Vinaigarette Dressing	1 packet	172	12g	16g	0g
Jalapeño Bites®	5 pieces (4 oz)	305	21g	29g	5g
Bronco Berry Sauce	57g	120	0g	30g	0g
Reg. Roast Beef Sandwich	1 sandwich	320	14g	34g	12g

Burger King®	Serving Size	Calories	Total Fat	Carbs	Protein
"Impossible Burger"	Regular (215g)	420	16g	46g	23g
Flame-Broiled Burger	1 sandwich	260	10g	27g	15g
BK Quad Stacker	1 sandwich	920	63g	31g	56g

sauce, you get what you get. Consider this a treat moment, then get back to regular eating!

Is it any wonder I like these so much? Twenty-eight of the 30 grams are from sugar, along with 21 grams of fat. What a way to ruin a girl's waistline. Ugh! Sure, if you were following that old calorie mindset, you might convince yourself that you can make 425 calories work in your daily amount of, let's say, 1500. Now you have a greater understanding of where all the calories come from, and you can be an informed consumer making selections that are going to help you reach your goals.

Now back to basics. The regular (beginning) option at most of the fast-food places are doable, especially if you toss away half of the bun and be aware of the sauces you are adding to it. Arby's regular roast beef sandwich has great protein (21 grams), decent fat (14 grams), and the meat is not deep-fried!

Burger King®

Here is the deal about veggie burgers, which are called "Impossible Burgers" at Burger King®. Those of us who've tried them believed we were making a good choice for weight loss. If you bought them because you are a member of P.E.T.A or you do not eat anything with a mom, then this was a perfect selection for you. But if you are selecting the veggie burger for weight loss, allow me to show you the holes.

The fat is managable and the protein is decent, but what's going on with the carbs? Eight grams are from sugar; that leaves 38 from something else. Are they 38 extra weight-loss worthy carbs? Are they from "grass of the lands" such as from broccoli, spinach or low-glycemic veggies? Nope, sorry! They make these burgers stick together with legumes. Legumes are very healthy but not weight-loss worthy. They will spike your blood sugar and they store quickly. You have a fat reserve tank, so you want to avoid these extra carbohydrates.

Taco Bell®

Oh, how I love Taco Bell®! If I could indulge in any drive-thru restaurant, this would be the one. I do not even want to evaluate what I might choose on a late night to take home, but here goes: Nachos BellGrande® with extra meat, extra cheese, extra side of sour cream, and I am in piglet heaven. Choices such as this one grew me into that 300-pound girl.

It has been a few years since I have indulged in Taco Bell®'s food, but for fun let's see how much damage I was doing. Oh my, 83 grams of fat and I asked for extra meat, cheese, and sour cream on top of that. What in the world was I thinking?

I know what I was thinking: I was thinking like a fluffy girl. Why couldn't I have just had a little taco versus blowing my fat grams out of the water? Why did I not just make a taco salad? I really love my taco salad, and I love fitting into my clothes even more than I love the nachos.

The challenge with the selections at Taco Bell® is most items are served with ground beef or grilled steak, both high in fat. Cheese is on everything, and sour cream is a must in most cases. To top it off, all the above ingredients are usually wrapped in some sort of tortilla or served with chips. Remember, in weight-loss mode you will need to forgo the filler carbs (breads, pasta, rice, potato, corn, tortillas, and chips).

Do not tell yourself that because the tortilla is thin it is a better choice. In most cases, those flat breads and tortilla have more filler carbs

Taco Bell®	Serving Size	Calories	Total Fat	Carbs	Protein
Nachos BellGrande®	11 oz	730	41g	69g	23g
Fully Loaded Nachos	481g	1,390	83g	128g	34g
Border Light Taco®	1 taco	140	5g	11g	11g
Taco Salad	1 salad	290	18g	17g	17g

than a regular slice of bread. The average slice of bread has about 20 grams from the filler column (Column B), while the usual tortilla or flat bread has about 45 grams. Yikes, almost the entire daily amount of filler carbs you budget in maintenance.

Let's take a look at what you *could* order at Taco Bell® when you are on a mission to have that big month of weight loss. You could work the Border Light Taco into your daily equation. One taco! But after that one, you will have NO wiggle room. The 11 carbs are from the shell (a grain). That is the amount I have found you can work with (preferably after the initial eight weeks) and still lose weight. This taco really does not have enough protein, but the low fats look good.

Let's see how Taco Bell®'s taco salad shakes out. The protein is good. I assume the carbs are "grass of the lands." See if you can order it with chicken and bring down the fat grams. Remember NO shell, beans, or red strips. Just meat and shredded lettuce.

Subway®

Yes, I know Jerrod lost a lot of weight eating at Subway®; however, Jerrod put a bunch back on. Just like anyone who changes the behaviors to get results in the first place, if you do not stick to those behaviors guess what happens? You will creep back in the wrong direction.

Let me give you a couple of thoughts to help you maneuver your way around Subway®. Subway® has some of the best selections for you to stay on game. Subway® also has some selections that, in your mind are healthy, and in the advertising they appear healthy. Jerrod lost a lot of weight with this mindset. However, in the big picture, the grains are what got us in trouble in the first place. I do not care how you slice it—white, wheat, rye, or pumpernickel—at the end of the day, they are all still bread. In maintenance mode, you can have 46 grams.

But if you are on a mission of fat loss, watch out. Lean on your "grass of the lands" and

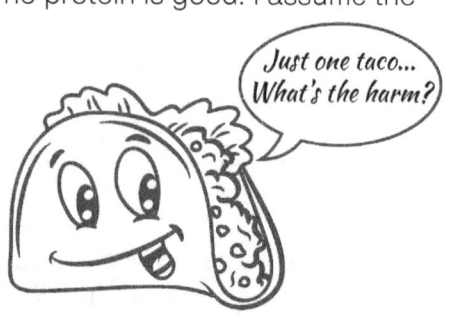

Just one taco... What's the harm?

Subway®	Serving Size	Calories	Total Fat	Carbs	Sugar	Protein
Oven Chicken Breast Salad	1 salad	130	2.5g	9g	4g	19g
Sweet Onion Foot-Long Sub	1 salad	760	9g	120g	34g	51g
Tuna Foot-Long Sub	1 salad	1,060	60g	90g	10g	42g

clean proteins, which are plentiful at Subway. Honestly, Subway® can be a breeze, but to get fast results, stay away from the fillers for the first eight weeks. I will show you how to bring the fillers (breads) back in later. At Subway® choose:

- Grilled chicken
- Deli Meats
- Salad (bring your own dressing)
- All the veggies you desire

Sit-Down Restaurants

What about the sit-down options? I kept racking my brain on how to explain this grouping of restaurants. Then, Angel Onion suggested we categorize them as chain restaurants. You probably do not drive through for take out. You may even take a moment to sit down and enjoy the food, and you might find yourself there a few times per week... choices, choices, choices.

Are you making a last-minute decision because you did not prep for the day? Or maybe your circle of friends has selected one of these locations to celebrate, or socialize. Either way, you need to be well informed. You will not derail the results you are seeking. These are restaurants such as: Applebee's, Bob Evans, Cracker Barrel, Olive Garden, and Red Lobster.

Be aware of the marketing strategies on the chain restaurants menus. Frequently, you will see sections of the menu specialized for weight loss. Don't get derailed by the latest buzz: the 500-calorie selection. Five hundred calories of what? If it is 500 calories from fat, or sugar, or filler carbohydrates such as rice or pasta (even if they are whole wheat), you will not get the results you are looking for.

I realize I could have listed many more selections; however, I felt you could get the essence from the following locations and plug in the information to restaurants that are similar. Also, keep in mind as you are learning how to eat versus starve, and how to eat and lose versus gain, my favorite desktop resource is a book called *Food Counts* by Corinne Netzer. She did all the research for us. All we need to do is plug in the numbers. Also visit https://nutritiondata.self.com. Here you'll find specialized menus for diabetic people, weight-conscious consumers, and others who have particular needs. I like the calculator that allows you to compare the nutritional values of two different foods. That's the easy way to make smart choices.

Bob Evans®

Breakfast Menu

Stuffed 3-Egg Omelets
The menu says, "We add all of the farm-fresh ingredients you love to a fluffy 3-egg omelet. Served with golden-brown home fries and two freshly baked biscuits, it's a country-sized breakfast hearty enough for even the biggest appetite. You can substitute Bob Evans Egg Lites™, our no-cholesterol egg blend, in any omelet for just 40¢ more."

Perfect! Ask for the egg blend version, skip the home fries and biscuit, and see if fresh berries or sliced tomatoes are available. Also, if you are extra hungry, ask for a side of sliced ham.

Turkey & Spinach Omelet
"Fresh baby spinach and diced tomatoes are cooked right in with the eggs. Then this fluffy omelet is stuffed with slow-roasted turkey and Monterey-Jack cheese and topped with shredded Cheddar cheese."

Western Omelet
"Diced smoked ham, onions, green and red peppers are cooked into the eggs, then stuffed and topped with shredded Cheddar cheese."

Ask the cook to go light on the cheese or do without it. Cheese is fat, and not heart-healthy fat.

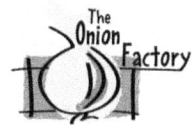

Are you making a last-minute decision to eat out because you did not prepare for the day?

Lunch Menu

Country Caesar Salad
According to Bob Evans' menu, "Fresh, hand-cut Romaine lettuce is tossed in our classic Caesar dressing, then topped with a hard-boiled egg, grape tomatoes, crispy bacon, croutons and shredded Parmesan cheese." Add slow-roasted chicken for $1.00.

Country Spinach Salad
"Tender chicken, bacon and a hard-boiled egg over a bed of fresh baby spinach. Topped with almond slivers, scallions and grape tomatoes or fresh strawberries when in season. Served with Hot Bacon dressing."

Get rid of the croutons. I am not sure I trust the bacon at restaurants (too many fat grams). Dump the yolk of the eggs (5 grams of fat) Ask for your dressing on the side. Remember: Blue cheese, Ranch, O & V, and Caesar are naturally sugar free. All you need to do is manage the amount. Use dressing sparingly. Most restaurants offer a light ranch. Or better yet, for your cleanest game, go to the Walden Farms website and order their to-go packets of dressings. Creamy Bacon, and Onion are my favorites. They do not taste diet-like.

Dinner Menu

Slow-Roasted Turkey Breast
The menu tempts us with this description: "Tender, hand-carved slices of turkey breast over our bread & celery dressing and topped with pan-roasted gravy. Served with mashed potatoes, glazed baby carrots and cranberry relish."

Salmon Fillet
"An 8-oz. portion of fork-tender Atlantic salmon with your choice of our Wildfire BBQ sauce or garlic herb butter. Served with a baked potato and garden vegetables."

Savory Sides

- Bob Evans® Signature coleslaw (drain off the excess dressing)
- Cottage cheese
- Fresh fruit dish (if berries and not loaded with sugar)
- Fresh garden salad (Menu says, "Add bacon and Cheddar cheese for only 50¢." NO! Fat, fat, fat.)
- Green vegetables (Be sure they're only green ones.)
- Green beans with ham
- Broccoli florets

Cracker Barrel®

Not too long ago, I went to a Cracker Barrel Old Country Store®. I had forgotten that their spicy grilled catfish is wonderful! During my peeling process, I leaned on Cracker Barrel® loads. During this particular visit, I was also quickly reminded why Type 2 Diabetes is in epidemic proportions, and why we have grown ourselves into 30, 40, and 50-plus percentages of fat.

I'd bet that many of the patrons need to take a nap after a helping of Cracker Barrel® biscuits. You can have as many as you like. They are "free." Every table seemed to have at least one person who ordered chicken and noodles. (Keep in mind this Midwestern delicacy is served over mashed potatoes.) To make matters worse, you get one more side. Hmmm, do you think these patrons choose yummy green beans? Nope, it's usually corn on the side.

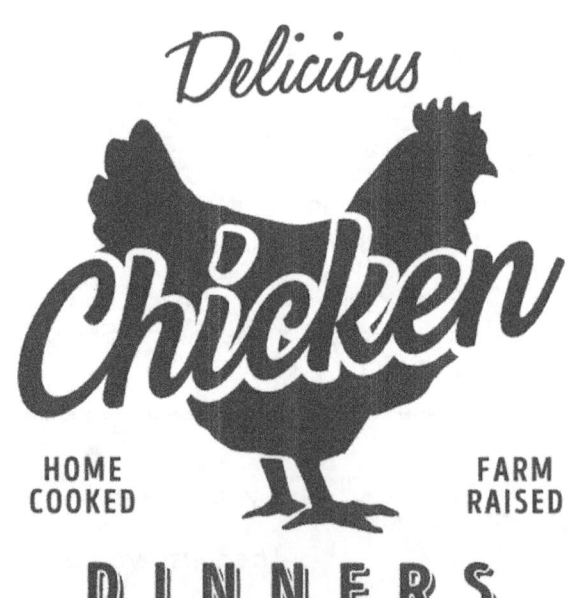

Cracker Barrel®	Serving Size	Calories	Total Fat	Carbs	Protein
Biscuit	1 biscuit	133	5.5g	30.9g	2.7g
Chicken and Dumplings	14 oz	731	34.4g	55g	47.6g
Hash-Brown Casserole	1 cup	499	38g	31g	0g
Fried Apples	1 cup	184	8.8g	28.4g	4g
Double Fudge Coca-Cola® Cake	1 slice	783	37.7g	110.3g	5.8g
Beef Stew	1 cup	120	4.5g	11g	9g
Grilled Chicken Tenderloins	4 pieces	170	4.5g	5g	27g
Grilled New Orleans Style Catfish	1 piece	270	18g	0g	4g
Meatloaf	1 order	386	10g	10g	21.3g
Vegetable Soup w/o Crackers	1 bowl	49	0g	13g	1g
Lemon Pepper Grilled Trout	1 fillet	163	9g	5g	17g
Green Beans (Low Carb Menu)	½ cup	70	2g	4g	2g
Side Salad	1 bowl	30	0g	6g	2g

I imagine that anyone who has visited the Cracker Barrel® restaurant has tried the hash-brown casserole and perhaps even asked for seconds. Would they enjoy it as much if they knew it had 38 grams of fat? And what healthy food did they eat with it?

The old saying goes, "An apple a day keeps the doctor away." Suppose that was about these fried apples? Nearly 9 grams of fat in a serving! Ouch!

And what better way to reward ourselves than with a piece of Cracker Barrel®'s signature chocolate cake, made with Coca-Cola®? Look at those calories and carbs!

Eighty-eight grams of those carbs in the cake come from sugar, and you get 38 grams of fat to boot. Is the delicious taste really worth this? Try the other Cracker Barrel® options instead.

Applebee's®
Maybe my friend Abby was right: The best way to avoid eating food that will cause you to lose weight is, Don't eat out, ever! I really thought I was in a groove with the restaurant section, but I hit a wall, a.k.a. Applebee's®. I am the guru of this stuff. You pick a protein like chicken, or fish, my favorites, because they give you a little wiggle room with fat grams. Then you pick "grass of the lands" such as a salad, a side of broccoli, maybe some coleslaw. Hopefully, you are getting the drill.

Applebee's	Serving Size	Calories	Total Fat	Carbs	Protein
Buffalo Wings w/ Bleu Cheese Dressing	1 portion	1,724	132g	30g	106g
Oriental Chicken Salad	1 salad	709	25g	72g	49g
Fiesta Lime Chicken	1 portion	1,285	47g	136g	74g
Honey Grilled Salmon	1 portion	555	10.1g	70.9g	47.7g
California Shrimp Salad	1 portion	860	70.5g	25.6g	34.3g
Quesadilla Burger	1 burger	520	25g	0g	44g
7 oz Steak Dinner	7 oz	330	10g	0g	44g

For years at Applebee's®, I would select a plate of romaine lettuce (plain). I would fuss about making sure they left off the extras: the croutons, grated cheese, and bacon bits with dressing on the side, adding just a dab. Then I would order a side of boneless buffalo chicken. I felt satisfied (satiated) when I ate anything made with buffalo sauce. I had NO idea of the amount of fat that went along with that selection.

I am not sure what possessed me to pull up the nutritional information on Applebee's® one day, but I did. The table above shows what I found. It seemed that every Applebee's® item I reviewed ran into speed bumps. What I thought would have a decent amount of nutrition was far from it. Let me show you. Here are some chicken and fish entrees. At first glance, they seem harmless. But look closer.

I had to go one step further when reviewing the salmon selection. I knew the 10 grams of fat were doable, but 71 grams of carbs threw me off. Were those "grass of the lands" carbs like a side of stir fried veggies? Was the dish served on rice? Or were these simple carbs (a.k.a. sugars)?

Bingo, the name "honey grilled" should have given it away: 67.8 grams of sugar. This was almost a three-day supply of sugar, even though the fats were in line and the protein was amazing. Maybe asking for NO sauce would solve the dilemma.

No wonder our eating habits are in such trouble. We do not even have a chance! How can a shrimp entrée contain 70 grams of fat? A shrimp entrée with more fat than a burger or a steak, how can that be?

I found irrational problems like this with all of my favorite items at Applebee's®. So let's check out a few other options.

We're looking for low-fat, clean-carb Applebee's® selections. Remember, with carbs you must analyze what type of carb. A. sugar, B. filler, or C. grass of the lands. And if you decide it is C, then you must see where it falls on the Glycemix index. We can make this work.

For example, if you order the 7-oz steak dinner, add a side of broccoli and a small dinner salad, and ask the server to make sure the chef doesn't finish the steak with a brush of butter over the top. This keeps your meal as clean as you possibly can.

Red Lobster®

Let's get right to the root of the evil on Red Lobster®'s menu. The moment you say, "Red

Lobster®," someone starts drooling over the Cheddar Bay Biscuits®. Don't do this! You will hate yourself in the morning.

There are many wonderful choices at Red Lobster®, so focus on what you *can* have, not on what you know full well you *do not* need. Start your Red Lobster® meal with shrimp.

Be careful choosing from Red Lobster®'s other popular entrées. A seafood dish is not necessarily weight-loss worthy. For example, the Ultimate Feast, Red Lobster Dinner, and Crab Alfredo each exceed a whole day's limit for FAT consumption. Yet there's hope. Look at the fat and carb grams for ten other Red Lobster® entrees, beginning with their flounder. (Just for the record, these ten choices are NOT deep-fried.) Eliminate the butter and ask your server to specify that you want your seafood GRILLED, and you will be good to go.

Finally, ask for broccoli as your side and choose Red Lobster® vinaigrette for salad dressing.

Red Lobster®	Serving Size	Calories	Total Fat	Carbs	Protein
Cheddar Bay Biscuits®	1 biscuit	150	8g	16g	-?-
Shrimp	1 oz	33	0.6g	0g	6.4g
Ultimate Feast	1 dinner	892	48.4g	13.3g	75.8g
Red Lobster® Dinner	1 dinner	1,388	86.18g	87g	
Crab Alfredo	1 dinner	1,170	66g		
Flounder	5 oz	100	1g	1g	21g
Lobster (No Butter)	1 tail	230	3g	2g	49g
King Crab Legs	1 serving	490		9g	
Deep Sea Scallops	5 oz	130	2g	2g	26g
Grouper	5 oz	110	1g	0g	26g
Tilapia (Grilled)	Lunch Portion (½ dinner)	186	6g	0g	30g
Halibut	5 oz	110	1g	1g	25g
Red Rockfish	5 oz	90	1g	1g	25g
Red Snapper	5 oz	110	1g	0g	25g
Rainbow Trout	5 oz	170	9g	0g	25g
Broccoli	3 oz	24	0.1g	47g	2.7g
Red Lobster® Vinaigrette	1 Tbsp	25	2g	249	2g

Olive Garden®	Serving Size	Calories	Total Fat	Carbs	Protein
Italian Salad	1 salad	201	6g	31g	0g
Breadstick (plain)	1 stick	150	2.5g	28g	5g
Fettucine Alfredo	1 lunch serving	780	18g	125g	24g
Tour of Italy	1 meal	1,450	74g	97g	0g
Minestrone Soup	1 bowl	164	1g	18g	5g
Chicken Giardino (dinner entrée)	1 meal	408	12g	0g	27g
Venetian Apricot Chicken	1 meal	448	11g	0g	27g
Pork Filletino w/ Vegetables	1 meal	340	9g	16g	20g

Olive Garden®

Once you get this nutritional formula down, eating out will be a breeze. You will be able to maintain your weight and even lose weight at one of the more tempting locations, Olive Garden®. How do you order weight-loss worthy at a pasta location? Anyone who has ever been to Olive Garden® realizes that it starts with a BIG bowl of salad and unlimited breadsticks. Let's see how the salad at Olive Garden® shakes out.

Anyone who has ever been to Olive Garden® knows that it starts with a BIG bowl of salad and unlimited breadsticks. You can start there. Make sure you save your breakfast and lunch fat grams so you will have a little more wiggle room with your fat grams for the evening. Maybe breakfast would look like an egg white omelet and lunch would be a salad with a chicken breast. That would give you almost 30 grams of fat for your night out at Olive Garden®.

Obviously, you'll need to stay away from the breadsticks. Those carbs are NOT from "grass of the lands," so they are going directly to your "assets." Whoever ate just one breadstick anyway? As a fluffy girl, I dipped my breadsticks in Alfredo sauce!

On the other hand, minestrone soup is an entrée that you can modify to work. The majority of its carbs come from "grass of the lands" (veggies) and you can pick out the little bit of noodles if you are super-focused. For your Olive Garden® entrées, try Chicken Giardino, Venetian Apricot Chicken, or Pork Filletino with vegetables.

Fine Dining

I mentioned earlier that I would be happy to enjoy fine dining every day of the week if my budget would allow, or if my business department would loosen the purse strings. Why do I feel that way? Because grilled chicken or fish is readily available at a fine restaurant and normally prepared very well.

I am less likely to be tempted there with deep-fried foods. A shrimp cocktail or tuna is easily found as an appetizer. The salads are usually creative, while fresh broccoli and asparagus are readily available.

Ruth's Chris Steakhouse®

For example, a night at Ruth's Chris Steakhouse® might look like this:

Appetizer

Shrimp Remoulade
"Jumbo Gulf shrimp dressed with your choice of our classic Creole remoulade sauce or our spicy New Orleans home-style cocktail sauce."

Salad

Vine Ripe Tomato & Buffalo Mozzarella Salad
"A sliced Beefsteak tomato, basil and fresh buffalo mozzarella cheese with balsamic vinaigrette." (NOTE: I would have budgeted the mozzarella to make sure I still had some fat grams.)

Entrée

Ahi-Tuna Stack
"Seared rare tuna topped with Colossal lump crab-meat and served sizzling with red pepper pesto."

Cold-Water Lobster Tail
"With blackening spice and topped with lemon and drizzled butter." (NOTE: Ask the chef to prepare with lemon only!)

Sides

Fresh Asparagus
With hollandaise (NOTE: Remember, a little dab goes a long way.)

Dessert

Fresh Seasonal Berries with Sweet Cream Sauce
"A celebration of natural flavors. Simple and simply sensational." (NOTE: Ask for the sweet cream sauce on the side and use it sparingly.)

DO NOT ORDER

Signature Steaks
"Our famous steaks are seared to perfection at 1800 degrees and topped with fresh butter so they sizzle all the way to your table."

Potatoes Au Gratin
"Idaho sliced potatoes with a three-cheese sauce"

Bread Pudding with Whiskey Sauce
"Our definitive version of a traditional New Orleans favorite"

Obviously, there is NO way you can stay on your game by ordering the above high-fat and high-sugar items "as is." Have I ever had their bread pudding or a steak there? Of course! Have I also cleaned up the last 20 pounds I gained, over and over? Yep! So the more you can learn to eat normally and only occasionally make high-fat, high-sugar selections is when you complete this weight management journey.

As you can see, I enjoy a full-course meal. When you choose wisely, you can enjoy all the courses you like. I enjoy food. I believe eating should be an experience for all of the senses. I am not necessarily looking for a big plate of food, but I am looking for the wow factor in food. Presentation is everything! Let's face it, food is fun.

When you order out, I think there's a psychological lure to treat yourself. You feel you need to select something that is a departure from the norm. If you are going to invest in someone else's culinary art, you are likely to desire an item that you would not normally prepare at home.

Eating out can become an escape, an indulgence, or a celebration. Food has even become our entertainment. If you are unsure of that thought, check out the menus and the atmosphere at Benihana®, Cheesecake Factory Bakery®, Cheeseburger in Paradise®, or the Rainforest Café®. We celebrate around food, and the atmosphere can enhance the experience. Occasionally, we even use food to attempt to fulfill some emotional void in our life.

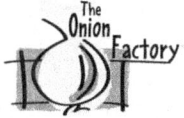

When I eat out,

I am looking for

the wow factor in food.

Can't Cook, But Can Grab at the Grocery

Of course I can cook! However, today I am not in the mood, I said to myself. *I can either cook today or I can write, but I cannot do both.* I am quickly learning I am not Superwoman. Today was a good thing, because it has been a very long time since I have walked into a grocery store and not been in the "What Can I Make?" mode, but the "What Can I Grab?" mode. This is what my grocery cart looked like:

- **2 bags lettuce** – Normally I would cut up my own but as I said, "I am not in the mood." I got lucky; my store was offering "buy one get one free" ($3.09 for 2). I can make that work. It's easy.

- **3 boxes Gorton's® Grilled Fillets** – I like the lemon pepper version; however, I picked up the new grilled Tilapia (lemon peppercorn); it should be good. Love the taste and the nutrition breakdown of this selection. I had forgotten that I leaned on this selection

	Gorton's® Grilled Fish Fillets
Serving Size	1 piece
Fat Grams	3g
Carbs	0g
Protein	19g

frequently when I was chipping away at the first 100 pounds I lost back in 2003. It never hurts to go back to what worked!

This fish tastes much more buttery than the stats would indicate. Perhaps that's why I like Gorton's so much. I always feel I am cheating when I eat these! I usually eat 2 pieces. While I could make them myself for a lot less, eating out would cost a lot more, so I feel like they are a good investment.

- **3 bags of Birdseye® Steamers** – These are a new selection for me. I normally get the boil-in veggie bags by Birdseye, but one of my Onions shared this idea with me. I got a great price at $1.29 per bag, since there are

	Broccoli w/ Cheese Sauce
Serving Size	1 cup
Fat Grams	1.5g
Carbs	7g
Sugar	3g
Protein	2g

3 servings per bag. They look good, and here is the nutrition breakdown for the broccoli cheese sauce version. Obviously, do not select the ones with potatoes or pasta in them. Think green, think "grass of the lands."

- **1 dozen eggs** – You can never go wrong with eggs. One dozen eggs have about 84 grams of clean protein. They are affordable, and you can make so many things out of them such as egg-white salad, omelets, soufflés, or hard-boiled eggs for your snacks. Just remember to dump the yolks, because that is where the fat and cholesterol are stored.

- **2 packages (7oz) Oscar Mayer® Deli fresh Roast Beef** – I use to get tripped up by the beef thought, but you can make this work, and it makes a great roast beef salad with tomatoes, green onions, fat-free feta, and a

	Deli Fresh Roast Beef
Serving Size	2 oz.
Fat Grams	2g
Protein	10g

light blue cheese dressing. If you ever get stuck and need a quick fix, run in the store and eat an entire package of Mayer Roast Beef on the fly. The whole box would give you 40 grams of protein for only 8 grams of fat. Not bad at all.

- **1 box of strawberries** – My latest fix if I am feeling like I need a treat, is cottage cheese with a few berries sliced on top. A dab of Walden Farms chocolate sauce and a few (I said a *few,* as in 3–4) slivered almonds. Yummy.

- **1 container 2% cottage cheese** – I detest eating fat-free cottage cheese. I do not mind cooking with it, but to eat fat-free alone...nope,

	2% Cottage Cheese
Serving Size	½ cup
Fat Grams	2g
Carbs	6g
Sugars	4g
Protein	12g

not going to do it. It has a taste that reminds me of something DIET, and that taste repels me. It is not something I would do for the rest of my life, so I have learned how to plug 2% cottage cheese into my daily equation.

- **1 bag of Crab Chunks** – I like these. Frequently, they become my hors de oeuvres before dinner or they make a quick snack. You just need to make sure you plug in the numbers. You cannot just eat the entire bag and get the results you are looking for. So pay attention to what you're doing.
You might be a little confused on the

	Crab Chunks
Serving Size	½ cup
Fat Grams	0g
Carbs	8g
Sugars	11g
Protein	3g

carbohydrates of the Crab Chunks. Once you subtract the sugars out of the carbs, it leaves you with 9 grams. You have to decide if the 9 grams are coming from "grass of the lands," which you can basically eat in unlimited quantities, or are they are coming from fillers, which you are trying to avoid because you have a fat reserve tank. And we are trying to get your body to use it, so you can get back into your skinny jeans and/or fix what ails you.

At this point, you can assume seafood is not a grass of the land. Crab meat is your source of protein, so the carbohydrates in this processed food must come from starch and other fillers. Is these tasty morsels worth ingesting 9 grams of filler carbohydrates? Obviously, eating fresh crab would be the cleanest option, but

I live on a cornfield, not by an ocean, so a girl must do what a girl must do. I had to read the ingredient label very carefully to figure out where the other 9 carb grams were coming from. Hmm... potato starches, modified tapioca starch, and a few other things I cannot pronounce.

On my best game, I would select fresh crab and leave Crab Chunks alone. But if you find yourself in maintenance mode, or this is a nine-month journey or longer, you can make a half-cup serving work occasionally. Honestly, you could do a lot worse. We have come a long way from pizza, popcorn, and bread sticks. Don't beat yourself up, just continue to make better choices and modify your behaviors. If you are working toward one of those killer 20-pound weight loss months, get the fresh crab!

- **1 bag Gel Bites®** – I hope you can find these in your area. I find them at Kroger®; in fact, Gel Bites® is a brand name. You can eat the entire bag and only consume 0 fat, 0 carbs, and get 9 grams of protein! Wow, wow, wow, what a great deal. Protein feeds the muscle. Take care of your muscle and you will maintain your metabolic rate. It's a win/win. This little bag is great to take to the movies. Even if you are not hungry, and you have had all your nutrition for the day, you may start craving a treat at the movies. These will save you! If these are not available in your area, you can always make some Jello jigglers (sugar-free, of course), which are essentially the same thing. But it's so much easier when you can just grab the bag.

- **1 tray of crab-stuffed portabella mushrooms** – What a great find! I found them ready-made in the fresh-foods section of my local grocery store. This is especially great for a Saturday night alone on the computer. Allow

	Stuffed Mushrooms
Serving Size	1 Mushroom
Fat Grams	3g
Protein	3g
Carbs	7g
Sugar	1g

me to explain that thought. If I get tempted later and feel the need to nurture with food, then I have my back-up plan, a mushroom. I will pop one of these in the oven, make a cup of tea, and realize be ready for my next appointment. The results will be worth it. I keep my mind on the big picture. I want to stay in control of my food. I know what it feels like to be out of control. I know what it takes to clean up 20 pounds of excess weight over and over again, and I want to find that happy landing place for my weight. I realize I am not totally there yet. I battle with my weight just like you do!

Writing this grocery section tonight, I was encouraged to think about the options we have. If you can't or won't cook, you can use these ideas to analyze the labels of quick-fix items, and you will be able to reinvent yourself. Or if you just need a break from the kitchen, as I sometimes do, then you can see how to do it. And guess what? All the above added up to less than $50. Whoever said eating right is expensive?

What to Do When You Don't Know What to Do

Health improvement starts with good shopping. What is in your grocery cart, and what is going to make it to your pantry?

I'll be the first to admit that grocery shopping is tough for me these days. Here we have obesity in epidemic proportions, and I see all the mistakes people are making right in front of me in the grocery aisle. I know they are unaware of what they do not know, and this is probably the most frustrating part of the equation. I also know they are trying, because, after they fill their carts with all the silly choices, they will add diet pop or skinny ice cream. They have NO idea what is hidden in the labels for those products. Sure, there might be a better choice than straight out soda pop and regular ice cream; however, there still might be just enough sugar or fat or filler carbs to impeded any weight loss.

Trader Joe's® Frozen Entrées

I want to give you a reminder from the grocery list in an earlier chapter. Thirty grams of fat per day is a lot to work with. And 24 grams of sugar goes along way when the baseline of your nutrition begins with what God gave us to work with. When you reach your goals and continue with your exercise efforts, you will even have more room to enjoy a few old favorites or a few extras of your new favorites.

In the meantime, here are a few quick and easy choices for the days when you do not have time to cook, you desire something really good, and you want to stay on your game. You can even make these work in weight-loss mode. You will just need to save a few extra fat grams for your evening meal.

Regardless of whether you can cook, I highly recommend you stash these six entrées away in your freezer for that moment when life gets too busy or you are just not in the mood to cook. They are affordable and taste better than most everyday restaurants out there. This is the short list:

- Tilapia Citronette
- Mojito Salmon
- Misoyaki Turbot
- Chicken Serenada
- Chicken Gorgonzola
- Chicken Pomodoro

Tilapia is fast and easy. If you add a serving of Trader Joe's® frozen asparagus or broccoli florets and a salad, you can be ready for dinner in five minutes. You cannot get any better than that.

Grocery Shopping Do's and Don'ts

Do Buy	Don't Buy
Green, Leafy Vegetables	Processed Foods
Fresh Berries	White Sugar
Lean Meats	White Flour
Egg Whites	Sodas (Regular or Diet)
Clean Yogurts	Chips
Water	Sweets

Trader Joe's® Entreés	Serving Size	Calories	Total Fat	Carbs	Protein
Tilapia Citronelle	1 serving	280	11g	6g	38g
Mojito Salmon	1 serving	310	16g	6g	32g
Misoyaki Turbot	1 serving	210	6g	6g	31g
Chicken Serenada	1 serving	290	12g	17g	29g
Chicken Gorgonzola	1 serving	320	16g	9g	32g
Chicken Pomodoro	1 serving	340	18g	9g	34g

However, the next one, Mojito Salmon, is my very favorite frozen seafood entrée from Trader Joe's. Yes, you must maneuver a few extra fat grams to enjoy this meal; however, if you keep your breakfast to omelets, you will have plenty of extra fat grams to utilize later in the day.

There you have it. Keep these six entreés stashed in your freezer and you will never need to miss a beat with your nutrition.

An After-Dinner Mint?

Why do many of us feel the need for an after-dinner mint? It has absolutely nothing to do with hunger. We've reached the end of the meal, and we should have filled up on our proteins and "grass of the lands." We have followed a strategic plan for our fats and been careful with our sugars, but dinner was not enough. Not enough nutritionally? Not enough emotionally? Not enough psychologically? You see, it all goes back to our own psychology. Why do we need, and want, a treat at the end of every meal? I have NO idea, but I do know the emotion is real. Perhaps for us Onions it goes back to how we were nurtured when we were young. Maybe we associate the after-dinner mint as a treat we've earned, or maybe our palate needs to be cleansed.

The French enjoy eating a sorbet between meals or cleansing their palates with wine between courses. Why do we still enjoy a dessert after the meal? Dessert is like the period at the end of the sentence. I think dessert means we have completed our meal, and until we have completed it we believe we are not done. We might even graze mindlessly an hour or so after dinner, looking for that completion. So check your behavior. Are you looking for a chocolate-chip cookie later?

If I am speaking directly to you, then you need to have a plan to deal with the your innate desire for something sweet. Maybe those gel bites will suffice. Maybe you'd like a protein shake for your morning snack. Or maybe you are that girl/guy who needs to save a berry or two for your evening treat. You will probably need to think about this and see what your tendencies are during your peeling journey.

Food is your missing link to change. You first need to understand what to eat versus what not to eat. Then you can take control of yourself, your health, your energy levels, your mental health, and your life.
You will have big weight-loss months, you will have small weight-loss months, and you will have months you get stuck. You need to consider how long it took you to grow into an Onion, and enjoy the journey of getting yourself back. Changing a size a month is very exciting. Ride that wave for a moment, instead of instantly gratifying yourself with food. The results are really worth it.

Your success is based on the knowledge, yes, but also the plan and loads of preparation. One stupid (lack of preparation) day can lead to another. Just like one day off your workouts can turn into two, and two can turn into three, and then a week. Before you realize it, you are off your game.

The big picture looks like this. If you get the results you desire, then all you need to do is manage your behaviors. If you ever go back to your old behaviors, then the old results are coming right back to you.

So this really is a long-term solution for what ails us, not a short-term quick fix. You need to be ready and have the desire to change, as well as the discipline to change!

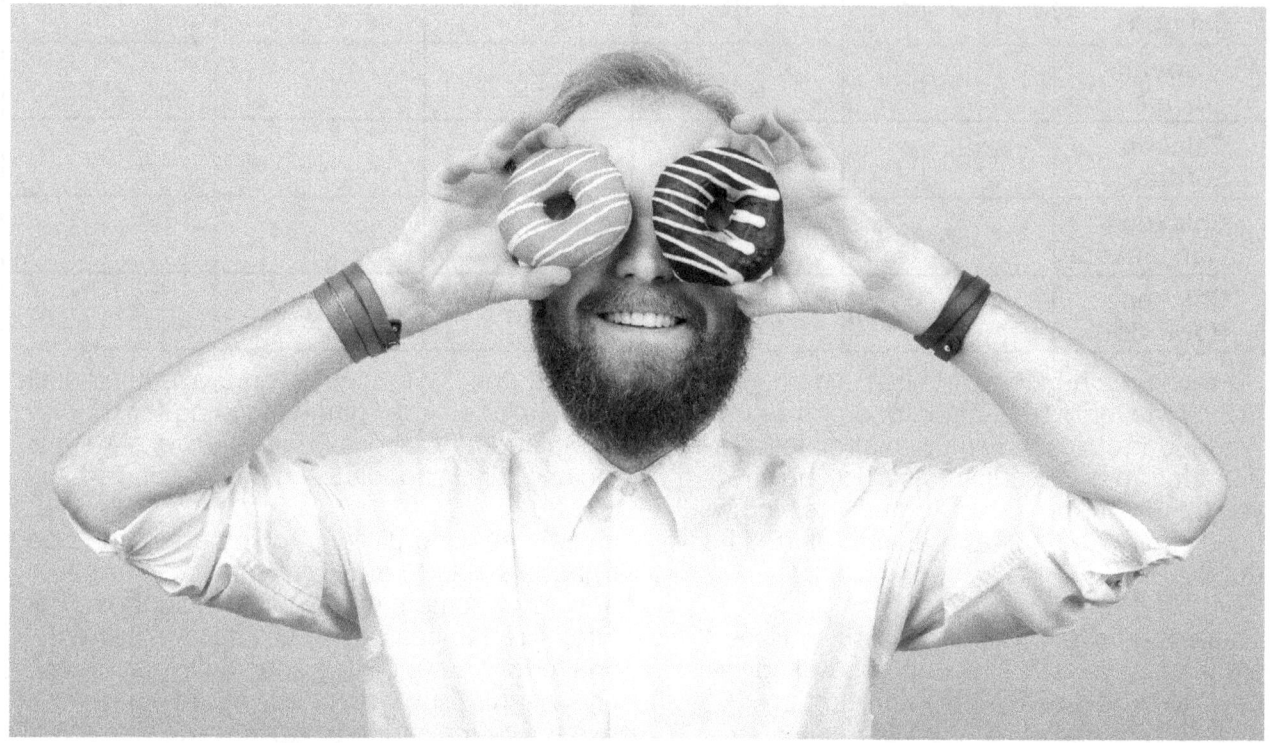

Everyday Don'ts

- Don't allow yourself to get too hungry, angry, or depressed. Food will not fix a bad day for you.

- Don't leave home without it—your back-up plan, that is. Take a snack just in case you find yourself "out and about" longer than you expected.

- Don't forget to nibble every 3 hours. Consistent eating will allow your blood sugar to stay steady.

- Do not feed into temptations or get distracted. If you make a less-than-worthy choice, forget about it and do not continue to sabotage yourself. Get right back on game.

- Don't succumb to pressure from your circle of influence. They may not love the fact that you have decided to make changes, especially if they are still eating like you used to. That "one bite" of what they're having might lead to a slippery slope in the wrong direction.

- Don't think food will fill an emotional void in your life or keep you entertained.

11. Eat Away!

I AM PASSIONATE ABOUT TAKING OLD IDEAS AND REINVENTING THEM INTO WEIGHT-LOSS WORTHY OPTIONS.

IF YOU DO NOT know what: A little bit

    A dash

        A dip

            A pinch

                Or a dollop is, you may have trouble with our recipes. However, I took a little extra time and put my mind to measuring the recipes' ingredients to give you my best guesstimate. So please THINK to taste what you're cooking and ADJUST to your liking!

I am a throw-and-go cook. In fact, if I remember correctly, I did not ace my Home Economics course. I thought, *Who needs a measuring cup?*

While I am not a formally trained chef, I am pretty creative and passionate about taking old ideas and reinventing them into weight-loss worthy options; I hope the results are recipes that the whole family will enjoy.

On the following page is an easy visual example of how you might start thinking about how to plan a meal that is weight-loss worthy.

Following that example page, you will find 62 recipes for breakfast, burgers, soups, salads, dinners, sides, desserts, beverages, and snacks. We have also added seven shortcuts and ideas for an emergency kit to take with you, so you won't be stuck without any weight-loss worthy food options available.

If you get the results you desire, then all you need to do is manage your behaviors.

If you go back to your old behaviors, you'll get your old results.

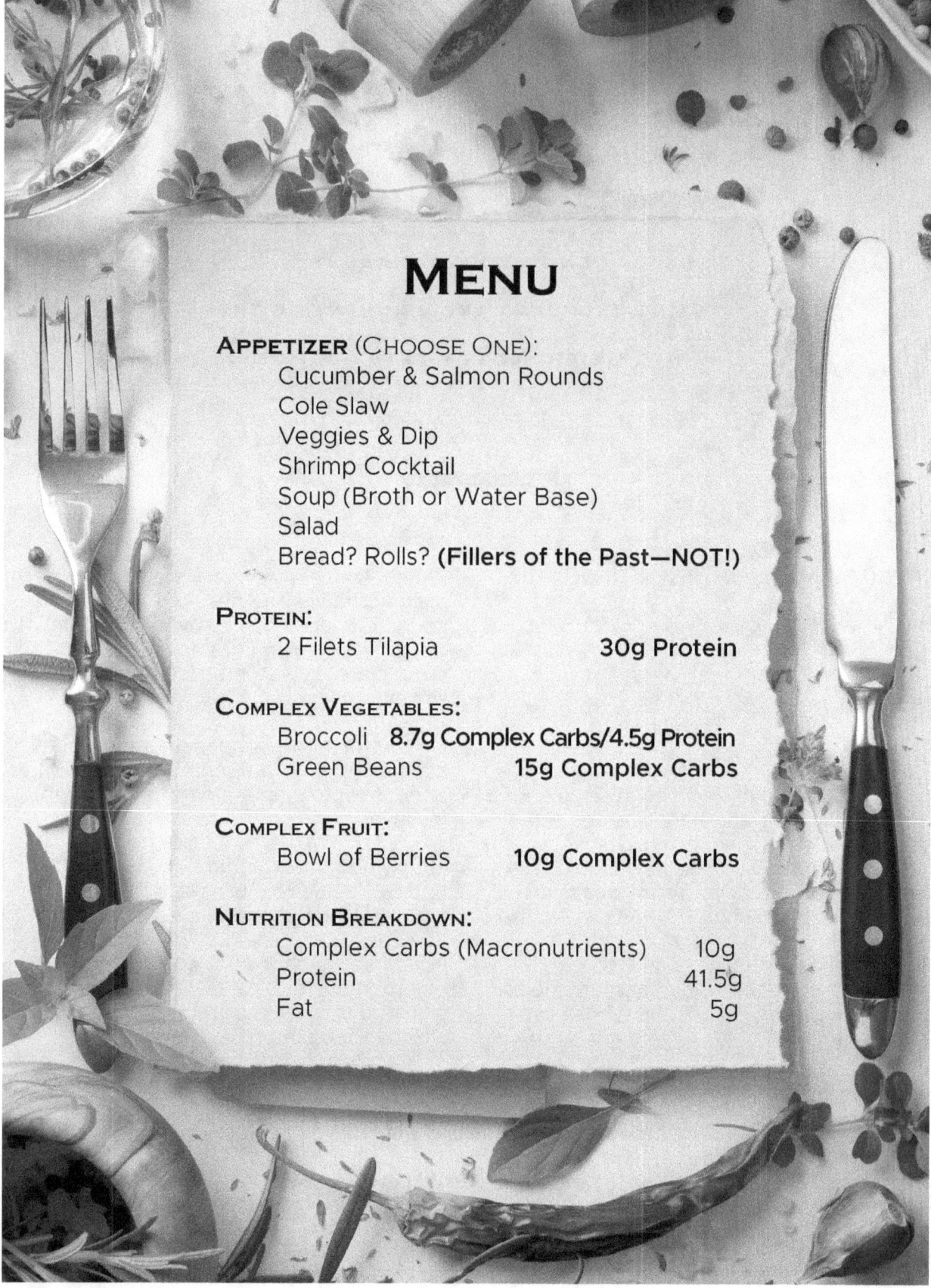

Menu

Appetizer (Choose One):
  Cucumber & Salmon Rounds
  Cole Slaw
  Veggies & Dip
  Shrimp Cocktail
  Soup (Broth or Water Base)
  Salad
  Bread? Rolls? **(Fillers of the Past—NOT!)**

Protein:
  2 Filets Tilapia   **30g Protein**

Complex Vegetables:
  Broccoli   **8.7g Complex Carbs/4.5g Protein**
  Green Beans   **15g Complex Carbs**

Complex Fruit:
  Bowl of Berries   **10g Complex Carbs**

Nutrition Breakdown:
  Complex Carbs (Macronutrients)   10g
  Protein   41.5g
  Fat   5g

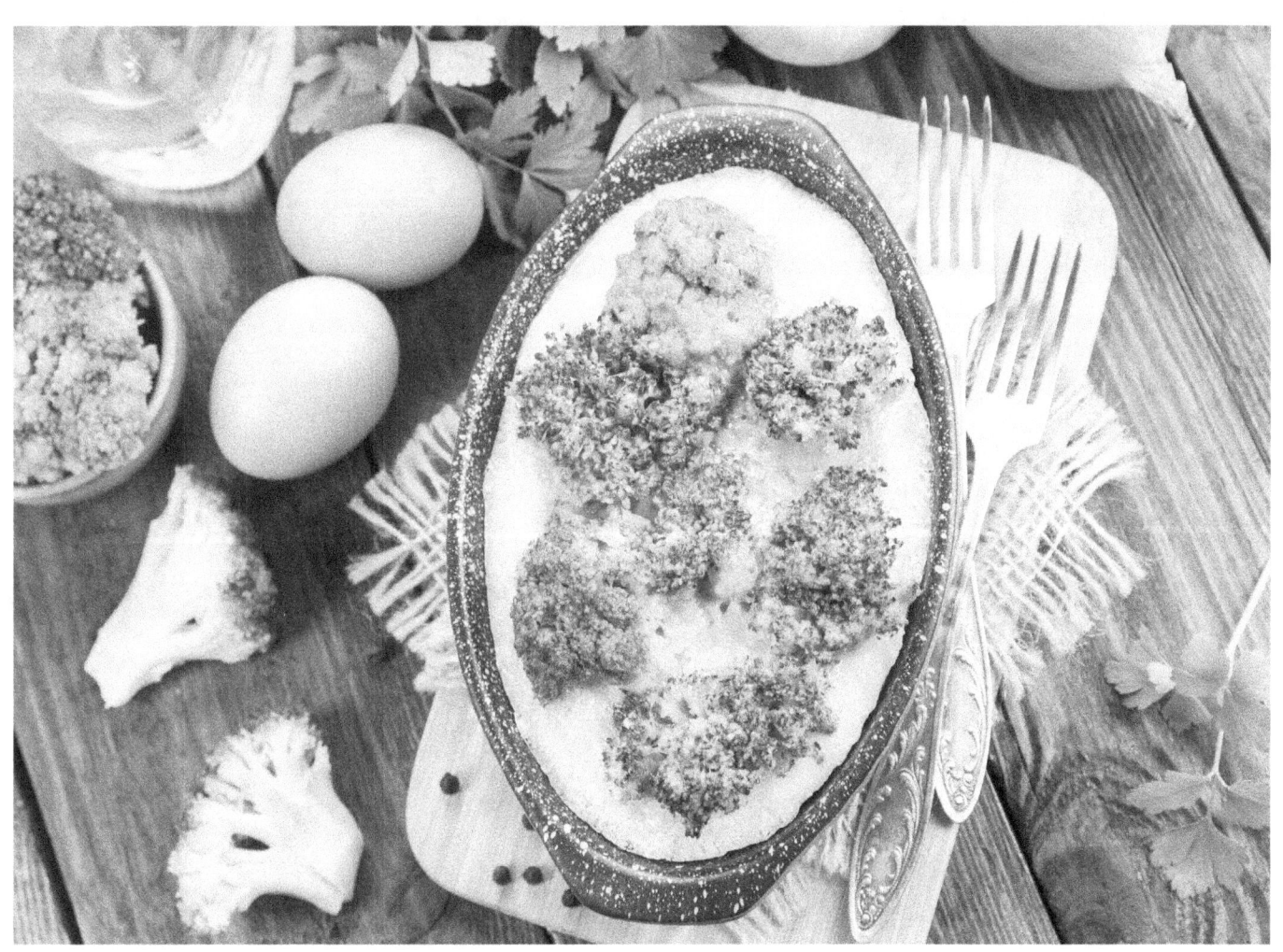

breakfasts

A SATISFYING BREAKFAST BEGINS EVERY SUCCESSFUL DAY.

EGG WHITE BREAKFAST BOWL

YIELDS: 1 serving

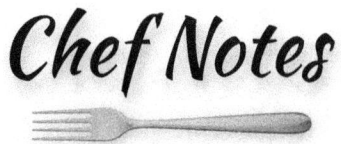

INGREDIENTS

- ½ cup egg whites
- ¼ cup frozen three-pepper blend
- 1 slice pepper jack cheese

DIRECTIONS

1. Spray a small fry pan with Pam®. Sauté the frozen three-pepper blend.
2. Spray an omelet pan with Pam®. Over medium heat, add the egg whites and scramble them.
3. Add the sautéed three-pepper blend.
4. Top with the slice of pepper jack cheese.

♦ Serving suggestion:

Serve with Parmesan Baked Tomato.

Nutrition Facts

Egg White Breakfast Bowl

Amount Per Serving	
Calories 130	Calories from Fat 50
	% Daily Value*
Total Fat 6g	9%
Saturated Fat 3.5g	18%
Trans Fat 0g	
Cholesterol 20mg	7%
Sodium 320mg	13%
Total Carbohydrate 2g	1%
Dietary Fiber 0g	0%
Sugars 2g	
Protein 18g	
Vitamin A 4% • Vitamin C 8%	
Calcium 15% • Iron 0%	

* Percent Daily Values are based on a 2,000 calorie diet. Your daily values may be higher or lower depending on your calorie needs:

	Calories:	2,000	2,500
Total Fat	Less than	65g	80g
Sat Fat	Less than	20g	25g
Cholesterol	Less than	300mg	300mg
Sodium	Less than	2,400mg	2,400mg
Total Carbohydrate		300g	375g
Dietary Fiber		25g	30g

INGREDIENTS: EGG WHITES, PEPPERS, ONION, PEPPER JACK CHEESE

ONION FACTORY: ANDERSON, IN

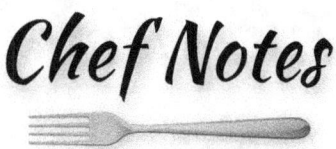

Chef Notes

- The remaining Knorr® Hollandaise sauce will keep in the refrigerator for 2 days.
- To upgrade, add grilled asparagus on the side. This is company worthy!

EGGS BENEDICT BOWL

YIELDS: 1 serving

INGREDIENTS

- ½ cup egg whites
- 1 egg
- 2 oz Black Forest ham, diced
- 1 Roma tomato, diced
- 1 pkg Knorr® Hollandaise sauce
- ½ cup fat-free cream
- ½ cup water
- parsley or green onion, to garnish

DIRECTIONS

1. To prepare Hollandaise sauce, combine:
   - Knorr® Hollandaise packet
   - ½ cup fat-free cream
   - ½ cup water

   Follow cooking directions on packet.

2. In small bowl, scramble together the egg whites and egg.

3. Spray a skillet with Pam®, then scramble the egg mixture. Do not overcook.

4. Top eggs with:
   - diced ham
   - diced tomato
   - ¼ cup prepared Hollandaise sauce

5. Garnish with parsley or green onion.

Nutrition Facts
Eggs Benedict Bowl

Amount Per Serving	
Calories 200	Calories from Fat 50
	% Daily Value*
Total Fat 6g	9%
Saturated Fat 2.5g	13%
Trans Fat 0g	
Cholesterol 175mg	58%
Sodium 1010mg	42%
Total Carbohydrate 7g	2%
Dietary Fiber 0g	0%
Sugars 5g	
Protein 28g	
Vitamin A 4% • Vitamin C 0%	
Calcium 6% • Iron 4%	

*Percent Daily Values are based on a 2,000 calorie diet. Your daily values may be higher or lower depending on your calorie needs:

	Calories:	2,000	2,500
Total Fat	Less than	65g	80g
Sat Fat	Less than	20g	25g
Cholesterol	Less than	300mg	300mg
Sodium	Less than	2,400mg	2,400mg
Total Carbohydrate		300g	375g
Dietary Fiber		25g	30g

INGREDIENTS: EGG WHITES, DICED HAM, EGG, FAT FREE CREAM

ONION FACTORY: ANDERSON, IN

BREAKFAST BURRITO

YIELDS: 1 serving

INGREDIENTS

- ½ cup egg whites
- ¼ cup frozen Cajun mirepoix, defrosted
- 1 Tbsp turkey sausage crumbles
- 1 Tbsp + 1 tsp shredded Cheddar
- 1 Tbsp salsa
- 1 Tbsp fat-free sour cream
- 1 tsp green onion, diced

DIRECTIONS

1. Saute frozen mirepoix in small frying pan.
2. In omelet pan over medium-high heat, sprayed with Pam®:
   - Add egg whites.
   - Top with mirepoix, sausage, and 1 Tbsp Cheddar cheese.
3. Cook until eggs are white and remove to cutting board.
4. To assemble:
   - Roll the burrito contents in egg whites and cut in half.
   - Top with 1 Tbsp salsa, 1 Tbsp sour cream, and 1 tsp shredded Cheddar.
   - Garnish with green onion.

Chef Notes

- Kroger® carries frozen Cajun mirepoix.
- To make your own Cajun mirepoix: Dice equal amounts of onions, celery, and green peppers.
- To make turkey sausage crumbles, put Banquet® turkey sausage in food processor and rough chop.

Nutrition Facts
Breakfast Burrito

Amount Per Serving

Calories 140 — Calories from Fat 35

	% Daily Value*
Total Fat 4g	6%
Saturated Fat 2.5g	13%
Trans Fat 0g	
Cholesterol 15mg	5%
Sodium 470mg	20%
Total Carbohydrate 7g	2%
Dietary Fiber 0g	0%
Sugars 4g	
Protein 18g	

| Vitamin A 15% | • | Vitamin C 2% |
| Calcium 15% | • | Iron 2% |

* Percent Daily Values are based on a 2,000 calorie diet. Your daily values may be higher or lower depending on your calorie needs:

	Calories:	2,000	2,500
Total Fat	Less than	65g	80g
Sat Fat	Less than	20g	25g
Cholesterol	Less than	300mg	300mg
Sodium	Less than	2,400mg	2,400mg
Total Carbohydrate		300g	375g
Dietary Fiber		25g	30g

INGREDIENTS: EGG WHITES, ONIONS, CELERY, GREEN PEPPERS, FAT FREE SOUR CREAM, SALSA, LOW FAT SHARP CHEDDAR CHEESE, GREEN ONIONS, TURKEY SAUSAGE

ONION FACTORY: ANDERSON, IN

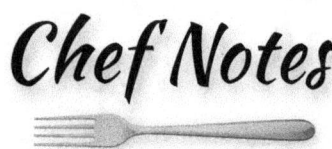

Chef Notes

♦ Serving suggestion:

Serve with a side of broccoli and a turkey sausage link.

CHEESY EGGS

YIELDS: 1 serving

INGREDIENTS

- ½ cup egg whites
- 1 egg
- 1 slice of 2% Velveeta® or ½ slice of regular Velveeta®

DIRECTIONS

1. In small bowl, scramble together egg whites and egg.
2. Cook eggs in omelet pan sprayed with Pam®. Do not overcook.
3. Top with cheese.

Nutrition Facts
Cheesy Eggs

Amount Per Serving	
Calories 130	Calories from Fat 40
	% Daily Value*
Total Fat 4.5g	7%
Saturated Fat 1.5g	8%
Trans Fat 0g	
Cholesterol 145mg	48%
Sodium 400mg	17%
Total Carbohydrate 3g	1%
Dietary Fiber 0g	0%
Sugars 1g	
Protein 18g	

Vitamin A 4%	•	Vitamin C 0%
Calcium 8%	•	Iron 4%

* Percent Daily Values are based on a 2,000 calorie diet. Your daily values may be higher or lower depending on your calorie needs:

	Calories:	2,000	2,500
Total Fat	Less than	65g	80g
Sat Fat	Less than	20g	25g
Cholesterol	Less than	300mg	300mg
Sodium	Less than	2,400mg	2,400mg
Total Carbohydrate		300g	375g
Dietary Fiber		25g	30g

INGREDIENTS: EGG WHITES, EGG, VELVEETA

ONION FACTORY: ANDERSON, IN

CRUSTLESS QUICHE

YIELDS: 8 servings

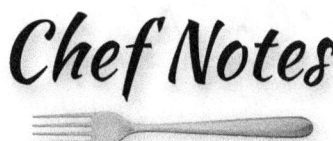

INGREDIENTS

- ❑ 8 eggs
- ❑ 4 cups egg whites
- ❑ 1 lb ground turkey sausage
- ❑ ½ cup shredded Cheddar cheese
- ❑ 2 green onions, chopped

DIRECTIONS

1. Preheat oven to 350 degrees.
2. In a large bowl, whip the eggs and egg whites until well blended.
3. Add remaining ingredients to the egg mixture.
4. Bake for 1 hr at 350 degrees.
5. Spoon on your choice of topping (see Chef Notes).
6. Spray a 9x13 pan with Pam®. Add egg mixture.
7. Bake for 50 minutes.

VARIATIONS

- ♦ Replace the ground turkey with diced ham.
- ♦ Add mushrooms and green peppers.
- ♦ Replace turkey and cheese with diced grilled chicken, feta chees, and spinach.

- ♦ Notice this recipe has 20 grams of protein per serving.
- ♦ Add sides of berries, tomatoes, or broccoli for a complete meal.

Nutrition Facts

Crustless Quiche

Amount Per Serving	
Calories 260	Calories from Fat 100
	% Daily Value*
Total Fat 11g	17%
Saturated Fat 3.5g	18%
Trans Fat 0g	
Cholesterol 235mg	78%
Sodium 770mg	32%
Total Carbohydrate 3g	1%
Dietary Fiber 0g	0%
Sugars 2g	
Protein 35g	
Vitamin A 10% • Vitamin C 4%	
Calcium 10% • Iron 10%	

* Percent Daily Values are based on a 2,000 calorie diet. Your daily values may be higher or lower depending on your calorie needs:

	Calories:	2,000	2,500
Total Fat	Less than	65g	80g
Sat Fat	Less than	20g	25g
Cholesterol	Less than	300mg	300mg
Sodium	Less than	2,400mg	2,400mg
Total Carbohydrate		300g	375g
Dietary Fiber		25g	30g

INGREDIENTS: EGG WHITES, TURKEY SAUSAGE, EGG, FAT FREE COTTAGE CHEESE, LOW FAT SHARP CHEDDAR CHEESE, GREEN ONION

ONION FACTORY: ANDERSON,IN

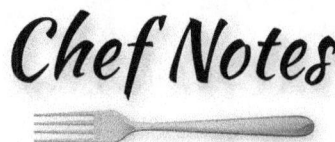

Chef Notes

♦ Kroger® Carbmaster® yogurt has a low carbohydrate content. Half a serving is a great afternoon snack.

BREAKFAST PARFAIT

YIELDS: 1 serving

INGREDIENTS

- ☐ 6 oz. container of Kroger® Strawberry Banana Carbmaster® yogurt
- ☐ ½ cup fat-free cottage cheese
- ☐ 5 strawberries, fresh or frozen

DIRECTIONS

1. Mix together Carbmaster® yogurt and cottage cheese.
2. Slice strawberries.
3. In clear 12 oz. plastic cup, layer:
   - ☐ 2 sliced strawberries
   - ☐ ½ yogurt mixture
   - ☐ 2 sliced strawberries
   - ☐ Remaining yogurt mixture
4. Top with remaining strawberry.

VARIATIONS

♦ Vanilla yogurt and raspberries

♦ Mixed-berry yogurt and raspberries

♦ Vanilla yogurt and blueberries

♦ Yogurt flavor of your choice and berries of your choice

Nutrition Facts
Breakfast Parfait

Amount Per Serving	
Calories 150	Calories from Fat 15

	% Daily Value*
Total Fat 1.5g	2%
Saturated Fat 1g	5%
Trans Fat 0g	
Cholesterol 15mg	5%
Sodium 500mg	21%
Total Carbohydrate 12g	4%
Dietary Fiber <1g	3%
Sugars 8g	
Protein 24g	

Vitamin A 4%	•		Vitamin C 40%
Calcium 10%	•		Iron 80%

*Percent Daily Values are based on a 2,000 calorie diet. Your daily values may be higher or lower depending on your calorie needs:

	Calories:	2,000	2,500
Total Fat	Less than	65g	80g
Sat Fat	Less than	20g	25g
Cholesterol	Less than	300mg	300mg
Sodium	Less than	2,400mg	2,400mg
Total Carbohydrate		300g	375g
Dietary Fiber		25g	30g

INGREDIENTS: CARBMASTER YOGURT, FAT FREE COTTAGE CHEESE, STRAWBERRIES

ONION FACTORY: ANDERSON, IN

VERDE OMELET

YIELDS: 1 serving

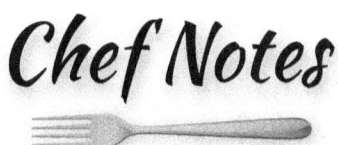

INGREDIENTS

- ½ cup egg whites
- 2 oz. diced, cooked chicken breast
- 2 Tbsp Verde sauce, divided
- ½ cup frozen Cajun mirepoix, divided
- 1 Tbsp shredded mozzarella cheese

♦ One 12 oz. bag of mirepoix will make 5–6 omelets.

♦ Kroger carries frozen Cajun mirepoix.

♦ To make your own Cajun mirapoix, dice equal amounts of celery, onion, and green pepper.

DIRECTIONS

1. Sauté frozen mirepoix in small frying pan.
2. Add sautéed egg whites to omelet pan sprayed with Pam® and cook over medium-high heat.
3. Add diced chicken, 1 Tbsp Verde sauce, and ¼ cup Cajun mirepoix.
4. When eggs become white, fold over into an omelet.
5. Immediately top with remaining mirepoix, 1 Tbsp Verde sauce, and mozzarella.

Nutrition Facts
Verde Omelet

Amount Per Serving

Calories 200   Calories from Fat 50

	% Daily Value*
Total Fat 6g	9%
Saturated Fat 3g	15%
Trans Fat 0g	
Cholesterol 50mg	17%
Sodium 700mg	29%
Total Carbohydrate 4g	1%
Dietary Fiber 0g	0%
Sugars 1g	
Protein 33g	

Vitamin A 10% • Vitamin C 0%
Calcium 20% • Iron 6%

* Percent Daily Values are based on a 2,000 calorie diet. Your daily values may be higher or lower depending on your calorie needs:

		Calories:	2,000	2,500
Total Fat	Less than		65g	80g
Sat Fat	Less than		20g	25g
Cholesterol	Less than		300mg	300mg
Sodium	Less than		2,400mg	2,400mg
Total Carbohydrate			300g	375g
Dietary Fiber			25g	30g

INGREDIENTS: EGG WHITES, CHICKEN BREAST, VERDE SAUCE, MOZZARELLA, ONIONS, CELERY, GREEN PEPPERS

ONION FACTORY: ANDERSON, IN

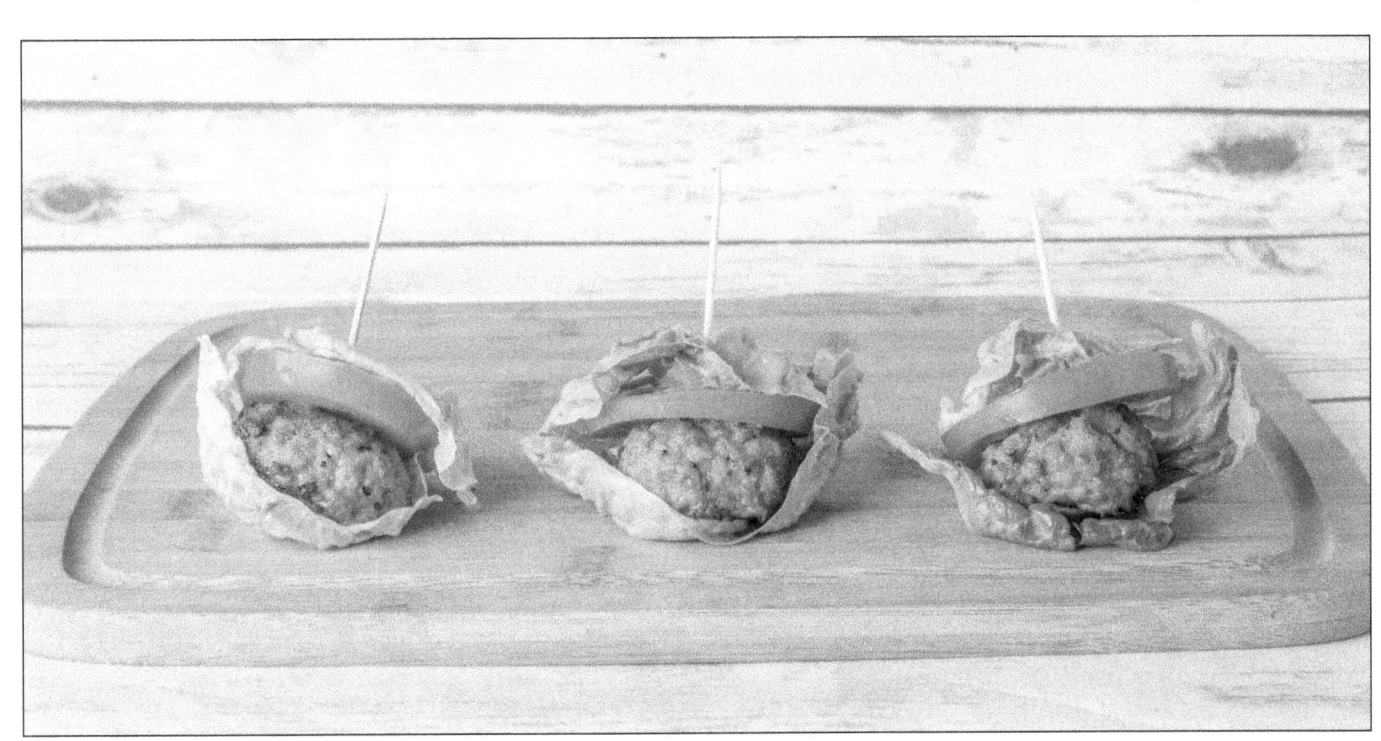

burgers

DON'T LET A BUN HIDE THE FLAVOR OF THESE DELICIOUS ENTRÉES

BACON AND CHEDDAR BURGER

YIELDS: 8 servings

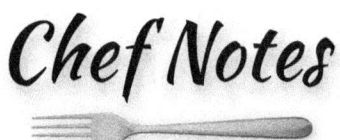

INGREDIENTS

- ❏ 2 lbs lean ground turkey 90/10
- ❏ 12 oz frozen mirepoix
- ❏ 1 pkg French onion soup mix
- ❏ 8 Tbsp shredded Cheddar cheese
- ❏ 8 tsp bacon bits

- ♦ May substitute lean ground beef 90/10 for turkey.
- ♦ Kroger carries frozen mirepoix.
- ♦ Mirepoix is equal parts of diced onion, celery, and carrots.

DIRECTIONS

1. Preheat oven to 350 degrees.
2. In large bowl, mix together the ground turkey, mirepoix, and French onion soup mix.
3. Form 8 burgers on 2 large rimmed cookie sheets (These will be large. They are quarter-pounders!)
4. Press your thumb into center of each burger to keep it from curling while it cooks.
5. Bake for 45 minutes until internal temperature reaches 165 degrees.
6. Top each burger with 1 Tbsp shredded Cheddar and 1 tsp bacon bits.

Nutrition Facts
Bacon and Cheddar Burger

Amount Per Serving

Calories 280 — Calories from Fat 130

	% Daily Value*
Total Fat 14g	22%
Saturated Fat 4.5g	23%
Trans Fat 0g	
Cholesterol 90mg	30%
Sodium 470mg	20%
Total Carbohydrate 5g	2%
Dietary Fiber 0g	0%
Sugars 2g	
Protein 25g	

Vitamin A 10% • Vitamin C 0%
Calcium 6% • Iron 45%

* Percent Daily Values are based on a 2,000 calorie diet. Your daily values may be higher or lower depending on your calorie needs:

	Calories:	2,000	2,500
Total Fat	Less than	65g	80g
Sat Fat	Less than	20g	25g
Cholesterol	Less than	300mg	300mg
Sodium	Less than	2,400mg	2,400mg
Total Carbohydrate		300g	375g
Dietary Fiber		25g	30g

INGREDIENTS: GROUND TURKEY, ONIONS, CELERY, GREEN PEPPERS, SHARP CHEDDAR CHEESE, ONION SOUP MIX, CRUMBLED BACON

ONION FACTORY: ANDERSON, IN

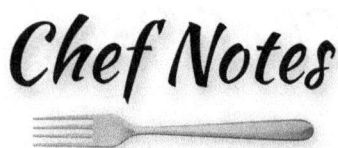

Chef Notes

- May substitute lean ground beef 90/10 for ground turkey.
- Kroger carries frozen three-pepper blend.

CHILI CHEESEBURGER

YIELDS: 8 servings

INGREDIENTS

- ☐ 2 lbs lean ground turkey 90/10
- ☐ 12 oz frozen three-pepper blend
- ☐ 15½ oz can Brooks® hot chili beans
- ☐ 1 pkg chili seasoning
- ☐ 4 slices Velveeta® cheese or 8 slices 2% Velveeta® cheese

DIRECTIONS

1. Preheat oven to 350 degrees.
2. In large bowl, mix the ground turkey, three-pepper blend, beans, and chili seasoning.
3. Form 8 burgers on 2 large rimmed cookie sheets (These will be large. They are quarter-pounders!)
4. Press your thumb into the center of each burger to keep it from curling while it cooks.
5. Bake for 45 minutes until internal temperature reaches 165 degrees.
6. Immediately top each burger with ½ slice Velveeta® cheese or 1 slice of Velveeta® 2% cheese.

Nutrition Facts

Chili Cheeseburger

Amount Per Serving

Calories 370	Calories from Fat 140

	% Daily Value*
Total Fat 15g	23%
Saturated Fat 5g	25%
Trans Fat 0g	
Cholesterol 100mg	33%
Sodium 980mg	41%
Total Carbohydrate 20g	7%
Dietary Fiber 5g	20%
Sugars 6g	
Protein 30g	

Vitamin A 6%	•	Vitamin C 15%
Calcium 20%	•	Iron 50%

* Percent Daily Values are based on a 2,000 calorie diet. Your daily values may be higher or lower depending on your calorie needs:

	Calories:	2,000	2,500
Total Fat	Less than	65g	80g
Sat Fat	Less than	20g	25g
Cholesterol	Less than	300mg	300mg
Sodium	Less than	2,400mg	2,400mg
Total Carbohydrate		300g	375g
Dietary Fiber		25g	30g

INGREDIENTS: GROUND TURKEY, BEANS, PEPPERS, ONION, VELVEETA, CHILI SEASONING

ONION FACTORY: ANDERSON, IN

FRENCH ONION BURGER

YIELDS: 8 servings

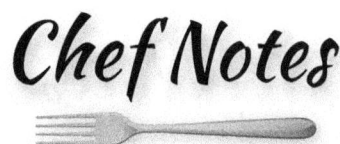

INGREDIENTS

- ❑ 2 lb lean ground turkey 90/10
- ❑ 12 oz frozen mirepoix
- ❑ 1 pkg French onion soup mix
- ❑ 8 slices mozzarella cheese
- ❑ 8 tsp crushed French's® Crispy Fried Onions

♦ May substitute lean ground beef 90/10 for turkey.

♦ Kroger® carries frozen mirepoix.

♦ Mirepoix is equal amounts of diced onion, celery, and carrots.

DIRECTIONS

1. Preheat oven to 350 degrees.
2. In large bowl, mix together the ground turkey, mirepoix, and French onion soup mix.
3. Form 8 equal-sized burgers. The burgers will be large. (They are quarter pounders!)
4. Make a thumbprint in the center of each burger to keep it from curling as it cooks.
5. Bake for 45 minutes until the internal temperature reaches 165 degrees.
6. Immediately place on each burger 1 slice mozzarella cheese and 1 tsp crushed crispy fried onions.

Nutrition Facts
French Onion Burger

Amount Per Serving

Calories 270 — Calories from Fat 120

	% Daily Value*
Total Fat 13g	20%
Saturated Fat 4g	20%
Trans Fat 0g	
Cholesterol 85mg	28%
Sodium 420mg	18%
Total Carbohydrate 6g	2%
Dietary Fiber 0g	0%
Sugars 2g	
Protein 24g	

Vitamin A 10% • Vitamin C 0%
Calcium 6% • Iron 45%

* Percent Daily Values are based on a 2,000 calorie diet. Your daily values may be higher or lower depending on your calorie needs:

	Calories:	2,000	2,500
Total Fat	Less than	65g	80g
Sat Fat	Less than	20g	25g
Cholesterol	Less than	300mg	300mg
Sodium	Less than	2,400mg	2,400mg
Total Carbohydrate		300g	375g
Dietary Fiber		25g	30g

INGREDIENTS: GROUND TURKEY, ONIONS, CELERY, GREEN PEPPERS, MOZZARELLA, ONION SOUP MIX, CRISPY FRIED ONIONS

ONION FACTORY: ANDERSON, IN

Chef Notes

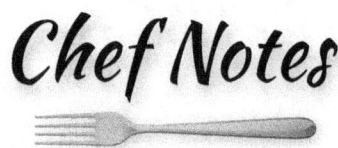

- May substitute lean ground beef 90/10 for ground turkey.
- Kroger® carries Cajun mirepoix.
- Mirepoix is equal amounts of diced onion, celery, and green peppers.

Nutrition Facts
Philly Cheesesteak Burger

Amount Per Serving	
Calories 330	Calories from Fat 140
	% Daily Value*
Total Fat 16g	25%
Saturated Fat 5g	25%
Trans Fat 0g	
Cholesterol 105mg	35%
Sodium 670mg	28%
Total Carbohydrate 8g	3%
Dietary Fiber 1g	4%
Sugars 4g	
Protein 31g	
Vitamin A 10% • Vitamin C 4%	
Calcium 8% • Iron 50%	

* Percent Daily Values are based on a 2,000 calorie diet. Your daily values may be higher or lower depending on your calorie needs:

	Calories:	2,000	2,500
Total Fat	Less than	65g	80g
Sat Fat	Less than	20g	25g
Cholesterol	Less than	300mg	300mg
Sodium	Less than	2,400mg	2,400mg
Total Carbohydrate		300g	375g
Dietary Fiber		25g	30g

INGREDIENTS: GROUND TURKEY, ONIONS, CELERY, GREEN PEPPERS, MUSHROOMS, DELI ROAST BEEF, ONION, PROVOLONE, ONION SOUP MIX, GARLIC SALT, SPRAY MARGARINE

ONION FACTORY: ANDERSON, IN

PHILLY CHEESESTEAK BURGER

YIELDS: 8 servings

INGREDIENTS

- ☐ 2 lbs lean ground turkey 90/10
- ☐ 12 oz frozen Cajun mirepoix
- ☐ 1 pkg French onion soup mix
- ☐ 1 lb deli roast beef, roughly chopped
- ☐ 12 oz fresh mushrooms, sliced
- ☐ 1 medium onion, chopped
- ☐ Garlic salt
- ☐ Spray butter
- ☐ 8 thin slices Provolone cheese

DIRECTIONS

1. Preheat oven to 350 degrees.
2. In large bowl, mix the ground turkey, Cajun mirepoix, and French onion soup mix.
3. Form 8 burgers on 2 large rimmed cookie sheets (These will be large. They are quarter-pounders!)
4. Press your thumb into the center of each burger to keep it from curling while it cooks.
5. Bake for 45 minutes until internal temperature reaches 165 degrees.
6. While burgers are baking, make topping: In medium non-stick frying pan sprayed with butter, sauté onion and mushrooms. Add chopped deli roast beef. Continue to sauté until mixture is hot. Add garlic salt to taste.
7. Top burgers with topping and Provolone cheese.

TERIYAKI BURGER

YIELDS: 8 servings

INGREDIENTS

- ☐ 2 lbs lean ground turkey 90/10
- ☐ 12 oz frozen mirepoix
- ☐ ⅓ cup Soy Vay® Very Very Teriyaki Sauce
- ☐ 8 Tbsp shredded mozzarella cheese

DIRECTIONS

1. In a large bowl, mix the ground turkey, mirepoix, and teriyaki sauce.
2. Form 8 burgers on 2 large rimmed cookie sheets (These will be large. They are quarter-pounders!)
3. Press your thumb into the center of each burger to keep it from curling while it cooks.
4. Bake for 45 minutes until internal temperature reaches 165 degrees.
5. Top hot burger with 1 Tbsp mozzarella.

Chef Notes

- ♦ May substitute lean ground beef 90/10 for ground turkey.
- ♦ Kroger® carries frozen mirepoix.
- ♦ Regular mirepoix is equal amounts of diced onion, celery, and carrots.

Nutrition Facts
Teriyaki Burger

Amount Per Serving	
Calories 260	Calories from Fat 110

	% Daily Value*
Total Fat 12g	18%
Saturated Fat 3.5g	18%
Trans Fat 0g	
Cholesterol 85mg	28%
Sodium 310mg	13%
Total Carbohydrate 6g	2%
Dietary Fiber 0g	0%
Sugars 5g	
Protein 22g	

Vitamin A 10%	•	Vitamin C 0%
Calcium 2%	•	Iron 45%

* Percent Daily Values are based on a 2,000 calorie diet. Your daily values may be higher or lower depending on your calorie needs:

	Calories:	2,000	2,500
Total Fat	Less than	65g	80g
Sat Fat	Less than	20g	25g
Cholesterol	Less than	300mg	300mg
Sodium	Less than	2,400mg	2,400mg
Total Carbohydrate		300g	375g
Dietary Fiber		25g	30g

INGREDIENTS: GROUND TURKEY, ONIONS, CELERY, GREEN PEPPERS, CARROTS, TERIYAKI ASIAN SAUCE, MOZZARELLA

ONION FACTORY: ANDERSON, IN

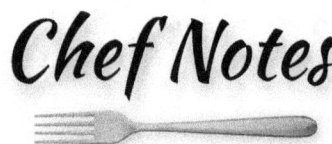
Chef Notes

MUSHROOM SWISS BURGER

YIELDS: 8 servings

INGREDIENTS

- ☐ 2 lbs lean ground turkey 90/10
- ☐ 1 small can sliced mushrooms or 1 cup fresh sliced mushrooms
- ☐ 1 pkg frozen 3-pepper-and-onion blend
- ☐ ¼ tsp onion powder
- ☐ ¼ tsp garlic powder
- ☐ ¼ tsp salt
- ☐ ¼ tsp pepper
- ☐ ¼ tsp Lawry's® seasoned salt
- ☐ 8 thin slices Swiss cheese

DIRECTIONS

1. Preheat oven to 350 degrees.
2. In large bowl, mix all ingredients together.
3. Form 8 burgers on 2 large rimmed cookie sheets (These will be large. They are quarter-pounders!)
4. Press your thumb into each burger to keep it from curling while it cooks.
5. Bake for 45 minutes until internal temperature reaches 165 degrees.
6. While burgers are baking, make topping: In medium non-stick frying pan sprayed with butter, sauté 3-pepper-and-onion. Season to taste.
7. Top burgers with topping and Swiss cheese.

Nutrition Facts
Mushroom Swiss Burger

Amount Per Serving

Calories 250	Calories from Fat 100

	% Daily Value*
Total Fat 11g	17%
Saturated Fat 3g	15%
Trans Fat 0g	
Cholesterol 80mg	27%
Sodium 400mg	17%
Total Carbohydrate 5g	2%
Dietary Fiber <1g	3%
Sugars 3g	
Protein 22g	

Vitamin A 10%	•	Vitamin C 0%
Calcium 2%	•	Iron 45%

*Percent Daily Values are based on a 2,000 calorie diet. Your daily values may be higher or lower depending on your calorie needs:

		Calories:	2,000	2,500
Total Fat	Less than		65g	80g
Sat Fat	Less than		20g	25g
Cholesterol	Less than		300mg	300mg
Sodium	Less than		2,400mg	2,400mg
Total Carbohydrate			300g	375g
Dietary Fiber			25g	30g

INGREDIENTS: GROUND TURKEY, ONIONS, CELERY, GREEN PEPPERS, MUSHROOMS, GREEN BEANS, ONION SOUP MIX, PROVOLONE

ONION FACTORY: ANDERSON, IN

TACO BURGER

YIELDS: 8 servings

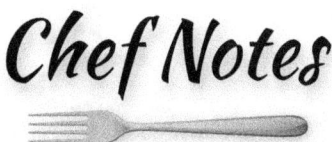

INGREDIENTS

- ❑ 2 lbs lean ground turkey 90/10
- ❑ 12 oz frozen Cajun mirepoix
- ❑ 1 pkg taco seasoning
- ❑ 4 slices pepper jack cheese

Chef Notes

- ♦ May substitute lean ground beef 90/10 for ground turkey.
- ♦ Kroger carries Cajun mirepoix.
- ♦ Cajun mirepoix is equal amounts of diced onion, celery, and green peppers.

DIRECTIONS

1. Preheat oven to 350 degrees.
2. In large bowl, mix the ground turkey, Cajun mirepoix, and taco seasoning.
3. Form 8 burgers on 2 large rimmed cookie sheets (These will be large. They are quarter-pounders!)
4. Press your thumb into the center of each burger to keep it from curling while it cooks.
5. Bake for 45 minutes until internal temperature reaches 165 degrees.
6. Immediately top each burger with ½ slice pepper jack cheese.

Nutrition Facts
Taco Burger

Amount Per Serving

Calories 280 — Calories from Fat 130

	% Daily Value*
Total Fat 14g	22%
Saturated Fat 5g	25%
Trans Fat 0g	
Cholesterol 90mg	30%
Sodium 440mg	18%
Total Carbohydrate 5g	2%
Dietary Fiber <1g	4%
Sugars 2g	
Protein 24g	

Vitamin A 15% • Vitamin C 0%
Calcium 8% • Iron 45%

* Percent Daily Values are based on a 2,000 calorie diet. Your daily values may be higher or lower depending on your calorie needs:

	Calories:	2,000	2,500
Total Fat	Less than	65g	80g
Sat Fat	Less than	20g	25g
Cholesterol	Less than	300mg	300mg
Sodium	Less than	2,400mg	2,400mg
Total Carbohydrate		300g	375g
Dietary Fiber		25g	30g

INGREDIENTS: GROUND TURKEY, ONIONS, CELERY, GREEN PEPPERS, PEPPER JACK CHEESE, TACO SEASONING

ONION FACTORY: ANDERSON, IN

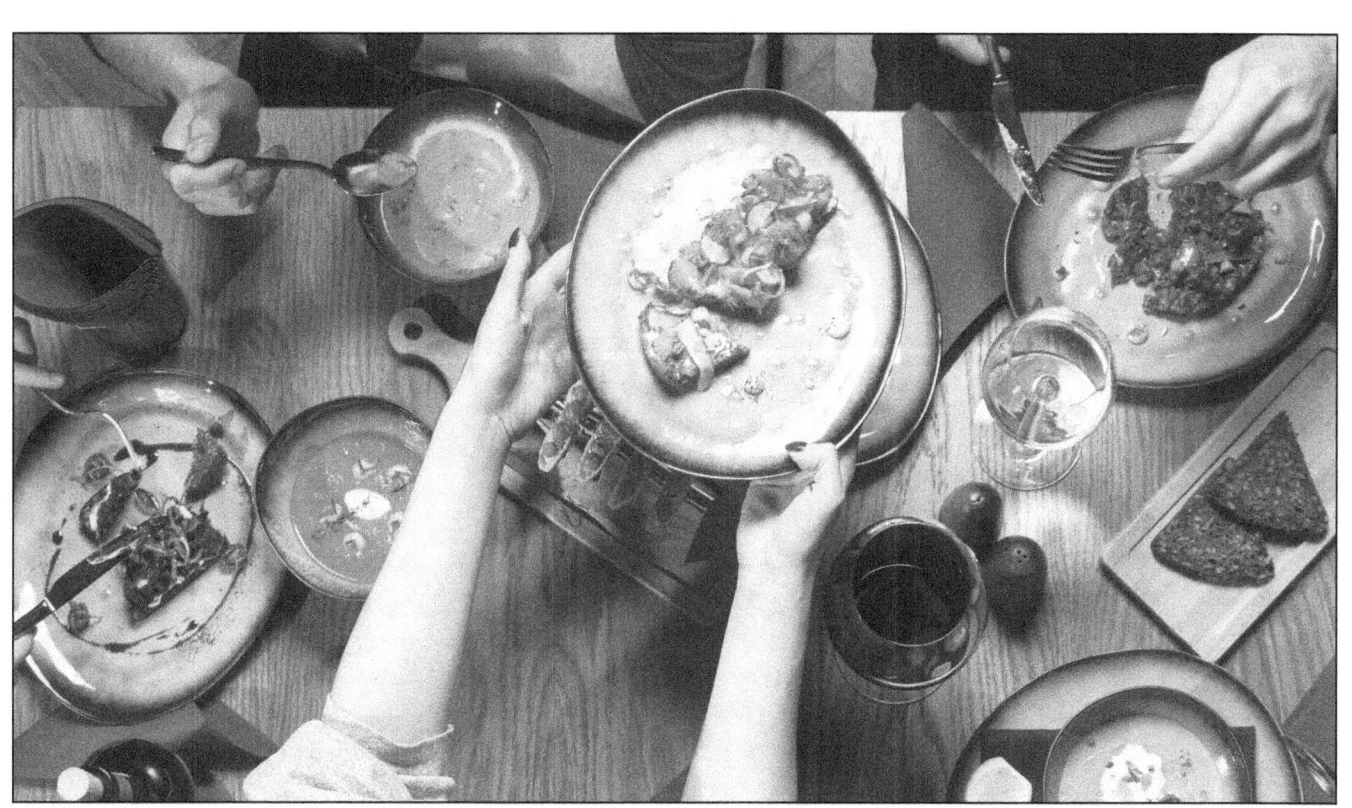

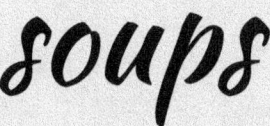

AMERICA'S FAVORITE COMFORT FOOD IS RICH WITH NUTRIENTS.

CHEESEBURGER SOUP

YIELDS: 8 servings (2 cups each)

INGREDIENTS

- ☐ 2 lbs ground turkey 90/10
- ☐ ¼ lb Bob Evans® hot ground sausage
- ☐ 4 oz 2% Velveeta® (¼ of block)
- ☐ 96 oz low-fat chicken broth
- ☐ 16 oz frozen riced cauliflower
- ☐ 12 oz frozen Cajun mirepoix
- ☐ 12 oz frozen regular mirepoix
- ☐ 1 Tbsp garlic powder
- ☐ 1 tsp garlic salt
- ☐ 1 tsp Creole seasoning

DIRECTIONS

1. Brown ground turkey and sausage.
2. Add cheese to cooked meat and stir until cheese melts.
3. Add broth, cauliflower, and mirepoix.
4. When hot, add rice and seasonings.
5. Simmer for at least 2 hours, seasoning to taste.

Chef Notes

- ♦ Kroger® carries frozen Cajun mirepoix.
- ♦ Regular mirepoix is equal amounts of diced celery, onion, and carrots.
- ♦ Cajun mirepoix is equal amounts of diced celery, onion, and green pepper.

Nutrition Facts
Cheeseburger Soup

Amount Per Serving	
Calories 380	Calories from Fat 160
	% Daily Value*
Total Fat 18g	28%
Saturated Fat 6g	30%
Trans Fat 0g	
Cholesterol 95mg	32%
Sodium 1780mg	74%
Total Carbohydrate 17g	6%
Dietary Fiber 2g	8%
Sugars 5g	
Protein 29g	
Vitamin A 25% • Vitamin C 35%	
Calcium 10% • Iron 50%	

* Percent Daily Values are based on a 2,000 calorie diet. Your daily values may be higher or lower depending on your calorie needs:

	Calories:	2,000	2,500
Total Fat	Less than	65g	80g
Sat Fat	Less than	20g	25g
Cholesterol	Less than	300mg	300mg
Sodium	Less than	2,400mg	2,400mg
Total Carbohydrate		300g	375g
Dietary Fiber		25g	30g

INGREDIENTS: CHICKEN BROTH, GROUND TURKEY, ONIONS, CELERY, GREEN PEPPERS, CARROTS, CAULIFLOWER, PORK SAUSAGE, VELVEETA 2%, ROYAL RICE BLEND, GARLIC POWDER, CREOLE SEASONING, GARLIC SALT

ONION FACTORY: ANDERSON, IN

Chef Notes

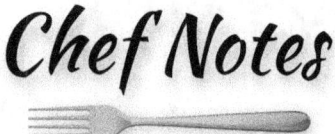

- Kroger® carries frozen Cajun mirepoix.
- Cajun mirepoix is equal amounts of diced onion, celery, and green peppers.
- Royal rice is equal amounts of white rice, brown rice, and wild rice.

BUFFALO CHICKEN CHOWDER

YIELDS: 8 servings (2 cups ea.)

INGREDIENTS

- ☐ 64 oz low-fat chicken broth
- ☐ 12 oz frozen Cajun mirepoix
- ☐ 24 oz riced cauliflower
- ☐ 16oz Chi Chi's® salsa
- ☐ 2 lbs shredded chicken breast or three 13-oz cans of canned chicken
- ☐ 16 oz fat-free cream
- ☐ 3 cups rough chopped celery
- ☐ ¼ cup Frank's® hot sauce
- ☐ ½ cup royal rice blend

DIRECTIONS

Combine all ingredients in a large pot and simmer for at least 1½ hours.

Nutrition Facts
Buffalo Chicken Chowder

Amount Per Serving	
Calories 270	Calories from Fat 30
	% Daily Value*
Total Fat 3.5g	5%
Saturated Fat 0g	0%
Trans Fat 0g	
Cholesterol 80mg	27%
Sodium 1980mg	83%
Total Carbohydrate 26g	9%
Dietary Fiber 4g	16%
Sugars 12g	
Protein 30g	
Vitamin A 20%	Vitamin C 80%
Calcium 10%	Iron 8%

* Percent Daily Values are based on a 2,000 calorie diet. Your daily values may be higher or lower depending on your calorie needs:

		Calories:	2,000	2,500
Total Fat	Less than		65g	80g
Sat Fat	Less than		20g	25g
Cholesterol	Less than		300mg	300mg
Sodium	Less than		2,400mg	2,400mg
Total Carbohydrate			300g	375g
Dietary Fiber			25g	30g

INGREDIENTS: CHICKEN BROTH, CHICKEN BREAST, CAULIFLOWER, SALSA, FAT FREE HALF AND HALF, ONIONS, CELERY, GREEN PEPPERS, CELERY, RICE, FRANK'S RED HOT SAUCE

ONION FACTORY: ANDERSON, IN

SWEET CHILI

YIELDS: 8 servings (2 cups ea.)

INGREDIENTS

- ❏ 2 lbs lean ground turkey 90/10
- ❏ 12 oz frozen Cajun mirepoix
- ❏ 28 oz diced tomatoes
- ❏ 28 oz crushed tomatoes
- ❏ 15½ oz Brooks® Hot Chili Beans
- ❏ 24 oz chili sauce

DIRECTIONS

1. Brown the ground turkey in a large pan.
2. Add remaining ingredients and simmer for 1 hour.

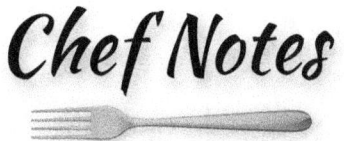

Chef Notes

- ♦ May substitute lean ground beef 90/10 for ground turkey.
- ♦ Kroger® carries Cajun mirepoix.
- ♦ Mirepoix is equal amounts of onion, celery, and green peppers.

Nutrition Facts
Sweet Chili

Amount Per Serving	
Calories 460	Calories from Fat 100
	% Daily Value*
Total Fat 11g	17%
Saturated Fat 3g	15%
Trans Fat 0g	
Cholesterol 80mg	27%
Sodium 1640mg	68%
Total Carbohydrate 52g	17%
Dietary Fiber 7g	28%
Sugars 30g	
Protein 26g	
Vitamin A 70% • Vitamin C 45%	
Calcium 4% • Iron 60%	

* Percent Daily Values are based on a 2,000 calorie diet. Your daily values may be higher or lower depending on your calorie needs:

	Calories:	2,000	2,500
Total Fat	Less than	65g	80g
Sat Fat	Less than	20g	25g
Cholesterol	Less than	300mg	300mg
Sodium	Less than	2,400mg	2,400mg
Total Carbohydrate		300g	375g
Dietary Fiber		25g	30g

INGREDIENTS: GROUND TURKEY, TOMATOES, TOMATOES, CHILI SAUCE, BEANS, ONIONS, CELERY, GREEN PEPPERS

ONION FACTORY: ANDERSON, IN

Chef Notes

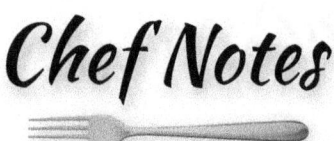

- May substitute lean ground beef 90/10 for lean ground turkey.
- Kroger® carries frozen mirepoix.
- Mirepoix is equal amounts of diced onion, celery and carrots.

ZESTY CHILI

YIELDS: 8 servings (2 cups ea.)

INGREDIENTS

- ☐ 2 lbs lean ground turkey 90/10
- ☐ 12 oz bag of frozen mirepoix
- ☐ 28 oz crushed tomatoes
- ☐ 28 oz diced tomatoes
- ☐ 28 oz tomato sauce
- ☐ 15½ oz Brooks® chili hot beans
- ☐ 4 oz Carroll Shelby's® chili mix

DIRECTIONS

1. Brown the ground turkey in a large pan.
2. Add the remaining ingredients.
3. Simmer for at least 1 hr.

Nutrition Facts
Zesty Chili

Amount Per Serving

Calories 450	Calories from Fat 110

	% Daily Value*
Total Fat 12g	18%
Saturated Fat 3g	15%
Trans Fat 0g	
Cholesterol 80mg	27%
Sodium 1690mg	70%
Total Carbohydrate 44g	15%
Dietary Fiber 10g	40%
Sugars 16g	
Protein 29g	

Vitamin A 80%	•	Vitamin C 40%
Calcium 4%	•	Iron 80%

* Percent Daily Values are based on a 2,000 calorie diet. Your daily values may be higher or lower depending on your calorie needs:

	Calories:	2,000	2,500
Total Fat	Less than	65g	80g
Sat Fat	Less than	20g	25g
Cholesterol	Less than	300mg	300mg
Sodium	Less than	2,400mg	2,400mg
Total Carbohydrate		300g	375g
Dietary Fiber		25g	30g

INGREDIENTS: TOMATOES, GROUND TURKEY, TOMATOES, BEANS, ONIONS, CELERY, GREEN PEPPERS, CHILI SEASONING

ONION FACTORY: ANDERSON, IN

ITALIAN SPINACH SAUSAGE SOUP

YIELDS: 12 servings (2 cups ea.)

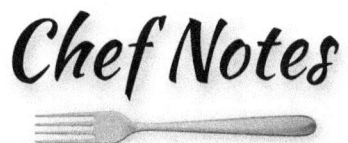

INGREDIENTS

- [ ] 1 lb. lean ground turkey 90/10
- [ ] 1.22 lb Jennie O® Sweet Italian Turkey Sausage
- [ ] 4 oz Bob Evans® hot sausage
- [ ] 96 oz fat-free chicken broth
- [ ] 24 oz frozen chopped spinach
- [ ] 32 oz fat-free cream
- [ ] 12 oz frozen riced cauliflower
- [ ] ½ cup Royal rice
- [ ] 1½ tsp garlic powder
- [ ] 1 tsp garlic salt
- [ ] 1 tsp salt
- [ ] ½ tsp pepper

DIRECTIONS

1. Brown the meats in a large pot.
2. Add chicken broth, spinach, cream, and riced cauliflower.
3. Simmer for 1 hour.
4. Add rice and seasonings.
5. Simmer an additional 45 minutes.
6. Add more garlic salt, salt, and pepper to taste.

Nutrition Facts
Italian Spinach Sausage Soup

Amount Per Serving	
Calories 290	Calories from Fat 110
	% Daily Value*
Total Fat 13g	20%
Saturated Fat 4g	20%
Trans Fat 0g	
Cholesterol 65mg	22%
Sodium 1650mg	69%
Total Carbohydrate 19g	6%
Dietary Fiber 2g	8%
Sugars 4g	
Protein 22g	
Vitamin A 35% • Vitamin C 25%	
Calcium 15% • Iron 20%	

* Percent Daily Values are based on a 2,000 calorie diet. Your daily values may be higher or lower depending on your calorie needs:

	Calories:	2,000	2,500
Total Fat	Less than	65g	80g
Sat Fat	Less than	20g	25g
Cholesterol	Less than	300mg	300mg
Sodium	Less than	2,400mg	2,400mg
Total Carbohydrate		300g	375g
Dietary Fiber		25g	30g

INGREDIENTS: CHICKEN BROTH, FAT FREE CREAM, SPINACH, TURKEY SAUSAGE, GROUND TURKEY, CAULIFLOWER, WILD RICE BLEND, PORK SAUSAGE, SALT, GARLIC, PEPPER

ONION FACTORY: ANDERSON,IN

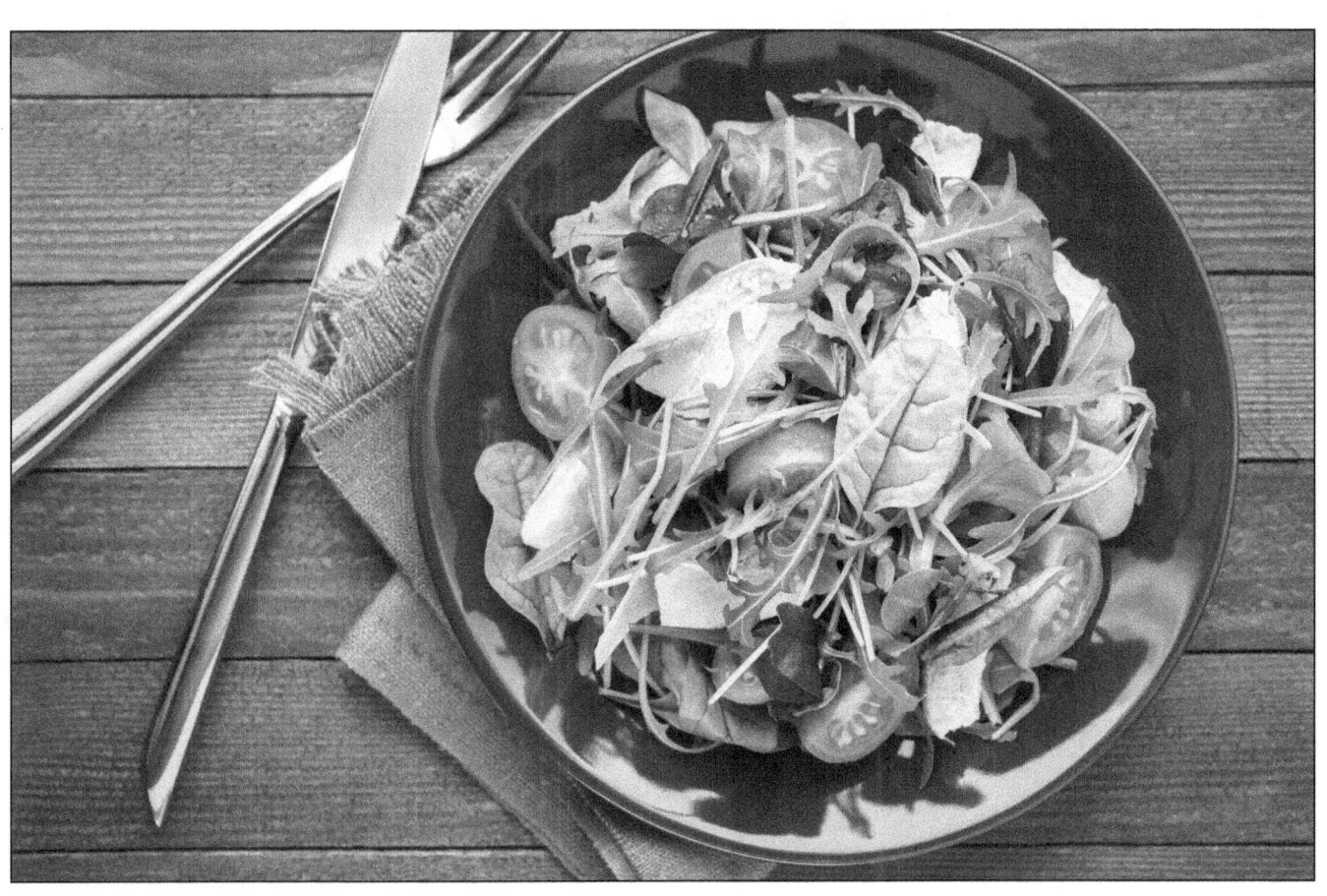

salads

THESE CRISP DISHES ARE ALWAYS IN SEASON

BUFFALO CHICKEN SALAD

YIELDS: 4 servings

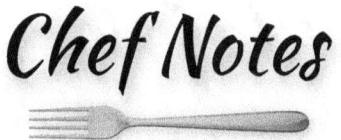

INGREDIENTS

- 1 lb chicken breast, cut into bite-size pieces
- 2 Tbsp Frank's® buffalo hot sauce
- 2 squirts spray margarine
- 12 cups shredded lettuce
- 1 cup diced celery
- ¼ cup shredded carrots
- 2 oz reduced fat blue cheese
- 4 Tbsp light Ranch dressing
- Pam®

DIRECTIONS

1. Sauté chicken breast in frying pan sprayed with Pam®.
2. When cooled, add 2 Tbsp Frank's® hot sauce and stir until coated.
3. Spray chicken evenly with 2 squirts of spray margarine.
4. Divide lettuce on four plates.
5. Top lettuce with prepared chicken.
6. Sprinkle each salad with ¼ cup celery and 2 Tbsp shredded carrots.
7. Sprinkle each salad with ½ oz blue cheese and 1 Tbsp light French dressing.

Nutrition Facts
Buffalo Chicken Salad

Amount Per Serving

Calories 230		Calories from Fat 70
		% Daily Value*
Total Fat 7g		11%
Saturated Fat 3g		15%
Trans Fat 0g		
Cholesterol 85mg		28%
Sodium 640mg		27%
Total Carbohydrate 11g		4%
Dietary Fiber 3g		12%
Sugars 5g		
Protein 33g		
Vitamin A 30%	•	Vitamin C 10%
Calcium 15%	•	Iron 10%

* Percent Daily Values are based on a 2,000 calorie diet. Your daily values may be higher or lower depending on your calorie needs:

	Calories:	2,000	2,500
Total Fat	Less than	65g	80g
Sat Fat	Less than	20g	25g
Cholesterol	Less than	300mg	300mg
Sodium	Less than	2,400mg	2,400mg
Total Carbohydrate		300g	375g
Dietary Fiber		25g	30g

INGREDIENTS: LETTUCE, CHICKEN BREAST, CELERY, REDUCED FAT RANCH DRESSING, BLUE CHEESE, SPICE, CARROTS, SPRAY MARGARINE

ONION FACTORY: ANDERSON, IN

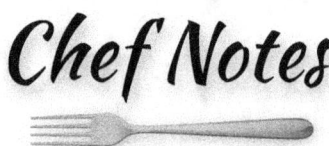

Chef Notes

VARIATION

- May substitute 4 oz grilled shrimp for chicken breast.
- This is company worthy—delicious and a beautiful presentation.

CHAMPAGNE PEAR SALAD

YIELDS: 1 serving

INGREDIENTS

- ❑ 3–4 cups spring lettuce mix
- ❑ 1 Tbsp Trader Joe's® Champagne Pear Vinaigrette with Gorgonzola
- ❑ 1 Tbsp fat-free feta cheese
- ❑ 4 oz grilled chicken breast, sliced
- ❑ 2 thin pear slices

DIRECTIONS

1. Toss lettuce with dressing.
2. Top with feta cheese and grilled chicken breast.
3. Garnish with thin pear slices.

Nutrition Facts
Champagne Pear Chicken Salad

Amount Per Serving

Calories 270 — Calories from Fat 20

	% Daily Value*
Total Fat 2.5g	4%
Saturated Fat 0g	0%
Trans Fat 0g	
Cholesterol 70mg	23%
Sodium 770mg	32%
Total Carbohydrate 26g	9%
Dietary Fiber 6g	24%
Sugars 9g	
Protein 36g	

Vitamin A 480% • Vitamin C 270%

Calcium 50% • Iron 110%

* Percent Daily Values are based on a 2,000 calorie diet. Your daily values may be higher or lower depending on your calorie needs:

	Calories:	2,000	2,500
Total Fat	Less than	65g	80g
Sat Fat	Less than	20g	25g
Cholesterol	Less than	300mg	300mg
Sodium	Less than	2,400mg	2,400mg
Total Carbohydrate		300g	375g
Dietary Fiber		25g	30g

INGREDIENTS: SPRING MIX, CHICKEN BREAST, PEAR, TRADER JOE'S CHAMPAGNE PEAR VINAIGRETTE, FAT FREE FETA CHEESE

ONION FACTORY: ANDERSON, IN

CHICKEN CAESAR SALAD

YIELDS: 1 serving

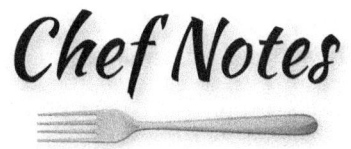

INGREDIENTS

- ❏ 3–4 cups Romaine lettuce, torn into bite-size pieces
- ❏ 4 oz grilled chicken breast, sliced
- ❏ 1 Tbsp Kens® Light Caesar dressing
- ❏ 1 Tbsp shaved Parmesan cheese

DIRECTIONS

1. Plate lettuce with chicken breast on top.
2. Pour 1 Tbsp dressing over all.
3. Garnish with 1 Tbsp shaved Parmesean cheese.

Nutrition Facts

Chicken Caesar Salad

Amount Per Serving

Calories 200	Calories from Fat 50

	% Daily Value*
Total Fat 5g	8%
Saturated Fat 1g	5%
Trans Fat 0g	
Cholesterol 75mg	25%
Sodium 210mg	9%
Total Carbohydrate 10g	3%
Dietary Fiber <1g	2%
Sugars 4g	
Protein 32g	

Vitamin A 0%	•		Vitamin C 2%
Calcium 2%	•		Iron 4%

* Percent Daily Values are based on a 2,000 calorie diet. Your daily values may be higher or lower depending on your calorie needs:

	Calories:	2,000	2,500
Total Fat	Less than	65g	80g
Sat Fat	Less than	20g	25g
Cholesterol	Less than	300mg	300mg
Sodium	Less than	2,400mg	2,400mg
Total Carbohydrate		300g	375g
Dietary Fiber		25g	30g

INGREDIENTS: ROMAINE, CHICKEN BREAST, LITE CAESAR DRESSING, PARMESAN

ONION FACTORY: ANDERSON, IN

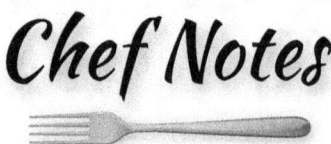

Chef Notes

You can divide the seasoned turkey into four packages. Use one now and freeze the rest for later. Great to have in the freezer for a quick lunch.

TACO SALAD

YIELDS: 4 servings

INGREDIENTS

- 1 lb lean ground turkey 90/10
- 1 pkg ChiChi's® or Taco Bell® taco seasoning
- 12–16 cups shredded lettuce
- 4 Tbsp shredded 2% sharp Cheddar cheese
- 8 oz medium salsa
- 4 Tbsp fat-free sour cream
- 1 green onion, sliced

DIRECTIONS

1. Sauté ground turkey. Add taco seasoning and follow directions on packet.
2. For each salad, plate:

- 3–4 cups shredded lettuce
- 4 oz seasoned ground turkey
- 1 Tbsp shredded cheese
- 2 oz salsa
- 1 Tbsp fat-free sour cream
- Sprinkle with sliced green onion

Nutrition Facts
Taco Salad

Amount Per Serving

Calories 350	Calories from Fat 120

	% Daily Value*
Total Fat 13g	20%
Saturated Fat 4g	20%
Trans Fat 0g	
Cholesterol 85mg	28%
Sodium 1160mg	48%
Total Carbohydrate 20g	7%
Dietary Fiber 5g	20%
Sugars 12g	
Protein 26g	

Vitamin A 40%	•	Vitamin C 15%
Calcium 15%	•	Iron 60%

* Percent Daily Values are based on a 2,000 calorie diet. Your daily values may be higher or lower depending on your calorie needs:

	Calories:	2,000	2,500
Total Fat	Less than	65g	80g
Sat Fat	Less than	20g	25g
Cholesterol	Less than	300mg	300mg
Sodium	Less than	2,400mg	2,400mg
Total Carbohydrate		300g	375g
Dietary Fiber		25g	30g

INGREDIENTS: LETTUCE, GROUND TURKEY, SALSA, FAT FREE SOUR CREAM, TACO SEASONING, LOW FAT SHARP CHEDDAR CHEESE, GREEN ONION

ONION FACTORY: ANDERSON, IN

DUMP SALAD

YIELDS: Vary

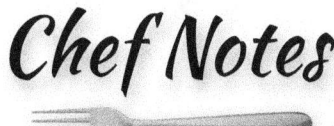

POSSIBLE INGREDIENTS

- ♦ Broccoli
- ♦ Cauliflower
- ♦ Cabbage
- ♦ Celery
- ♦ Cucumber
- ♦ Green pepper
- ♦ Green onion
- ♦ Tomatoes

☐ Trader Joe's® Cranberry Walnut Gorgonzola Salad Dressing

☐ Bacon bits

☐ Fat-free Feta cheese

☐ Lean protein

DIRECTIONS

1. In large bowl, cut vegetables into bite-size pieces.
2. Toss with Trader Joe's Cranberry Walnut Gorgonzola Salad Dressing (about 1 Tbsp per 2 cups of chopped vegetables in bowl).
3. To make a meal, add 4 oz grilled chicken or grilled shrimp.

Chef Notes

- ♦ Origin of this salad was on Sundays when I would clean out the unused vegetables in my refrigerator, chop them into bite-size pieces, add my favorite dressing, then put everything in a large bowl and eat from it throughout the next week.
- ♦ We have not provided Nutrition Facts for this recipe because the nutrients will vary, depend on the ingredients you use.

VARIATIONS

- ♦ Bacon bits: Add 1 tsp per 2 cups chopped vegetables.
- ♦ Fat-free feta cheese: Add 1 Tbsp per 2 cups chopped vegetables.

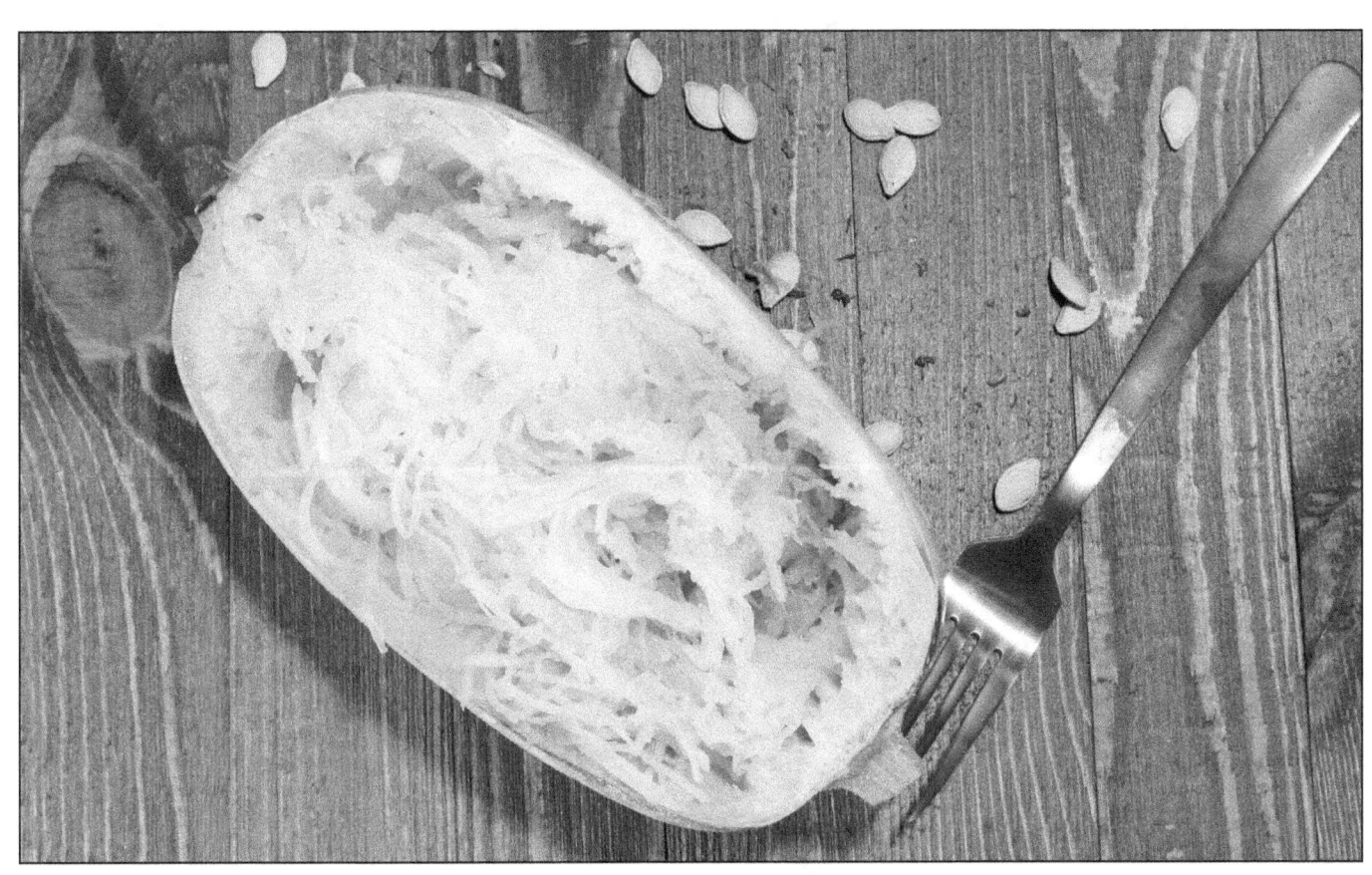

dinners

THESE MEALS BRING FAMILY AND FRIENDS TOGETHER

BEEF TIPS

YIELDS: 8 servings

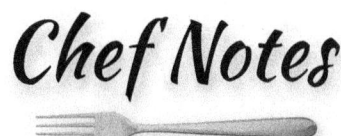

INGREDIENTS

- ❏ 2 lbs lean beef round, cut into chunks
- ❏ 1 pkg French onion soup mix
- ❏ 8 oz mushroom stems and pieces, not drained
- ❏ 1 Tbsp arrowroot
- ❏ ¼ cup water

DIRECTIONS

1. In crockpot, combine lean beef chunks, soup mix, and mushrooms.
2. Simmer on high for 4 hours.
3. Stir together arrowroot and water to make a rue.
4. Add arrowroot rue to crockpot. This will thicken the liquid.
5. Continue on low heat for 30 minutes.

- ♦ This is an expensive recipe, but good for a change of pace.
- ♦ Be careful to choose lean meat, 90/10 or better.
- ♦ Serve with smashed cauliflower and green beans.

Nutrition Facts
Beef Tips

Amount Per Serving	
Calories 160	Calories from Fat 30
	% Daily Value*
Total Fat 3.5g	5%
Saturated Fat 1.5g	8%
Trans Fat 0g	
Cholesterol 70mg	23%
Sodium 340mg	14%
Total Carbohydrate 4g	1%
Dietary Fiber 0g	0%
Sugars 1g	
Protein 27g	
Vitamin A 0% • Vitamin C 0%	
Calcium 2% • Iron 15%	

* Percent Daily Values are based on a 2,000 calorie diet. Your daily values may be higher or lower depending on your calorie needs:

	Calories:	2,000	2,500
Total Fat	Less than	65g	80g
Sat Fat	Less than	20g	25g
Cholesterol	Less than	300mg	300mg
Sodium	Less than	2,400mg	2,400mg
Total Carbohydrate		300g	375g
Dietary Fiber		25g	30g

INGREDIENTS: LEAN BEEF ROUND, MUSHROOMS, ONION SOUP MIX, ARROWROOT

ONION FACTORY: ANDERSON, IN

Chef Notes

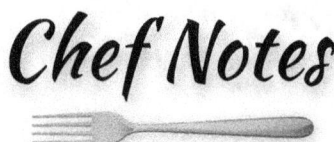

- May substitute lean ground beef 90/10 for ground turkey.
- Kroger has frozen three-pepper blend.

SPAGHETTI

YIELDS: 8 servings

INGREDIENTS

- ☐ 2 lbs lean ground turkey 90/10
- ☐ 1 Tbsp Mrs. Dash® seasoning
- ☐ 12 oz frozen three-pepper blend
- ☐ 64 oz Ragú® Traditional pasta sauce
- ☐ 24 oz Classico® Spicy Tomato and Basil pasta sauce
- ☐ 2 Nerf-football-size spaghetti squash
- ☐ ½ cup shredded mozzarella cheese

DIRECTIONS

1. In large pan, brown ground turkey and season with Mrs. Dash®.
2. Add frozen peppers and two pasta sauces. Simmer for 45 minutes.
3. Preheat oven to 350 degrees.
4. Cut spaghetti squash in half lengthwise. Scoop out seeds.
5. Place squash flat side down in large roasting pan with 2" of water. Bake in oven for 1 hour.
6. When squash are cool to touch, scrape out strands of squash.
7. To serve, top 5 oz of hot squash with 1 cup spaghetti sause and 1 Tbsp shredded mozzarella cheese.

Nutrition Facts

Spaghetti

Amount Per Serving

Calories 470 — Calories from Fat 160

	% Daily Value*
Total Fat 18g	28%
Saturated Fat 4g	20%
Trans Fat 0g	
Cholesterol 85mg	28%
Sodium 1290mg	54%
Total Carbohydrate 40g	13%
Dietary Fiber 8g	32%
Sugars 23g	
Protein 29g	

Vitamin A 40% • Vitamin C 40%
Calcium 15% • Iron 60%

* Percent Daily Values are based on a 2,000 calorie diet. Your daily values may be higher or lower depending on your calorie needs:

	Calories:	2,000	2,500
Total Fat	Less than	65g	80g
Sat Fat	Less than	20g	25g
Cholesterol	Less than	300mg	300mg
Sodium	Less than	2,400mg	2,400mg
Total Carbohydrate		300g	375g
Dietary Fiber		25g	30g

INGREDIENTS: SPAGHETTI SAUCE, GROUND TURKEY, SPAGHETTI SQUASH, PEPPERS, ONION, MOZZARELLA, MRS. DASH

ONION FACTORY: ANDERSON, IN

LASAGNA

YIELDS: 12 servings

INGREDIENTS

- ☐ 3 lbs lean ground turkey 90/10
- ☐ 1 Tbsp Mrs. Dash® seasoning
- ☐ 12 oz bag frozen three-pepper blend
- ☐ 64 oz Ragú® Traditional pasta sauce
- ☐ 24 oz Classico® Spicy Tomato and Basil pasta sauce
- ☐ 24 oz fat-free cottage cheese
- ☐ ½ cup egg whites
- ☐ 2 12-oz bags frozen chopped broccoli
- ☐ 2 cups shredded mozzarella, divided evenly

DIRECTIONS

1. In large saucepan, brown ground turkey and season with Mrs. Dash®.
2. Add frozen peppers and two pasta sauces. Simmer for 45 minutes.
3. In medium bowl, combine cottage cheese and egg whites.
4. Preheat oven to 350 degrees.
5. Spray a 9x13 pan with Pam® and assemble in layers:
   - ♦ ½ meat sauce
   - ♦ frozen chopped broccoli
   - ♦ cottage cheese and egg mixture
   - ♦ 1 cup shredded mozzarella
   - ♦ remaining meat sauce
6. Place 9x13 pan on cookie sheet to catch spills.
7. Bake for 1½ hours.
8. Sprinkle with remaining mozzarella.
9. Return to oven 5–10 minutes to melt cheese.
10. Let set 15–30 minutes before serving.

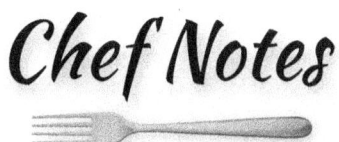

Nutrition Facts
Lasagna

Amount Per Serving

Calories 440 — Calories from Fat 140

	% Daily Value*
Total Fat 16g	25%
Saturated Fat 4g	20%
Trans Fat 0g	
Cholesterol 90mg	30%
Sodium 1140mg	48%
Total Carbohydrate 27g	9%
Dietary Fiber 6g	24%
Sugars 16g	
Protein 38g	

Vitamin A 40% • Vitamin C 80%
Calcium 15% • Iron 60%

* Percent Daily Values are based on a 2,000 calorie diet. Your daily values may be higher or lower depending on your calorie needs:

	Calories:	2,000	2,500
Total Fat	Less than	65g	80g
Sat Fat	Less than	20g	25g
Cholesterol	Less than	300mg	300mg
Sodium	Less than	2,400mg	2,400mg
Total Carbohydrate		300g	375g
Dietary Fiber		25g	30g

INGREDIENTS: SPAGHETTI SAUCE, GROUND TURKEY, FAT FREE COTTAGE CHEESE, BROCCOLI, PEPPERS, ONION, EGG WHITES, MOZZARELLA, MRS. DASH

ONION FACTORY: ANDERSON, IN

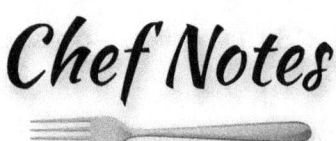

Chef Notes

- May use fresh or frozen filets.
- Serve with a 1 cup serving of your favorite vegetable medley for a complete meal.

TILAPIA

YIELDS: 1 serving

INGREDIENTS

- ❑ 4–6 oz Tilapia filet
- ❑ 2 squirts spray margarine
- ❑ 1 tsp Mrs. Dash® seasoning
- ❑ 1 Tbsp Kraft® Parmesan, Romano, and Asiago cheese

DIRECTIONS

1. Spray a skillet with Pam®.
2. Place fish in pan, spray with margarine.
3. Sprinkle with Mrs. Dash® and Kraft® cheese.
4. Bake at 425 degrees for 12 minutes.

Nutrition Facts
Tilapia

Amount Per Serving

Calories 190 — Calories from Fat 45

	% Daily Value*
Total Fat 5g	8%
Saturated Fat 3.5g	18%
Trans Fat 0g	
Cholesterol 80mg	27%
Sodium 250mg	10%
Total Carbohydrate 0g	0%
Dietary Fiber 0g	0%
Sugars 0g	
Protein 37g	

| Vitamin A 0% | • | Vitamin C 4% |
| Calcium 20% | • | Iron 4% |

* Percent Daily Values are based on a 2,000 calorie diet. Your daily values may be higher or lower depending on your calorie needs:

	Calories:	2,000	2,500
Total Fat	Less than	65g	80g
Sat Fat	Less than	20g	25g
Cholesterol	Less than	300mg	300mg
Sodium	Less than	2,400mg	2,400mg
Total Carbohydrate		300g	375g
Dietary Fiber		25g	30g

INGREDIENTS: TILAPIA, PARMESAN CHEESE, MRS. DASH, SPRAY MARGARINE

ONION FACTORY: ANDERSON, IN

SPINACH FETA MEATLOAF

YIELDS: 12 servings

INGREDIENTS

- ½ lb Bob Evans Hot Italian Sausage
- 3 lbs lean ground turkey
- 12 oz frozen three-pepper blend
- 64 oz Ragú® Traditional pasta sauce; reserve 1 cup for topping
- 24 oz Classico® Spicy Tomato Basil pasta sauce
- ½ cup Italian-style bread crumbs
- ¼ cup egg whites
- 1 Tbsp Mrs. Dash® seasoning
- 5 oz fat-free or reduced-fat Feta cheese
- 24 oz frozen chopped spinach
- 1 Tbsp Splenda® granules
- 2 Tbsp yellow mustard

DIRECTIONS

1. Brown sausage in skillet and set aside.
2. In large bowl, combine ground beef, three-pepper blend, pasta sauces, bread crumbs, and egg whites. Do not overmix. Mixture should be crumbly. Set aside.
3. In microwave, defrost spinach in bag for 3 minutes. Place in colander to drain, then squeeze until dry.
4. Preheat oven to 350 degrees.
5. Spray a 9x13 pan with Pam®, then assemble these layers in the pan:
   - ½ meat mixture
   - dry spinach
   - feta cheese
   - browned sausage
   - remaining meat mixture
6. Place this pan on a larger cookie sheet to catch possible overrun. Bake at 350 degrees for 1 hour, then drain meatloaf of juices.
7. In small bowl, make topping of 1 cup reserved pasta sauce, 1 Tbsp Splenda® granules, and 2 Tbsp yellow mustard.
8. Spread topping evenly over hot meatloaf. Return to oven for 10 minutes to warm.
9. Drain again and serve.

Nutrition Facts
Spinach Feta Meatloaf

Amount Per Serving

Calories 490	Calories from Fat 190

	% Daily Value*
Total Fat 21g	32%
Saturated Fat 5g	25%
Trans Fat 0g	
Cholesterol 95mg	32%
Sodium 1250mg	52%
Total Carbohydrate 28g	9%
Dietary Fiber 5g	20%
Sugars 14g	
Protein 34g	

Vitamin A 60%	•	Vitamin C 25%
Calcium 15%	•	Iron 60%

* Percent Daily Values are based on a 2,000 calorie diet. Your daily values may be higher or lower depending on your calorie needs:

	Calories:	2,000	2,500
Total Fat	Less than	65g	80g
Sat Fat	Less than	20g	25g
Cholesterol	Less than	300mg	300mg
Sodium	Less than	2,400mg	2,400mg
Total Carbohydrate		300g	375g
Dietary Fiber		25g	30g

INGREDIENTS: SPAGHETTI SAUCE, GROUND TURKEY, SPINACH, PEPPERS, ONION, PORK SAUSAGE, FAT FREE FETA CHEESE, EGG WHITES, BREAD CRUMBS, YELLOW MUSTARD, MRS. DASH, SPLENDA

ONION FACTORY: ANDERSON, IN

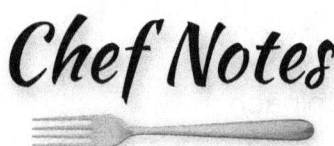
Chef Notes

- This recipe makes four generous servings and includes lean protein and vegetables.

- The recipe may be doubled. The doubled recipe would fit in a lasagna pan.

Nutrition Facts
Chicken Primavera

Amount Per Serving	
Calories 360	Calories from Fat 100
	% Daily Value*
Total Fat 11g	17%
Saturated Fat 5g	25%
Trans Fat 0g	
Cholesterol 105mg	35%
Sodium 870mg	36%
Total Carbohydrate 31g	10%
Dietary Fiber 6g	24%
Sugars 6g	
Protein 36g	
Vitamin A 40%	Vitamin C 150%
Calcium 15%	Iron 10%

* Percent Daily Values are based on a 2,000 calorie diet. Your daily values may be higher or lower depending on your calorie needs:

	Calories:	2,000	2,500
Total Fat	Less than	65g	80g
Sat Fat	Less than	20g	25g
Cholesterol	Less than	300mg	300mg
Sodium	Less than	2,400mg	2,400mg
Total Carbohydrate		300g	375g
Dietary Fiber		25g	30g

INGREDIENTS: CHICKEN BREAST, ALFREDO SAUCE, BROCCOLI, CAULIFLOWER, CARROTS, STIR FRY VEGETABLES WITH NOODLES, CRISPY FRIED ONIONS

ONION FACTORY: ANDERSON, IN

CHICKEN PRIMAVERA

YIELDS: 4 servings

INGREDIENTS

- ☐ 1 lb chicken breast
- ☐ Mrs. Dash® seasoning
- ☐ 12 oz frozen broccoli florets
- ☐ 12 oz frozen California blend vegetables
- ☐ 12 oz frozen stir fry vegetables with noodles
- ☐ 15 oz Classico® Creamy Alfredo Sauce, reserve 1 cup for final step
- ☐ ½ cup crushed French's® Crispy Fried Onions; reserve ¼ cup for final step

DIRECTIONS

1. Preheat oven to 350 degrees.

2. Spray pan with Pam®, season chicken with Mrs. Dash®, and bake in oven for 1 hour.

3. Cut the baked chicken into bite-size pieces.

4. Crush French's® Crispy Fried onions and divide into two ¼-cup measures.

5. In large bowl:, combine the chicken breast, thawed vegetables, 1 cup Alfredo Sauce, 1and ¼ cup crushed fried onions.

6. Spray 9 x 10 pan. Spread mixture evenly in pan. Bake for 1 hour.

7. Remove from oven and stir in remaining Alfredo sauce.

8. Garnish with remaining ¼ cup crushed fried onions.

STUFFED PEPPERS

YIELDS: 8 servings (2 pepper halves each)

INGREDIENTS

- ❑ 8 medium green peppers
- ❑ 2 lbs lean ground turkey 90/10
- ❑ 1 Tbsp Mrs. Dash® seasoning
- ❑ 12 oz frozen three-pepper blend
- ❑ 12 oz frozen riced cauliflower
- ❑ 64 oz Ragú® Traditional pasta sauce
- ❑ 24 oz Classico® Spicy Tomato and Basil pasta sauce
- ❑ ½ cup shredded mozzarella

DIRECTIONS

1. Fill a roaster pan halfway with water. Bring to boil.
2. Split peppers lengthwise. Scoop out seeds and stem.
3. Boil for 8–10 minutes until peppers change color.
4. In a large saucepan, brown ground turkey. Season with Mrs. Dash®.
5. Add frozen pepper, riced cauliflower, and two pasta sauces. Simmer for 45 minutes.
6. Preheat oven to 350 degrees.
7. Place peppers on 2 large rimmed cookie sheets.
8. Evenly distribute the meat sauce on peppers.
9. Bake 30 minutes, until filling is hot.
10. Sprinkle mozzarella evenly over hot peppers.
11. Return to oven for 5–10 minutes for cheese to melt.

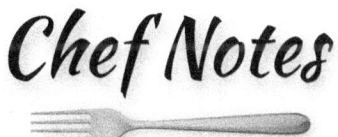

Chef Notes

♦ May substitute lean ground beef, 90/10 for turkey.

Nutrition Facts
Stuffed Peppers

Amount Per Serving	
Calories 490	Calories from Fat 150
	% Daily Value*
Total Fat 17g	26%
Saturated Fat 4g	20%
Trans Fat 0g	
Cholesterol 85mg	28%
Sodium 1280mg	53%
Total Carbohydrate 44g	15%
Dietary Fiber 10g	40%
Sugars 25g	
Protein 31g	
Vitamin A 35%	Vitamin C 430%
Calcium 10%	Iron 90%

* Percent Daily Values are based on a 2,000 calorie diet. Your daily values may be higher or lower depending on your calorie needs:

	Calories:	2,000	2,500
Total Fat	Less than	65g	80g
Sat Fat	Less than	20g	25g
Cholesterol	Less than	300mg	300mg
Sodium	Less than	2,400mg	2,400mg
Total Carbohydrate		300g	375g
Dietary Fiber		25g	30g

INGREDIENTS: SPAGHETTI SAUCE, GREEN PEPPER, GROUND TURKEY, PEPPERS, ONION, CAULIFLOWER, MOZZARELLA, MRS. DASH

ONION FACTORY: ANDERSON, IN

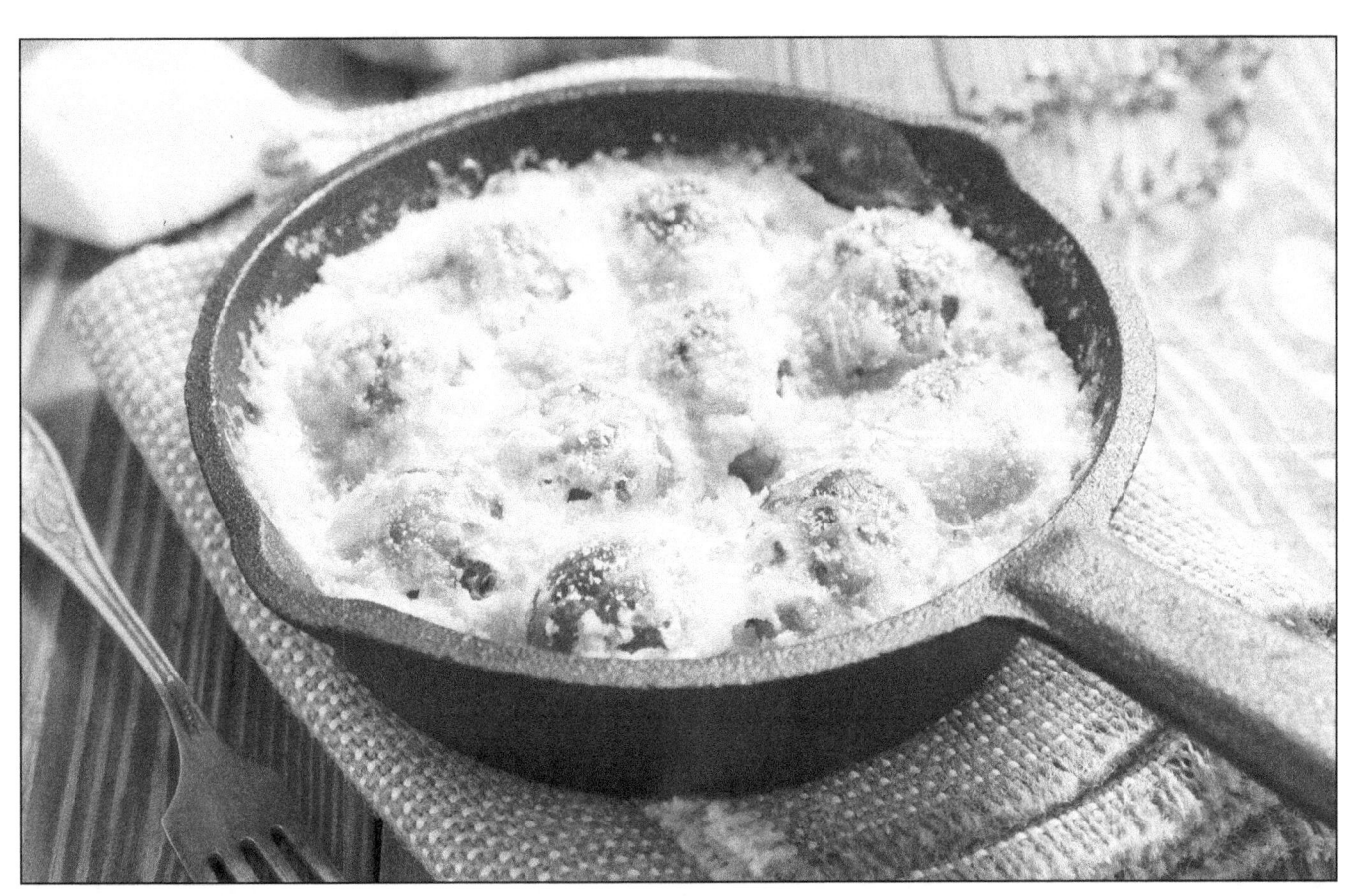

sides

WHY SETTLE FOR FILLERS WHEN YOU CAN HAVE DELICIOUS?

ALFREDO BRUSSEL SPROUTS

YIELDS: 4 servings

Chef Notes

INGREDIENTS

- ❑ 12 oz frozen Brussel Sprouts
- ❑ ⅓ cup Classico® Creamy Alfredo Sauce

DIRECTIONS

1. Microwave brussel sprouts for 5 minutes.
2. Add Alfredo sauce and toss.
3. Finish in 350-degree oven for 6–7 minutes.

-or-

1. Mix together frozen brussel sprouts and Alfredo sauce.
2. Bake at 350 degrees for 30 minutes. (This method provides a more roasted flavor.)

Nutrition Facts
Alfredo Brussel Sprouts

Amount Per Serving	
Calories 50	Calories from Fat 15
	% Daily Value*
Total Fat 1.5g	2%
Saturated Fat 1g	5%
Trans Fat 0g	
Cholesterol 5mg	2%
Sodium 160mg	7%
Total Carbohydrate 8g	3%
Dietary Fiber 3g	12%
Sugars 2g	
Protein 4g	

Vitamin A 10%	•	Vitamin C 110%	
Calcium 4%	•	Iron 4%	

* Percent Daily Values are based on a 2,000 calorie diet. Your daily values may be higher or lower depending on your calorie needs:

	Calories:	2,000	2,500
Total Fat	Less than	65g	80g
Sat Fat	Less than	20g	25g
Cholesterol	Less than	300mg	300mg
Sodium	Less than	2,400mg	2,400mg
Total Carbohydrate		300g	375g
Dietary Fiber		25g	30g

INGREDIENTS: BRUSSELS SPROUTS, ALFREDO SAUCE

ONION FACTORY: ANDERSON, IN

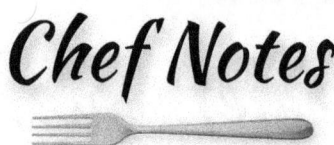

Chef Notes

- Great five-minute fix!
- All-in-one pan meal.

Nutrition Facts
Hoosier Jambalaya

Amount Per Serving	
Calories 360	Calories from Fat 150

	% Daily Value*
Total Fat 16g	25%
Saturated Fat 5g	25%
Trans Fat 0g	
Cholesterol 100mg	33%
Sodium 2350mg	98%
Total Carbohydrate 22g	7%
Dietary Fiber 10g	40%
Sugars 6g	
Protein 36g	

Vitamin A 35%	•	Vitamin C 30%
Calcium 25%	•	Iron 20%

* Percent Daily Values are based on a 2,000 calorie diet. Your daily values may be higher or lower depending on your calorie needs:

	Calories:	2,000	2,500
Total Fat	Less than	65g	80g
Sat Fat	Less than	20g	25g
Cholesterol	Less than	300mg	300mg
Sodium	Less than	2,400mg	2,400mg
Total Carbohydrate		300g	375g
Dietary Fiber		25g	30g

INGREDIENTS: CANNED GREEN BEANS, SPICY ITALIAN CHICKEN SAUSAGES, MUSHROOMS, TOMATOES WITH GREEN CHILIES, PAM SPRAY

ONION FACTORY: ANDERSON, IN

HOOSIER JUMBALAYA

YIELDS: 1 serving

INGREDIENTS

- ☐ 2 links spicy jalapeno chicken sausages
- ☐ 2 oz canned sliced mushrooms, drained
- ☐ 1 Tbsp diced tomatoes with chilies
- ☐ 14 oz can green beans

DIRECTIONS

1. Brown chicken sausages in medium fry pan with spray butter.
2. Add small amount of liquid from green beans.
3. Drain green beans, add to sausage.
4. Sauté until flavors blend
5. Add mushrooms and diced tomatoes.

SMASHED CAULIFLOWER

YIELDS: 4 servings

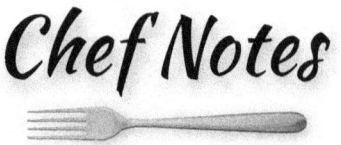

INGREDIENTS

- ❑ 2-12 oz packages frozen cauliflower
- ❑ ⅓ cup Kraft® Italian Mozzarella & Parmesean cheese
- ❑ large onion, cut in half
- ❑ 1 Tbsp Mrs. Dash® seasonin®g
- ❑ 1 Tbsp butter
- ❑ Garlic salt, to taste
- ❑ Salt and pepper, to taste

DIRECTIONS

1. Cut cauliflower in segments. Place in salt water.
2. Add diced onion and garlic cloves.
3. Boil until soft. Drain.
4. Place softened veggies in a bowl. Chop until the mixture looks like mashed potatoes.
5. Add butter and seasonings to taste.

Nutrition Facts
Smashed Cauliflower

Amount Per Serving

Calories 35 — Calories from Fat 0

	% Daily Value*
Total Fat 0g	0%
Saturated Fat 0g	0%
Trans Fat 0g	
Cholesterol 0mg	0%
Sodium 360mg	15%
Total Carbohydrate 7g	2%
Dietary Fiber 5g	20%
Sugars 2g	
Protein 3g	

Vitamin A 0%	•	Vitamin C 90%
Calcium 4%	•	Iron 4%

*Percent Daily Values are based on a 2,000 calorie diet. Your daily values may be higher or lower depending on your calorie needs:

	Calories:	2,000	2,500
Total Fat	Less than	65g	80g
Sat Fat	Less than	20g	25g
Cholesterol	Less than	300mg	300mg
Sodium	Less than	2,400mg	2,400mg
Total Carbohydrate		300g	375g
Dietary Fiber		25g	30g

INGREDIENTS: CAULIFLOWER, ONION, MRS. DASH, GARLIC SALT

ONION FACTORY: ANDERSON, IN

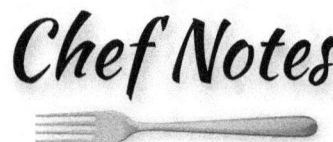

Chef Notes

BROCCOLI COLESLAW

YIELDS: 4 servings

INGREDIENTS

- ☐ 12 oz. Broccoli slaw mix
- ☐ 12 oz broccoli florets
- ☐ 2 Tbsp Hormel® bacon bits
- ☐ ⅛ cup raisins or Craisins®
- ☐ ½ cup diced red onion
- ☐ 2 Tbsp apple cider vinegar
- ☐ 2 Tbsp light Miracle Whip®
- ☐ 2 Tbsp Splenda®
- ☐ Splash of milk

DIRECTIONS

1. Marinate red onion in apple cider vinegar and sugar.
2. In large bowl mix, together broccoli slaw and florets, bacon bits and raisins.
3. Mix together marinated onion mixture with Miracle Whip®, Splenda®, and a splash of milk.
4. Place in refrigerator for 2 hours before serving.

Nutrition Facts
Broccoli Coleslaw

Amount Per Serving

Calories 100	Calories from Fat 15

	% Daily Value*
Total Fat 1.5g	2%
Saturated Fat 0g	0%
Trans Fat 0g	
Cholesterol <5mg	1%
Sodium 200mg	8%
Total Carbohydrate 16g	5%
Dietary Fiber 4g	16%
Sugars 8g	
Protein 6g	

Vitamin A 90%	•	Vitamin C 250%
Calcium 8%	•	Iron 10%

* Percent Daily Values are based on a 2,000 calorie diet. Your daily values may be higher or lower depending on your calorie needs:

	Calories:	2,000	2,500
Total Fat	Less than	65g	80g
Sat Fat	Less than	20g	25g
Cholesterol	Less than	300mg	300mg
Sodium	Less than	2,400mg	2,400mg
Total Carbohydrate		300g	375g
Dietary Fiber		25g	30g

INGREDIENTS: BROCCOLI, BROCCOLI SLAW, ONION, LIGHT SALAD DRESSING, APPLE CIDER VINEGAR, RAISINS, BACON BITS, MILK, SPLENDA

ONION FACTORY: ANDERSON, IN

CUCUMBER AND ONION SALAD

YIELDS: 4-6 servings

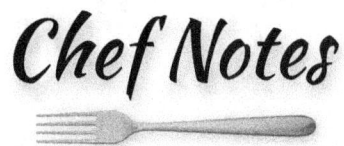

INGREDIENTS

- ☐ 4 cups thinly sliced cucumbers
- ☐ 1 large white onion, thinly sliced
- ☐ ⅓ cup white wine vinegar
- ☐ 1⅓ cups water
- ☐ 2 packets Splenda® or other artificial sweetener
- ☐ 1 tsp salt
- ☐ ½ tsp pepper

DIRECTIONS

1. In medium size bowl, place cucumbers and onions.
2. In small bowl, vigorously mix together vinegar, water, Splenda®, salt and pepper.
3. Pour dressing mixture over vegetables.
4. Refrigerate for 2 hrs.

♦ Serving suggestion:

Add ½ cup ice cubes to get the salad icy cold if you need to serve it soon.

Nutrition Facts
Cucumber and Onion Salad

Amount Per Serving

Calories 35 — Calories from Fat 0

	% Daily Value*
Total Fat 0g	0%
Saturated Fat 0g	0%
Trans Fat 0g	
Cholesterol 0mg	0%
Sodium 580mg	24%
Total Carbohydrate 8g	3%
Dietary Fiber 1g	4%
Sugars 4g	
Protein 1g	

| Vitamin A 2% | • | Vitamin C 10% |
| Calcium 2% | • | Iron 2% |

* Percent Daily Values are based on a 2,000 calorie diet. Your daily values may be higher or lower depending on your calorie needs:

	Calories:	2,000	2,500
Total Fat	Less than	65g	80g
Sat Fat	Less than	20g	25g
Cholesterol	Less than	300mg	300mg
Sodium	Less than	2,400mg	2,400mg
Total Carbohydrate		300g	375g
Dietary Fiber		25g	30g

INGREDIENTS: CUCUMBER, ONION, WHITE WINE VINEGAR, SPLENDA

ONION FACTORY: ANDERSON, IN

Chef Notes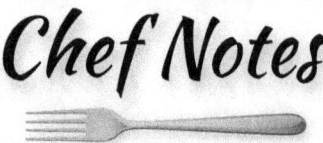

PARMESAN BAKED TOMATO

YIELDS: 1 serving

INGREDIENTS

- ☐ Roma tomato
- ☐ Mrs. Dash® seasoning
- ☐ 2 tsp Parmesan cheese

DIRECTIONS

1. Preheat oven to Broil.
2. Split tomato lengthwise.
3. Season with Mrs. Dash®.
4. Sprinkle each half with 1 tsp Parmesan cheese.
5. Broil until cheese bubbles, about one minute.

Nutrition Facts

Parmesean Baked Tomato

Amount Per Serving

Calories 45	Calories from Fat 15

% Daily Value*

Total Fat 1.5g	2%
Saturated Fat 1g	5%
Trans Fat 0g	
Cholesterol <5mg	1%
Sodium 80mg	3%
Total Carbohydrate 6g	2%
Dietary Fiber 2g	8%
Sugars 4g	
Protein 3g	

Vitamin A 25%	•	Vitamin C 30%
Calcium 8%	•	Iron 2%

* Percent Daily Values are based on a 2,000 calorie diet. Your daily values may be higher or lower depending on your calorie needs:

	Calories:	2,000	2,500
Total Fat	Less than	65g	80g
Sat Fat	Less than	20g	25g
Cholesterol	Less than	300mg	300mg
Sodium	Less than	2,400mg	2,400mg
Total Carbohydrate		300g	375g
Dietary Fiber		25g	30g

INGREDIENTS: TOMATOES, PARMESAN CHEESE, MRS. DASH

ONION FACTORY: ANDERSON, IN

LETTUCE WRAPS

YIELDS: 4 servings

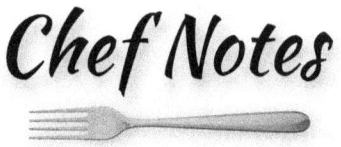

INGREDIENTS

- 1 lb chicken breast, cut in thin strips
- Mrs. Dash® seasoning
- ⅓ cup Soy Vay® Veri Veri Teriyaki sauce
- Package of burger-size lettuce leaves
- 4 Tbsp fat-free sour cream
- Sesame seeds for garnish

DIRECTIONS

1. In a frying pan sprayed with Pam®, cook thin strips of chicken breast. Season with Mrs. Dash®.
2. Add the teriyaki sauce to glaze the chicken.
3. To assemble, put 4 oz chicken breast on a lettuce leaf, top with 1 Tbsp fat-free sour cream and a sprinkle of sesame seeds.

Nutrition Facts
Lettuce Wraps

Amount Per Serving

Calories 160 — Calories from Fat 10

	% Daily Value*
Total Fat 1g	2%
Saturated Fat 0g	0%
Trans Fat 0g	
Cholesterol 75mg	25%
Sodium 410mg	17%
Total Carbohydrate 12g	4%
Dietary Fiber 0g	0%
Sugars 7g	
Protein 29g	

Vitamin A 50% • Vitamin C 6%
Calcium 4% • Iron 6%

* Percent Daily Values are based on a 2,000 calorie diet. Your daily values may be higher or lower depending on your calorie needs:

	Calories:	2,000	2,500
Total Fat	Less than	65g	80g
Sat Fat	Less than	20g	25g
Cholesterol	Less than	300mg	300mg
Sodium	Less than	2,400mg	2,400mg
Total Carbohydrate		300g	375g
Dietary Fiber		25g	30g

INGREDIENTS: CHICKEN BREAST, LETTUCE, FAT FREE SOUR CREAM, TERIYAKI ASIAN SAUCE, SESAME SEEDS

ONION FACTORY: ANDERSON, IN

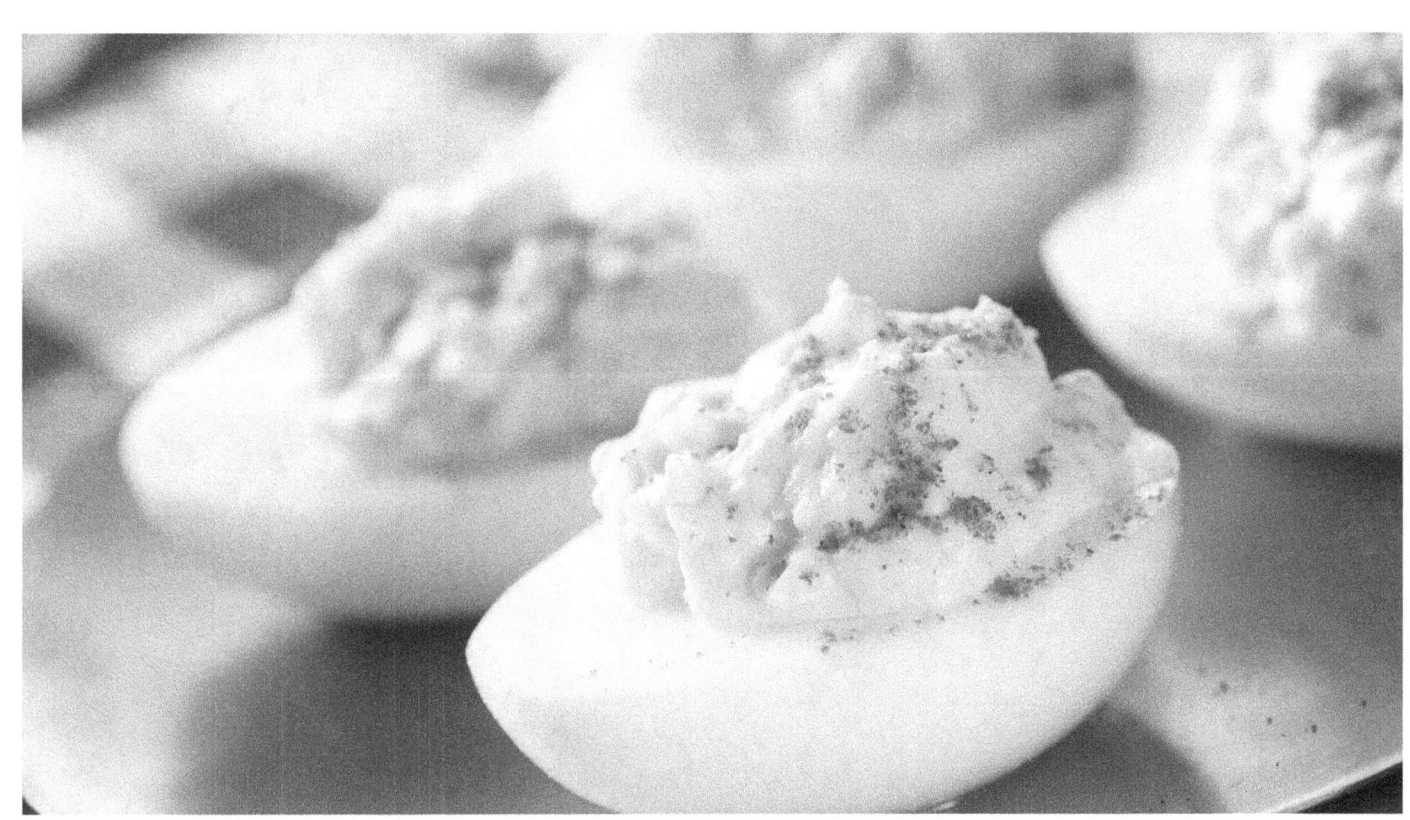

snacks

EAT SMALL AMOUNTS OFTEN TO KEEP YOUR CAMPFIRE BURNING

ASPARAGUS WRAPS

YIELDS: 3 servings (4 spears ea.)

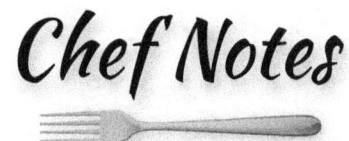

INGREDIENTS

- Half of 5-oz jar Kraft® pimento cheese spread
- 12 fresh asparagus spears
- 7 oz deli thin-sliced roast beef

DIRECTIONS

1. Wash asparagus. While slightly wet, wrap in paper towel.
2. Microwave in paper towel for 2 minutes.
3. Do not overcook. The asparagus should still have a crunch.
4. Spread a small amount of pimento cheese spread on roast beef slice.
5. Place on asparagus spear on one end of beef slice and roll.

♦ Great holiday appetizer!

Nutrition Facts
Asparagus Wraps

Amount Per Serving	
Calories 170	Calories from Fat 80
	% Daily Value*
Total Fat 9g	14%
Saturated Fat 5g	25%
Trans Fat 0g	
Cholesterol 55mg	18%
Sodium 530mg	22%
Total Carbohydrate 5g	2%
Dietary Fiber 1g	4%
Sugars 3g	
Protein 17g	
Vitamin A 15% •	Vitamin C 10%
Calcium 4% •	Iron 15%

* Percent Daily Values are based on a 2,000 calorie diet. Your daily values may be higher or lower depending on your calorie needs:

	Calories:	2,000	2,500
Total Fat	Less than	65g	80g
Sat Fat	Less than	20g	25g
Cholesterol	Less than	300mg	300mg
Sodium	Less than	2,400mg	2,400mg
Total Carbohydrate		300g	375g
Dietary Fiber		25g	30g

INGREDIENTS: DELI ROAST BEEF, ASPARAGUS, PIMENTO CHEESE SPREAD

ONION FACTORY: ANDERSON, IN

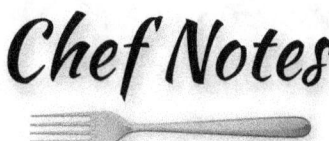

DEVILED EGGS

YIELDS: 6 servings (2 egg halves ea.)

INGREDIENTS

- ☐ One dozen hard boiled eggs
- ☐ Mrs. Dash® seasoning
- ☐ ¼ cup finely chopped celery leaves
- ☐ Squirt of yellow mustard
- ☐ 1 Tbsp Light Miracle Whip®

DIRECTIONS

1. Halve 6 of the hard boiled eggs and remove 6 yolks. Set aside the egg whites to stuff.
2. Chop very fine remaining 6 hard boiled eggs.
3. Add chopped celery leaves, Mrs. Dash®, yellow mustard, and Light Miracle Whip® to the chopped eggs.
4. Stuff the egg halves.

Nutrition Facts
Deviled Eggs

Amount Per Serving

Calories 90	Calories from Fat 45

% Daily Value*

Total Fat 5g	8%
Saturated Fat 1.5g	8%
Trans Fat 0g	
Cholesterol 185mg	62%
Sodium 150mg	6%
Total Carbohydrate 1g	0%
Dietary Fiber 0g	0%
Sugars 0g	
Protein 10g	

Vitamin A 6%	•	Vitamin C 0%	
Calcium 4%	•	Iron 6%	

* Percent Daily Values are based on a 2,000 calorie diet. Your daily values may be higher or lower depending on your calorie needs:

	Calories:	2,000	2,500
Total Fat	Less than	65g	80g
Sat Fat	Less than	20g	25g
Cholesterol	Less than	300mg	300mg
Sodium	Less than	2,400mg	2,400mg
Total Carbohydrate		300g	375g
Dietary Fiber		25g	30g

INGREDIENTS: EGG, EGG WHITES, CELERY, LIGHT SALAD DRESSING, MRS. DASH, YELLOW MUSTARD

ONION FACTORY: ANDERSON, IN

SALMON & CUCUMBER ROUNDS

YIELDS: 2 servings

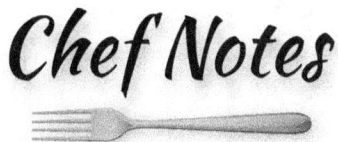

INGREDIENTS

- ☐ 4 slices of cucumber
- ☐ 1 tsp light garden vegetable cream cheese
- ☐ 2½ oz packet of salmon
- ☐ 1 Tbsp light Ranch dressing
- ☐ Thinly sliced radish

Chef Notes

- ♦ May substitute salmon with tuna or chicken.
- ♦ Great for holiday entertaining.

DIRECTIONS

1. On each cucumber, spread a dab of cream cheese.
2. In small bowl, mix salmon with ranch dressing.
3. Spread salmon mixture over cucumbers with cream cheese.
4. Garnish with radish.

Nutrition Facts

Salmon and Cucumber Rounds

Amount Per Serving	
Calories 60	Calories from Fat 30

	% Daily Value*
Total Fat 3.5g	5%
Saturated Fat 1g	5%
Trans Fat 0g	
Cholesterol 15mg	5%
Sodium 210mg	9%
Total Carbohydrate 2g	1%
Dietary Fiber 0g	0%
Sugars 1g	
Protein 7g	

Vitamin A 0%	•	Vitamin C 2%
Calcium 0%	•	Iron 2%

* Percent Daily Values are based on a 2,000 calorie diet. Your daily values may be higher or lower depending on your calorie needs:

		Calories:	2,000	2,500
Total Fat		Less than	65g	80g
Sat Fat		Less than	20g	25g
Cholesterol		Less than	300mg	300mg
Sodium		Less than	2,400mg	2,400mg
Total Carbohydrate			300g	375g
Dietary Fiber			25g	30g

INGREDIENTS: SALMON, CUCUMBER, LITE RANCH DRESSING, LOWFAT CREAM CHEESE, RADISHES

ONION FACTORY: ANDERSON, IN

Chef Notes

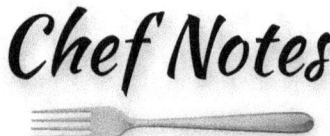

STUFFED PORTABELLO MUSHROOMS

YIELDS: 4 servings

INGREDIENTS

- ❏ 4 Portabella mushrooms (approx. 6" diameter)
- ❏ ½ cup pizza sauce
- ❏ 16 turkey pepperoni slices, diced
- ❏ ¼ cup cooked turkey sausage
- ❏ ¼ cup mozzarella cheese
- ❏ ⅛ tsp garlic powder
- ❏ ⅛ tsp onion powder
- ❏ salt and pepper to taste

DIRECTIONS

1. Preheat oven to 375 degrees.
2. Cook turkey sausage in skillet.
3. Add pizza sauce and diced pepperoni.
4. Sprinkle with garlic and onion powders, salt and pepper to taste.
5. Add ¼ mixture to each mushroom.
6. Bake for 20 minutes or until filling is hot.
7. Add mozzarella immediately after removing mushrooms from oven.
8. Return mushrooms to oven for 5 minutes until cheese melts.

Nutrition Facts
Stuffed Portabella Mushrooms

Amount Per Serving

Calories 80	Calories from Fat 35

	% Daily Value*
Total Fat 3.5g	5%
Saturated Fat 1.5g	8%
Trans Fat 0g	
Cholesterol 20mg	7%
Sodium 310mg	13%
Total Carbohydrate 5g	2%
Dietary Fiber 1g	4%
Sugars 3g	
Protein 7g	

Vitamin A 4%	•	Vitamin C 4%
Calcium 6%	•	Iron 4%

*Percent Daily Values are based on a 2,000 calorie diet. Your daily values may be higher or lower depending on your calorie needs:

	Calories:	2,000	2,500
Total Fat	Less than	65g	80g
Sat Fat	Less than	20g	25g
Cholesterol	Less than	300mg	300mg
Sodium	Less than	2,400mg	2,400mg
Total Carbohydrate		300g	375g
Dietary Fiber		25g	30g

INGREDIENTS: PORTABELLA MUSHROOMS, PIZZA SAUCE, TURKEY PEPPERONI, TURKEY SAUSAGE, MOZZARELLA, ONION POWDER, GARLIC POWDER

ONION FACTORY: ANDERSON, IN

RELISH TRAY WITH DIP

YIELDS: Vary

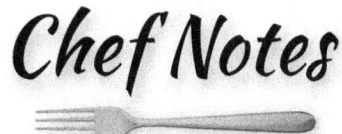

INGREDIENTS

- A variety of fresh vegetables, such as:
  - Celery
  - Cucumbers
  - Broccoli
  - Cauliflower
  - Peppers
  - Zucchini
  - Cherry tomatoes
- 16 oz fat-free cottage cheese
- 16 oz fat-free sour cream
- 1 pkg Knorr® vegetable dip mix

DIRECTIONS

1. Blend cottage cheese in blender.
2. Fold in sour cream and vegetable mix.

—or—

Mix all ingredients in a bowl. (This makes a chunkier alternative.)

- A red pepper has 5 grams of sugar; a green pepper has only 2 grams of sugar. Choose wisely!
- Stay on track at parties and volunteer to bring the vegetable tray!

NOTE: No Nutrition Facts for this recipe because the nutrients will vary, depending on which vegetables you choose.

Chef Notes

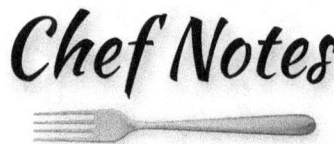

TUNA SALAD

YIELDS: 5 servings (2 oz each)

INGREDIENTS

- ☐ 12½-oz can of tuna in water
- ☐ 1½ Tbsp Light Miracle Whip®
- ☐ 1 tsp Mrs. Dash® seasoning
- ☐ ¼ cup rough chopped celery leaves
- ☐ ¼ cup finely chopped green onion

DIRECTIONS

1. Drain tuna. Use fork to break up the meat.
2. Mix all ingredients together in bowl.

Nutrition Facts
Tuna Salad

Amount Per Serving	
Calories 60	Calories from Fat 10
	% Daily Value*
Total Fat 1g	2%
Saturated Fat 0g	0%
Trans Fat 0g	
Cholesterol 25mg	8%
Sodium 200mg	8%
Total Carbohydrate 1g	0%
Dietary Fiber 0g	0%
Sugars 0g	
Protein 12g	
Vitamin A 2% • Vitamin C 2%	
Calcium 2% • Iron 6%	

* Percent Daily Values are based on a 2,000 calorie diet. Your daily values may be higher or lower depending on your calorie needs:

	Calories:	2,000	2,500
Total Fat	Less than	65g	80g
Sat Fat	Less than	20g	25g
Cholesterol	Less than	300mg	300mg
Sodium	Less than	2,400mg	2,400mg
Total Carbohydrate		300g	375g
Dietary Fiber		25g	30g

INGREDIENTS: CANNED TUNA, GREEN ONION, CELERY, LIGHT SALAD DRESSING, MRS. DASH

ONION FACTORY: ANDERSON, IN

EGG SALAD

YIELDS: 4 servings (2 oz each)

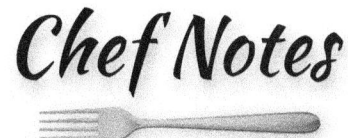

INGREDIENTS

- 6 hardboiled eggs, minus 2 egg yolks
- 1½ Tbsp Light Miracle Whip®
- 1 tsp Mrs. Dash® seasoning
- ¼ cup rough chopped celery leaves
- ¼ cup finely chopped green onion

DIRECTIONS

1. Finely chop 4 whole hardboiled eggs and 2 egg whites.
2. Mix all ingredients together in bowl.

♦ Nourishing and economical snack.

♦ Keep in refrigerator for those times you need to "grab and go."

Nutrition Facts

Egg Salad

Amount Per Serving

Calories 100	Calories from Fat 50

% Daily Value*

Total Fat 6g	9%
Saturated Fat 1.5g	8%
Trans Fat 0g	
Cholesterol 185mg	62%
Sodium 150mg	6%
Total Carbohydrate 3g	1%
Dietary Fiber <1g	3%
Sugars 1g	
Protein 8g	

Vitamin A 6%	•	Vitamin C 4%
Calcium 4%	•	Iron 4%

* Percent Daily Values are based on a 2,000 calorie diet. Your daily values may be higher or lower depending on your calorie needs:

	Calories:	2,000	2,500
Total Fat	Less than	65g	80g
Sat Fat	Less than	20g	25g
Cholesterol	Less than	300mg	300mg
Sodium	Less than	2,400mg	2,400mg
Total Carbohydrate		300g	375g
Dietary Fiber		25g	30g

INGREDIENTS: EGG, EGG WHITES, GREEN ONION, CELERY, LIGHT SALAD DRESSING, MRS. DASH

ONION FACTORY: ANDERSON, IN

CHICKEN SALAD

YIELDS: 5 servings (2 oz each)

INGREDIENTS

- ☐ 12½ oz can chicken breast
- ☐ 1½ Tbsp Light Miracle Whip®
- ☐ 1 tsp Mrs. Dash® seasoning
- ☐ ¼ cup rough chopped celery leaves
- ☐ ¼ cup finely chopped green onion

DIRECTIONS

1. Drain chicken. Use fork to break up the meat.
2. Mix all ingredients together in bowl.

Nutrition Facts
Chicken Salad

Amount Per Serving	
Calories 80	Calories from Fat 15
	% Daily Value*
Total Fat 2g	3%
Saturated Fat 0g	0%
Trans Fat 0g	
Cholesterol 40mg	13%
Sodium 290mg	12%
Total Carbohydrate 1g	0%
Dietary Fiber 0g	0%
Sugars 0g	
Protein 12g	

Vitamin A 0%	•	Vitamin C 4%
Calcium 0%	•	Iron 2%

* Percent Daily Values are based on a 2,000 calorie diet. Your daily values may be higher or lower depending on your calorie needs:

		Calories:	2,000	2,500
Total Fat	Less than		65g	80g
Sat Fat	Less than		20g	25g
Cholesterol	Less than		300mg	300mg
Sodium	Less than		2,400mg	2,400mg
Total Carbohydrate			300g	375g
Dietary Fiber			25g	30g

INGREDIENTS: CHICKEN BREAST, GREEN ONION, CELERY, LIGHT SALAD DRESSING, MRS. DASH

ONION FACTORY: ANDERSON, IN

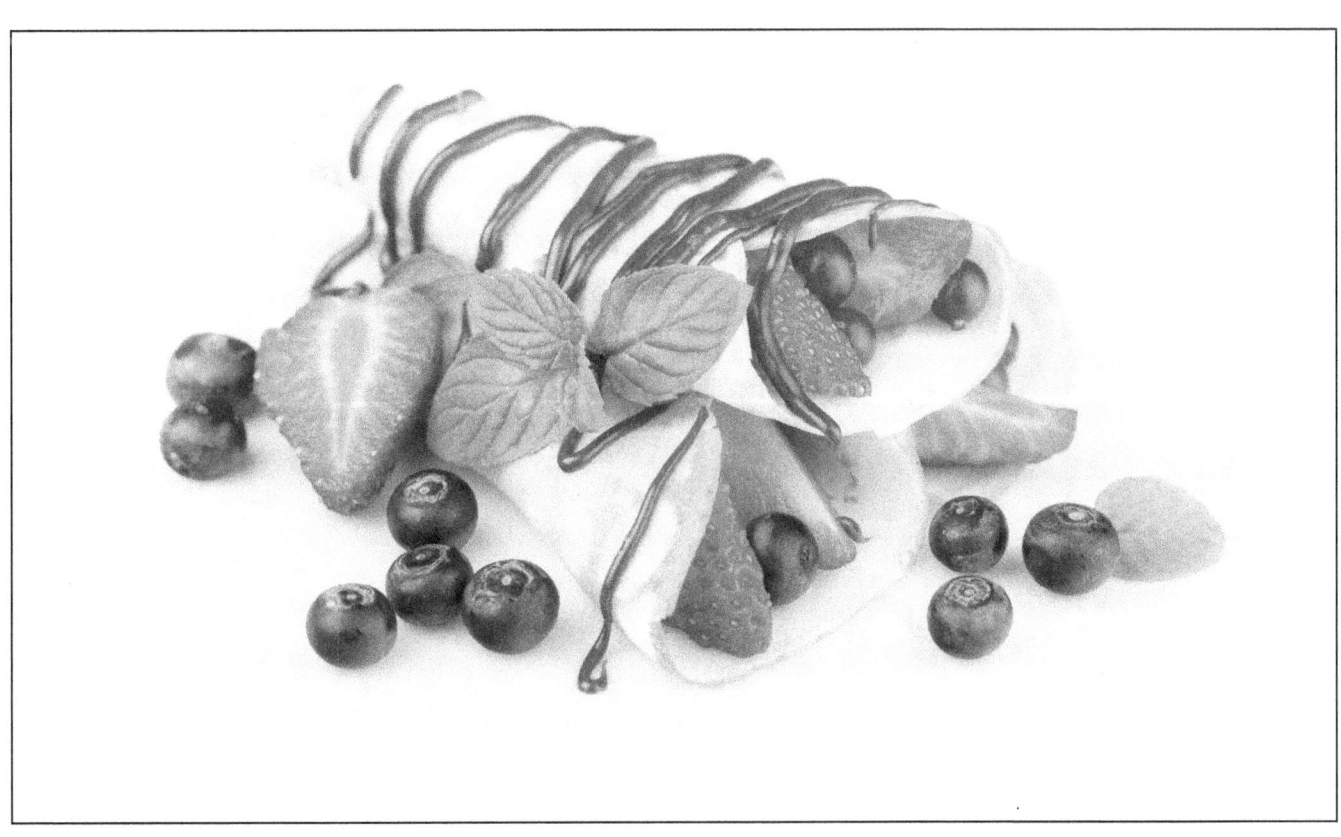

desserts

ALL OF THE ENJOYMENT WITHOUT THE SUGAR

CARAMEL APPLE CRÊPES

YIELDS: 1 serving

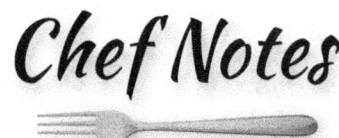

INGREDIENTS

- ½ cup egg whites
- ¼ small apple, thinly sliced
- 1 Tbsp Walden Farms® Pancake Syrup
- 1 Tbsp + 1 tsp Walden Farms® Caramel Sauce
- Cinnamon to taste
- Splenda® to taste
- 1 dollop light whipped topping

DIRECTIONS

1. Peel and quarter apple. Cut into thin slices.
2. In a small frying pan, place apples and pancake syrup. Cook until apples are tender.
3. Pour egg whites into omelet pan that has been sprayed with Pam®.
4. Drizzle egg whites with I Tbsp caramel sauce and sprinkle with cinnamon and Splenda®.
5. Cook until egg whites are firm, roll onto a plate.
6. Top with apples, drizzle with ½ tsp caramel sauce, sprinkle with cinnamon.
7. Accent with 1 small dollop of light whipped topping.

Chef Notes

- Satisfies a sweet tooth craving.
- Makes a beautiful presentation.
- Variation: Substitute frozen apple slices for easier preparation.

Nutrition Facts

Caramel Apple Crêpes

Amount Per Serving

Calories 90	Calories from Fat 0

	% Daily Value*
Total Fat 0g	0%
Saturated Fat 0g	0%
Trans Fat 0g	
Cholesterol 0mg	0%
Sodium 280mg	12%
Total Carbohydrate 7g	2%
Dietary Fiber <1g	4%
Sugars 4g	
Protein 13g	

Vitamin A 0%	•		Vitamin C 2%
Calcium 2%	•		Iron 0%

* Percent Daily Values are based on a 2,000 calorie diet. Your daily values may be higher or lower depending on your calorie needs:

	Calories:	2,000	2,500
Total Fat	Less than	65g	80g
Sat Fat	Less than	20g	25g
Cholesterol	Less than	300mg	300mg
Sodium	Less than	2,400mg	2,400mg
Total Carbohydrate		300g	375g
Dietary Fiber		25g	30g

INGREDIENTS: EGG WHITES, APPLES, FAT FREE PANCAKE SYRUP, FAT FREE CARAMEL SYRUP, FAT FREE WHIPPED TOPPING, CINNAMON, SPLENDA

ONION FACTORY: ANDERSON, IN

Chef Notes

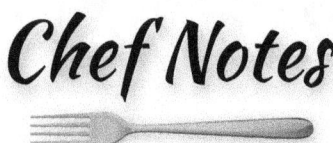

- The blueberry sauce keeps well in the refrigerator for two weeks. This sauce can also be frozen.

BLUEBERRY COBBLER

YIELDS: 1 serving

INGREDIENTS

- ½ cup fat-free cottage cheese
- 2 Tbsp blueberry sauce (see below)
- ¼ cup blueberries
- 1 tsp slivered almonds

DIRECTIONS

In small bowl, layer:

- cottage cheese
- blueberry sauce
- blueberries
- slivered almonds

BLUEBERRY SAUCE

YIELDS: 24 servings

INGREDIENTS

- 12 oz Walden Farms® Pancake Syrup
- 12 oz water
- 3 cups fresh or frozen blueberries
- 1 Tbsp arrowroot

DIRECTIONS

1. In medium saucepan, cook syrup, water, and blueberries. Bring to a boil.
2. In small cup or bowl, mix 1 Tbsp arrowroot with 1 Tbsp water.
3. Gradually add to blueberry sauce to thicken.

Nutrition Facts
Blueberry Cobbler

Amount Per Serving

Calories 70	Calories from Fat 0

	% Daily Value*
Total Fat 0g	0%
Saturated Fat 0g	0%
Trans Fat 0g	
Cholesterol 5mg	2%
Sodium 220mg	9%
Total Carbohydrate 11g	4%
Dietary Fiber 1g	4%
Sugars 7g	
Protein 8g	

Vitamin A 2%	•	Vitamin C 6%	
Calcium 4%	•	Iron 0%	

* Percent Daily Values are based on a 2,000 calorie diet. Your daily values may be higher or lower depending on your calorie needs:

	Calories:	2,000	2,500
Total Fat	Less than	65g	80g
Sat Fat	Less than	20g	25g
Cholesterol	Less than	300mg	300mg
Sodium	Less than	2,400mg	2,400mg
Total Carbohydrate		300g	375g
Dietary Fiber		25g	30g

INGREDIENTS: FAT FREE COTTAGE CHEESE, BLUEBERRIES, FAT FREE PANCAKE SYRUP, ARROWROOT, ALMONDS

ONION FACTORY: ANDERSON, IN

FRUIT FLAN

YIELDS: 8 servings

INGREDIENTS

- ☐ 8 oz low-fat cream cheese
- ☐ 32 oz Dannon Light & Fit® vanilla yogurt
- ☐ 8 oz Cool Whip®
- ☐ 2 Tbsp sugar-free apricot jam
- ☐ strawberries for garnish
- ☐ blueberries for garnish

DIRECTIONS

1. In mixing bowl, combine cream cheese, yogurt, and Cool Whip®. Whisk together, blending well.
2. Divide mixture evenly into 8 medium-size ramekins.
3. Cut strawberries in half and then into thin pieces.
4. Garnish the outside of the ramekin with a circle of strawberries. Then make a circle of blueberries.
5. Place a flat sliced strawberry in the middle of each ramekin.
6. Microwave apricot jam for 15–30 seconds. Brush glaze over top of the flan.
7. Refrigerate for 1 hour before serving.

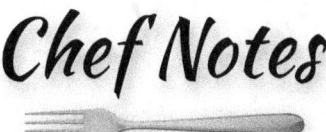

Chef Notes

- ♦ Although the recipe makes 8 ramekins, do not eat 8 in one day!
- ♦ This recipe has NO NUTRITIONAL VALUE, just empty calories.
- ♦ However, it is a festive dessert for the holidays and guests.

Nutrition Facts
Fruit Flan

Amount Per Serving

Calories 130	Calories from Fat 0

	% Daily Value*
Total Fat 0g	0%
Saturated Fat 0g	0%
Trans Fat 0g	
Cholesterol <5mg	2%
Sodium 190mg	8%
Total Carbohydrate 24g	8%
Dietary Fiber 1g	4%
Sugars 12g	
Protein 7g	

Vitamin A 0%	•		Vitamin C 20%
Calcium 2%	•		Iron 0%

* Percent Daily Values are based on a 2,000 calorie diet. Your daily values may be higher or lower depending on your calorie needs:

	Calories:	2,000	2,500
Total Fat	Less than	65g	80g
Sat Fat	Less than	20g	25g
Cholesterol	Less than	300mg	300mg
Sodium	Less than	2,400mg	2,400mg
Total Carbohydrate		300g	375g
Dietary Fiber		25g	30g

INGREDIENTS: NONFAT VANILLA YOGURT, LOW FAT COTTAGE CHEESE, COOL WHIP, STRAWBERRIES, BLUEBERRIES, SUGAR FREE JAM

ONION FACTORY: ANDERSON, IN

Chef Notes

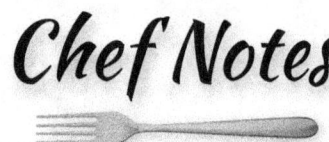

PEANUT BUTTER AND JELLY ROLL-UPS

YIELDS: 1 serving

INGREDIENTS

- ½ cup egg whites
- 2 tsp peanut butter
- 1 Tbsp sugar-free strawberry jelly or jam
- cinnamon to taste
- Splenda® to taste

DIRECTIONS

1. Spray omelet pan with Pam®. Add egg whites, then sprinkle with cinnamon and Splenda®.
2. When egg whites begin to set, add 2 tsp peanut better to melt and spread.
3. Warm jelly in microwave, drizzle over peanut butter.
4. Finish cooking until egg whites are set.
5. Roll and place on plate. Drizzle with a little jelly, add a sprinkle of cinnamon.

Nutrition Facts
Peanut Butter and Jelly Roll-Ups

Amount Per Serving

Calories 120	Calories from Fat 35

	% Daily Value*
Total Fat 4g	6%
Saturated Fat 1g	5%
Trans Fat 0g	
Cholesterol 0mg	0%
Sodium 220mg	9%
Total Carbohydrate 8g	3%
Dietary Fiber 3g	12%
Sugars <1g	
Protein 14g	

Vitamin A 0%	•	Vitamin C 0%	
Calcium 2%	•	Iron 2%	

* Percent Daily Values are based on a 2,000 calorie diet. Your daily values may be higher or lower depending on your calorie needs:

	Calories:	2,000	2,500
Total Fat	Less than	65g	80g
Sat Fat	Less than	20g	25g
Cholesterol	Less than	300mg	300mg
Sodium	Less than	2,400mg	2,400mg
Total Carbohydrate		300g	375g
Dietary Fiber		25g	30g

INGREDIENTS: EGG WHITES, SUGAR FREE JAM, PEANUT BUTTER, CINNAMON, SPLENDA

ONION FACTORY: ANDERSON, IN

SNICKERS® FIX

YIELDS: 1 serving

INGREDIENTS

- ½ small Gala apple
- 1 tsp peanut butter
- 1 tsp finely chopped peanuts

DIRECTIONS

1. Cut apple in half and core.
2. Warm peanut butter in microwave for 3–5 seconds until it melts.
3. Dip apple half in warm peanut butter and dip in peanuts.

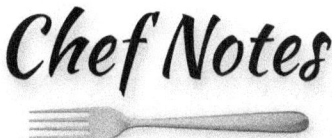

- Snickers® Fix is for a day when you are craving a candy bar and need more than berries.
- Be careful! An apple has 22 grams of sugar and berries are much lower in sugar.

Nutrition Facts
Snickers® Fix

Amount Per Serving	
Calories 80	Calories from Fat 30
	% Daily Value*
Total Fat 3.5g	5%
Saturated Fat 0.5g	3%
Trans Fat 0g	
Cholesterol 0mg	0%
Sodium 20mg	1%
Total Carbohydrate 12g	4%
Dietary Fiber 2g	8%
Sugars 8g	
Protein 2g	
Vitamin A 0% • Vitamin C 6%	
Calcium 0% • Iron 2%	

* Percent Daily Values are based on a 2,000 calorie diet. Your daily values may be higher or lower depending on your calorie needs:

	Calories:	2,000	2,500
Total Fat	Less than	65g	80g
Sat Fat	Less than	20g	25g
Cholesterol	Less than	300mg	300mg
Sodium	Less than	2,400mg	2,400mg
Total Carbohydrate		300g	375g
Dietary Fiber		25g	30g

INGREDIENTS: APPLE, PEANUT BUTTER, PEANUT

ONION FACTORY: ANDERSON,IN

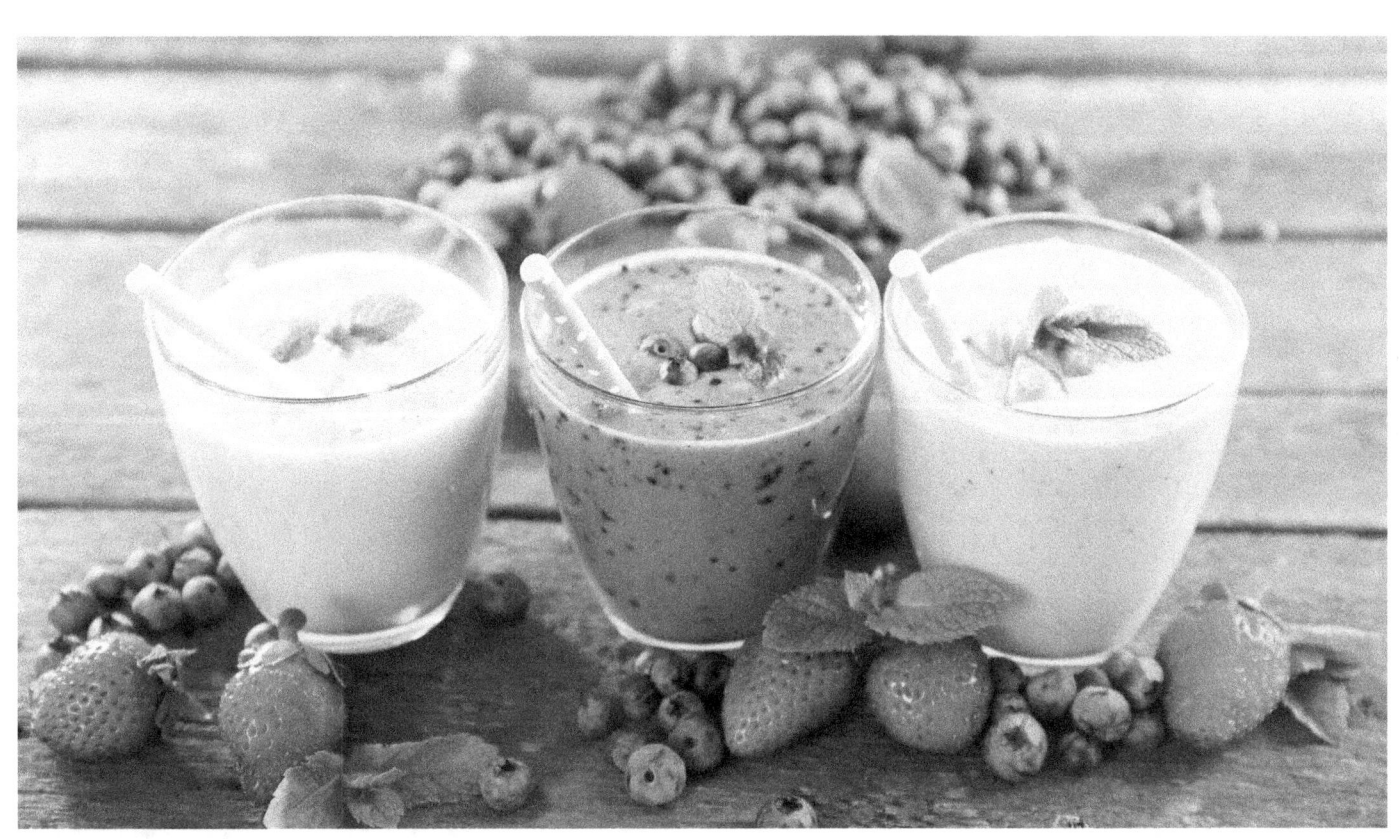

beverages

SHARE A CUP OF HOSPITALITY

CAPPUCCINO

YIELDS: 1 serving

INGREDIENTS

- ☐ 1 scoop Nectar® Cappuccino protein powder
- ☐ 1 cup water

DIRECTIONS

1. Fill 1 cup measure with water and heat in microwave for 1 minute 20 seconds.
2. Pour hot water in blender and add Nectar® protein powder.
3. Blend on high until frothy.

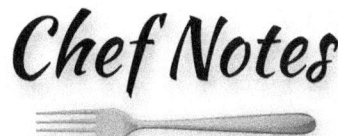

Chef Notes

♦ If your cappuccino curdles, the water is too hot. Reduce heating time.

Nutrition Facts

Cappuccino

Amount Per Serving

Calories 100	Calories from Fat 0

% Daily Value*

Total Fat 0g	0%
Saturated Fat 0g	0%
Trans Fat 0g	
Cholesterol 0mg	0%
Sodium 55mg	2%
Total Carbohydrate 0g	0%
Dietary Fiber 0g	0%
Sugars 0g	
Protein 23g	

Vitamin A 0%	•	Vitamin C 0%
Calcium 8%	•	Iron 0%

* Percent Daily Values are based on a 2,000 calorie diet. Your daily values may be higher or lower depending on your calorie needs:

		Calories:	2,000	2,500
Total Fat	Less than		65g	80g
Sat Fat	Less than		20g	25g
Cholesterol	Less than		300mg	300mg
Sodium	Less than		2,400mg	2,400mg
Total Carbohydrate			300g	375g
Dietary Fiber			25g	30g

NGREDIENTS: NECTAR CAPPUCCINO

ƆNION FACTORY: ANDERSON.IN

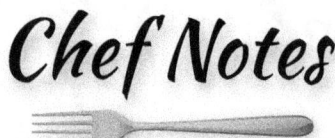

Chef Notes

CHOCOLATE MILK

YIELDS: 1 serving

INGREDIENTS

- ☐ 1 scoop Matrix® Perfect Chocolate protein powder
- ☐ 1 cup ice and cold water

DIRECTIONS

1. Fill one cup measure with ice. Add water to the I-cup line.
2. Pour in blender and add Matrix® protein powder.
3. Blend on high for 15–30 seconds.

Nutrition Facts
Chocolate Milk

Amount Per Serving

Calories 120	Calories from Fat 20

	% Daily Value*
Total Fat 2g	3%
Saturated Fat 1g	5%
Trans Fat 0g	
Cholesterol 40mg	13%
Sodium 140mg	6%
Total Carbohydrate 3g	1%
Dietary Fiber 1g	4%
Sugars 2g	
Protein 23g	

Vitamin A 0%	•	Vitamin C 0%	
Calcium 0%	•	Iron 4%	

* Percent Daily Values are based on a 2,000 calorie diet. Your daily values may be higher or lower depending on your calorie needs:

	Calories:	2,000	2,500
Total Fat	Less than	65g	80g
Sat Fat	Less than	20g	25g
Cholesterol	Less than	300mg	300mg
Sodium	Less than	2,400mg	2,400mg
Total Carbohydrate		300g	375g
Dietary Fiber		25g	30g

INGREDIENTS: MATRIX CHOCOLATE

ONION FACTORY: ANDERSON, IN

LEMON SHAKE-UP

YIELDS: 1 serving

INGREDIENTS

- 1 scoop Nectar® lemonade protein powder
- 1 cup ice and cold water

DIRECTIONS

1. Fill 1 cup measure with ice, add water to fill to 1-cup line.
2. Pour water into blender. Pulse in Nectar® for 30 seconds.

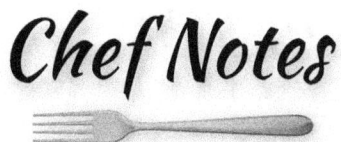

- An old State Fair favorite without the guilt of sugar!

Nutrition Facts
Lemon Shake-Up

Amount Per Serving	
Calories 100	Calories from Fat 0
	% Daily Value*
Total Fat 0g	0%
Saturated Fat 0g	0%
Trans Fat 0g	
Cholesterol 0mg	0%
Sodium 70mg	3%
Total Carbohydrate 0g	0%
Dietary Fiber 0g	0%
Sugars 0g	
Protein 23g	
Vitamin A 0% • Vitamin C 0%	
Calcium 8% • Iron 0%	

* Percent Daily Values are based on a 2,000 calorie diet. Your daily values may be higher or lower depending on your calorie needs:

	Calories:	2,000	2,500
Total Fat	Less than	65g	80g
Sat Fat	Less than	20g	25g
Cholesterol	Less than	300mg	300mg
Sodium	Less than	2,400mg	2,400mg
Total Carbohydrate		300g	375g
Dietary Fiber		25g	30g

INGREDIENTS: NECTAR ROADSIDE LEMONADE

ONION FACTORY: ANDERSON, IN

Chef Notes

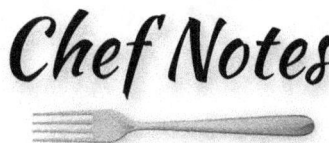

STRAWBERRY SHAKE

YIELDS: 1 serving

INGREDIENTS

- ❏ 1 cup frozen whole strawberries
- ❏ water to make 1 cup
- ❏ 1 scoop Matrix® vanilla protein powder
- ❏ light whipped cream

DIRECTIONS

1. Place 1 cup frozen strawberries in measuring cup.
2. Add water to 1-cup line.
3. Place in blender with 1 scoop Matrix® protein powder.
4. Blend on high for 15–30 seconds.
5. Top with a dollop of light whipped cream.

Nutrition Facts

Strawberry Shake

Amount Per Serving

Calories 140 — Calories from Fat 20

	% Daily Value*
Total Fat 2g	3%
Saturated Fat 1.5g	8%
Trans Fat 0g	
Cholesterol 40mg	13%
Sodium 90mg	4%
Total Carbohydrate 9g	3%
Dietary Fiber 2g	8%
Sugars 6g	
Protein 23g	

Vitamin A 2%	•	Vitamin C 50%
Calcium 15%	•	Iron 4%

* Percent Daily Values are based on a 2,000 calorie diet. Your daily values may be higher or lower depending on your calorie needs:

	Calories:	2,000	2,500
Total Fat	Less than	65g	80g
Sat Fat	Less than	20g	25g
Cholesterol	Less than	300mg	300mg
Sodium	Less than	2,400mg	2,400mg
Total Carbohydrate		300g	375g
Dietary Fiber		25g	30g

INGREDIENTS: STRAWBERRIES, MATRIX SIMPLY VANILLA, WHIPPED CREAM

ONION FACTORY: ANDERSON, IN

7 Shortcuts

- Chili Lime chicken burgers
- Turkey meatballs (Trader Joe's® or Aldi's®)
- Ahi Tuna (Trader Joe's®)
- Wendy's® chili
- Deli meat (the easiest and cleanest quarter-pound of protein you can find)
- Celery & Better 'N Peanut Butter® (1 Tbsp = 1g fat, 6.5g carbs, 2g sugar, 2g protein)
- Hardboiled eggs (Check any gas station's convenience section.)

Emergency Kit

- Ostrim® meat jerky sticks
- Protein drinks (e.g., Muscle Milk Light® or EAS)
- Snack pack pickles (not the sweet ones)
- V8® vegetable juice
- Edamame (¼ cup = 4g fat, 10g carbs, 14g protein)
- Turkey pepperoni
- 2% light mozzarella cheese sticks (1 stick = 2.5g fat, 8g protein)
- Kroger® Gel Bites® (Enjoy the entire bag if you like. They are all protein.)

12. Circle of Influence

HAVE YOU EVER NOTICED that fluffy people tend to hang out with other fluffy people and fit people tend to hang out with other fit people? We feel more comfortable with those people who are most like us. However, if you've noticed, it only takes one person, who is losing weight, to influence the rest of the fluffy crowd. Then, everyone wants to know what you are doing to lose. Sometimes the influence is wacky. Like why is it that the moment you decide to start that "diet" or begin that fitness program your thin friends and family want to invite you out for lunch?

What I love about Onions' leadership is how they do not force others into changes. They lead by example. As a fluffy girl, I remember the pressure of getting "the look" if I ordered a dessert. When something is taken away, or forbidden, we seem to desire it more. When we cannot have something, even if we did not desire it in the first place, suddenly we are starving for it. If we embrace the understanding that we are in trouble with obesity, then we must influence others carefully.

With our kids, we must not sabotage them by the look, or the negative imprints we give with "the look." We must lead them with our own nutritional changes. You will be amazed how your family will graze on the good stuff if there is no bad stuff available. Whatever happened to the relish tray? When you are hungry, fresh berries, or broccoli and dip taste amazing! Who does the grocery shopping in the house? Who is the enabler? It is up to us to lead our children into healthy living.

Women Set the Pace

As moms, daughters, and wives, we have a huge opportunity to fix the state our families are in. As 30-, 40-, 50-, and 60-plus-year-olds, we know just how hard the battle has been fighting our own weight. But if we look back to our size and appearance when we were in our teens, or our twenties, we can see that we weren't in as bad of shape as our youth are now. Like most moms, I loved the convenience of fast food. But I think fast food was meant to be the exception to the rule, not the mainstay of our nutrition.

It's pretty well accepted that in most American households, women do the cooking and the grocery shopping. Imagine, as you take this journey of finding the woman within, the woman behind layers of fat, layers of myths, and oodles of old behaviors, not only will you change your life, but your new habits will be contagious.

In essence, we have the ability to change the course of obesity right in our homes. The first step is to teach you how to eat versus starve, and the next step will be to make simple adjustments in your shopping and cooking, so your family can enjoy the same results. I can't tell you how many Onions come in and tell me that their husband, or daughter has lost as much, or more, during her camp just from a few modifications. The biggest hurdle is getting the fillers out of your daily nutrition. Remember, we are already full, over-full in fact.

The current generation does not have pass away before us. By making the commitment to change, we can alter the understanding of food for our children and grandchildren. I fear if we don't, obesity might be society's demise.

As you increase your understanding and you learn that you can get great nutrition from food choices that will not go straight to your butt, you will not be hungry. The dynamics of good nutrition for everyone in your household can change. Just ask Gail.

All in the Family

I have had many people come in and out of my life during the past few years of putting this guide together. Surprisingly, it seems that the people I need, the information, and the confirmation of thoughts seem to be in front of me right when I need them most. Gail has been with me now for a while. She is another amazing woman from Anderson, Indiana. Gail is a BSN, RN, and IBCLC, which is short for International Board Certified Lactation Consultant, very impressive credentials.

The part I love about meeting Gail is she came in thinking, "I know this stuff," even though at 50-years-old she had grown into a size 28. She understood the value of protein. She was trained in nursing school on basic nutrition. Okay, maybe she really never loved exercising, but she is an intelligent woman. I thought: *How did she grow into a size 28?*

As she was learning how to peel her body, we shared many aha moments, especially when

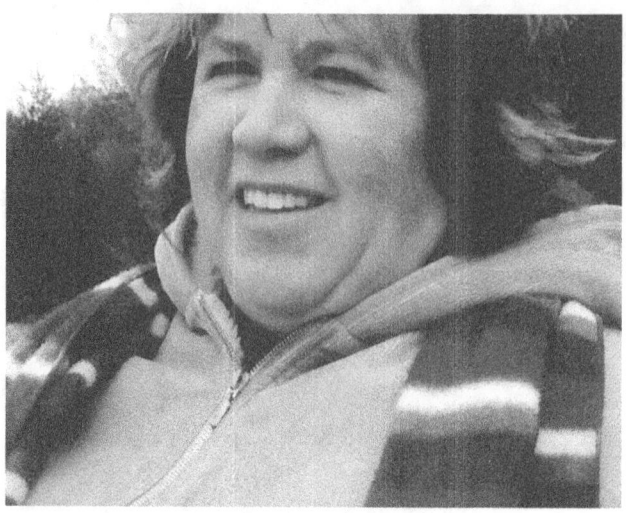

Gail BEFORE

we discussed the need to add more protein to her nutrition. Adequate protein was one of the missing links for Gail.

As we adjusted her body composition each week, I kept noticing she would lose fat, but she would also lose lean mass. We would continue to tweak her nutritional needs until she could just lose fat. Who cares if you can lose five pounds of water this week? But, wow, if you can lose five pounds of fat. Impressive! If you sacrificed five pounds of muscle this week, then you have just worked against yourself. Gail needed more protein.

Today, Gail and I had another personal training session. Last week, we worked out a few bugs in her nutrition, and she was able to peel off another six pounds, reaching 79 pounds lost. She is still losing a little lean in the equation, however, we are heading in the right direction.

December was not a big month, results-wise, for Gail. She recently accepted a promotion at the hospital and found herself invited to many holiday events. And we know all "events" are always surrounded by food especially around the holidays. I think she was excited to get through the holidays without any weight gains, but she also did not move closer to her goal.

Last week was monumental for her, because we figured out what she was adding to her daily nutrition (the food plan) that was throwing her into stuck mode; too many berries and a few animal crackers, ouch.

She was only burning off the extras she had consumed during her cardio sessions. Even though berries are healthy, too much fructose is still too much fructose. The body can only burn off so much. I think she is really ready for the next peel.

It is amazing what a great week will do for the psyche. I also think the tough times force you to learn about your body, and the good weeks inspire a person to go all the way, or at least one more week.

As Gail moves closer to her goals, her daughters are getting nervous. Mom was always a size 28. Now Mom is a 16. The thought that Mom is getting closer to the size of clothes they wear, as she gets smaller and smaller, is unacceptable. She isn't allowed to get smaller than they are.

I know this because Gail started her first camp with her daughter Katie, who was getting ready to be married. Unfortunately, Katie fell out halfway through camp due to a car accident. The accident, and all the stress of getting married, probably did not facilitate the right time to change and learn how to be on her game nutritionally and physically. She would need all of her energy just to enjoy the most important day of her life. A year later, she is settled. Now she is ready. Tonight, I had her in part two of the camp she started almost a year ago. Katie is fed up. The time is right, and she is ready to peel.

In addition to Katie, Gail has another daughter, Natalie, who is 15. Although Natalie did not join an Onion camp, she lost 30 pounds during Gail's journey.

It was funny when Gail explained the success today. She said, "All I started doing was replacing old recipes with new ones. My family did not even notice the fillers were gone. We replaced pasta with broccoli in our lasagna dish. We replaced spaghetti noodles with spaghetti squash, and before I knew it, Natalie was 30 pounds lighter."

Family Influence

Let me tell you a story about family, community, relationships, and influence. The story begins with wife and mom, Brenda. Brenda proved my theory about women and their opportunity to produce change. She decided, last fall, that she was not going to spend another winter sitting on the couch.

Brenda started an Onion camp, changed the way she was eating and started strengthening her heart and stimulating her muscles to prevent atrophy. She began peeling and turned back the clock of time. Guess what also happened? With the changes in her cooking, Brenda's husband, Ron, lost 25 pounds!

Ron soon got the itch to get more results; so, Brenda sent him to Onion camp. She was so excited to see her husband change. And she is so disciplined. Brenda never set any records, but slow and steady always wins the race. She finished! To date, she has lost 50 pounds.

Family Influence Continues

I remember the day Brenda looked at me and said, "I wish my daughter Tammy would do this." Brenda is the coolest mom ever. She leads by example and she is soft spoken, but the greatest impact on her family comes from the choices she's made. Instead of demanding change, she facilitates change.

Around the time Ron had lost 50 pounds, Brenda announced, "I think my daughter is coming to your next seminar." I thought I could see tears welling in her eyes. You could see how proud and excited she was. Her daughter, Tami, started the

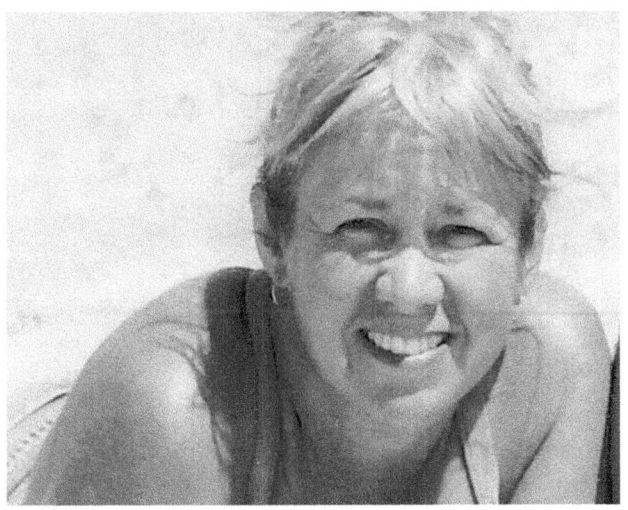

Gail AFTER

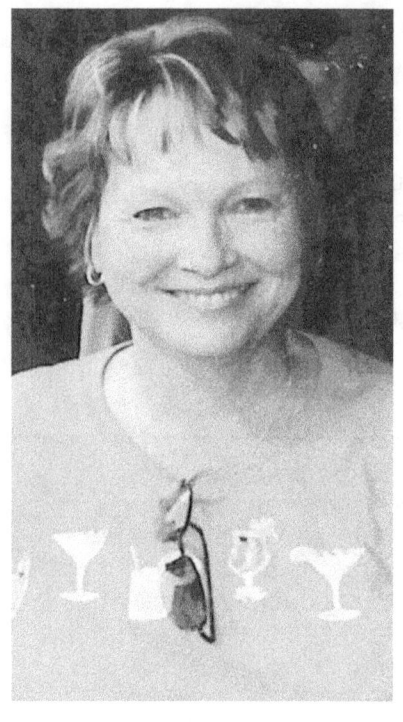
Brenda BEFORE

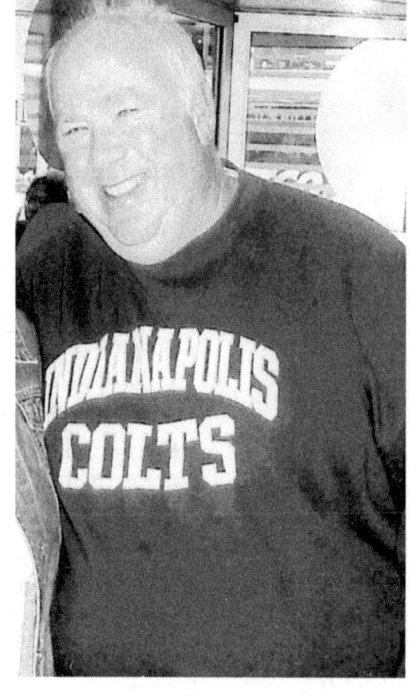
Ron BEFORE

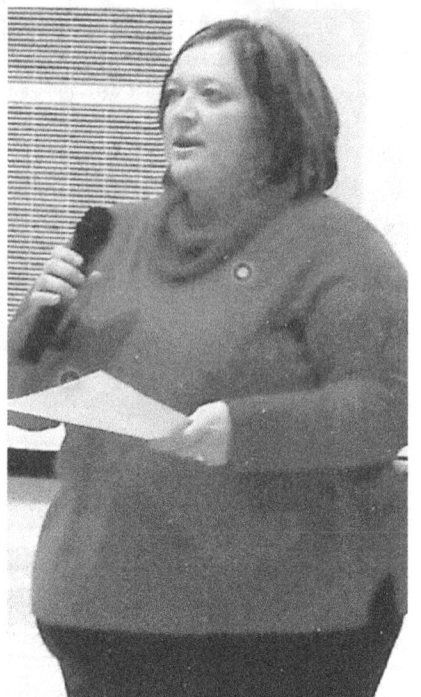
Tammy BEFORE

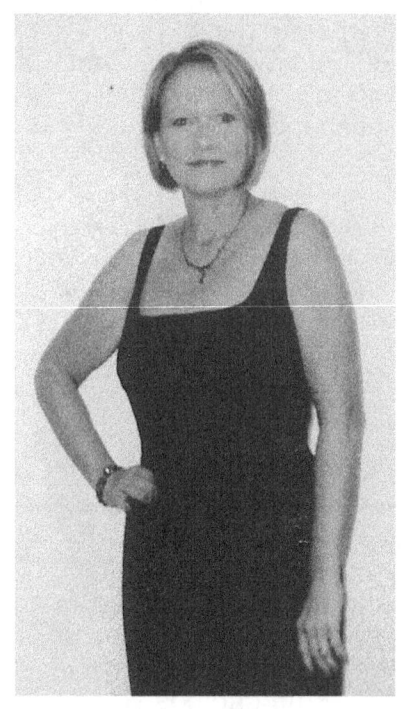
Brenda AFTER

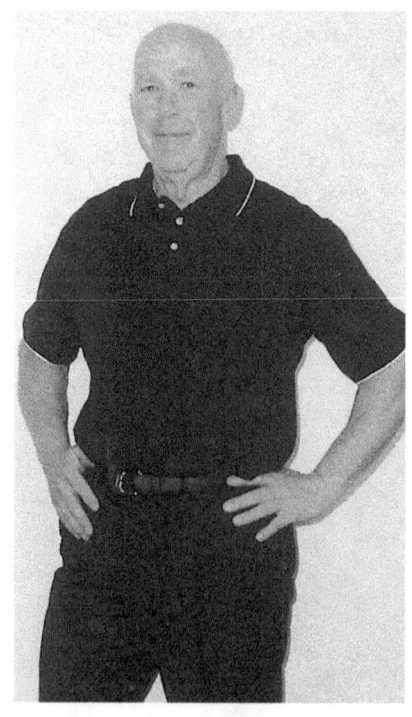
Ron AFTER

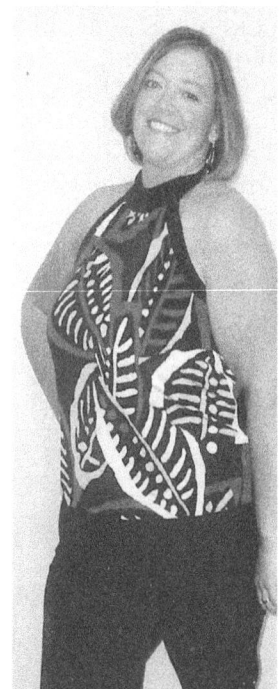
Tammy AFTER

following camp, and she came in with determination and drive. Tammy has been setting new records! She has lost almost 100 pounds in seven months! Everyone who walks into their family business is amazed at the success of Brenda, Ron, and Tammy. This family doesn't just amaze others. They are spreading their new knowledge about nutrition and health into the community.

Community Influence Spreads

The best thoughts in this guide are shared from the girls in my community. This is real life happening, and the girls have worked very hard at finding their way to create a new version of themselves.

Recently, a client shared her revelation with me. She stated boldly, "I told my husband no more BLT's." I thought to myself: *Of course no BLT's. They are on bread, and we are already full.* I must have appeared confused, because she clarified, "No more Bites, Licks, or Tastes!" She knew those bites, licks, and tastes would derail off her game and get in the way of her realizing a great week of results. She is focused on the science of peeling. And she is influencing everyone around her.

Remember Chris? She was the first Onion to reach the goal of 100 pounds lost, and she is the angel on my shoulder. She has kept me on-task, both personally and professionally, since her camp back in 2005. Chris has been a wonderful spokesperson and billboard as she checks in patients in a busy doctor's office. My story of community and relationships continues with Chris's influence.

Anna first learned about the Onion system by going to her doctor, where Chris works, and seeing how much weight Chris had lost. Around that same time, Anna and her husband, Larry, happened to go into Brenda and Ron's place of business. After seeing Brenda, Ron, and Tami, Anna was impressed with their family's new healthy bodies and lifestyle changes. Soon, Anna signed up and started Onion Camp.

Anna lost 26 pounds, 26 inches and 3-percent body fat in just eight weeks. More importantly, Anna found herself. She had spent a lifetime taking care of the school cafeteria. After retiring, she still filled in as a substitute whenever the school needed her.

One of Anna's big victories was how she improved her posture. From the beginning, I noticed how much she leaned over. It's not uncommon for individuals who have a desk job, work over a counter, or even medical professionals, who lean over patients all day, to have poor posture. I am passionate about good posture.

When I work with clients, I give extra attention to the shoulder area and to the front and the back of the deltoid (shoulder). The back of the deltoid is called the posterior deltoid. It is the body part that in usually underdeveloped, or shortened, from lack of use; thus the slouch. When you lose weight via good nutrition and strength training, two things will happen. First, a woman's bra straps will get loose and saggy, so I frequently suggest that the girls shorten their straps. The second thing is your posture will improve.

Posture is a key to great appearance and a lean look. One of the easiest things you can do to strengthen your core is sit up straight, stand up straight, and do not slouch! Anna noticed her back feeling better, and she says she had never before realized that she did not sit up straight.

The cafeteria kept calling for Anna's help. Anna kept telling them that not only was she retired, but also, the constant standing and slouching was getting to her. The more she improved her health, the more lifestyle changes she wanted to make. She was feeling good. No more backaches, loads more energy, and a dress size or two smaller all at the age of 58.

Her final epiphany, and decision, came when she told the school cafeteria that she would no longer fill in. Helping them out was getting in the way of her feeling better.

Like Brenda influenced Ron, Anna's new choices influenced her husband Larry, who struggles with sugar diabetes and heart problems. He has a pacemaker. I have often wondered if Anna's determination stems more from not feeling well, or from watching her husband struggle with his health. Larry began following Anna's new food choices and lifestyle changes.

One day, Larry went in for a doctor's appointment. Chris (Angel Onion) checked him in. As the doctor was completing Larry's exam, he noticed that some open sores were healing. I mentioned earlier that Larry has diabetes. One of the manifestations of diabetes is wounds have a difficult time healing. Larry's doctor is amazed with how well the sores were healing and says, "Whatever you are doing, keep doing it, keep

> ### When Someone Loses Weight,
> ### Why Don't We Ask How They Did It?
>
> ♦ Are we afraid that they really haven't lost weight, and we do not want to be wrong?
>
> ♦ Are we afraid to imply that they were fat before?
>
> ♦ Is it because we are struggling with weight loss ourselves, and seeing someone else lose weight puts pressure on us?
>
> ♦ Is it too personal of a question to ask?

it up!" It's amazing what a little solid nutrition can do for a body. All Larry did was follow Anna's lead in removing white flour and white sugar from his nutrition and paying attention to lean proteins and veggies.

The best part of these community relationships and influence stories is how I learned about the connections. One day, the wife of the doctor—the office where Chris works—came into my office and shared with me how well Larry was doing. To which I replied, "Is everyone in this town interconnected?"

I love learning how we are making a difference, not just with the women who come to an eight-week course at The Onion Factory℠, but how we are truly impacting our community.

A few other patients, who saw Chris's transformation, later shared that they were afraid to ask if she was losing weight. I need to think deeper about that thought, because there must be loads of psychology as to why we do not inquire about it when we see someone is losing weight.

We need to discover the answers to these questions, so our nutritional recovery plan is available to more of the community and reach out beyond our current universe of 1,500+ camp graduates.

What about the Men?

While seminars are not a carbon copy of each other, I am confident that each one is fairly close to the past one. Although men attend the same seminars as women, I often question whether they grasp the same information.

I finally asked a male Onion, Bill, if he had indeed attended a seminar, or did he have a selective-listening disorder? He responded that he'd learned a long time ago how to tune women out. Bill is a blast. If all goes as planned, he will be the first male Onion to reach 100 pounds lost. Never in a million years would I have thought I would be working with the male segment of our population. I quickly learned that obesity is not gender specific, and it is universal. As soon as women started making changes and achieving weight loss and good health, the men desired to follow suit, copycats that they are.

Let's get something off your mind really quick. You are sitting there thinking, *But don't men lose faster then women?* Guess what? One pound of fat equals 3,500 calories, whether it's stored on a man or a woman. The difference between the sexes can only be found in their beginning metabolic rates. Because men have more lean mass (muscle), they naturally have a higher metabolic rate and can burn up their reserve tank quicker.

A side factor may be that women crave breads and sweets while men tend to crave meats. Lucky them, as long as their meat choices are lean and not high in saturated fat. Men crave food that feeds the muscle, and we crave food that is sent quickly to our assets. We have a problem with our male Onions forgetting some of the information they learned from their seminar. They fail to remember the following:

- Protein shakes are mixed with water, not milk, saving 12 grams of sugar per serving.
- Saturday night cocktails must be put on hold.
- Scotch is a cocktail, so it also goes on hold.
- Not eating because you are not hungry is not an option.
- Drinking enough water is crucial.

For our guy Onions, we call their camp Man Camp; sort of like the latest real estate offerings of man caves. I would like to share a newspaper article with you about an Onion from one of our Man Camps.

Man Camp's "Biggest Loser"

The Onion Factory recently awarded 64-year-old Walter B. the distinction of "Biggest Loser." To date, he has lost 75 pounds and is reclaiming his life.

Once an avid outdoorsman who loved to tromp through the woods, hunt, and go fishing, Walter had gained too much weight to move around comfortably. With high blood pressure, he tired easily and was experiencing shortness of breath. Teetering on the edge of a serious health crisis, Walter recalls, "I was not at all happy with the way I was feeling and looking. I couldn't enjoy outdoor, or even indoor, activities like I wished."

Battling extra pounds for years, he'd tried other avenues of losing weight. While enjoying success for a time, "it never lasted, and I would end up gaining back more than I'd lost."

One day, a customer who'd lost weight walked into his place of business. "I hardly knew what to say about his weight loss," Walter recalls. The customer explained that he had achieved success through The Onion Factory^{SM}. Walter considered the visit a "wake up call." He attended the very next seminar, joined The Onion Factory^{SM}'s **Man Camp** and found a system that worked. "After using The Onion Factory^{SM}

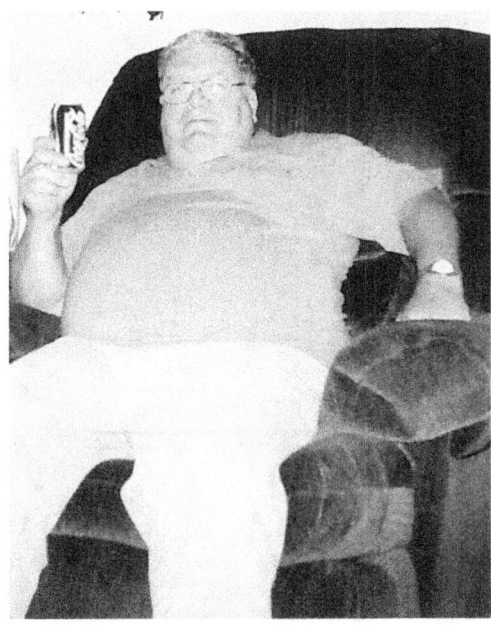
Walter BEFORE

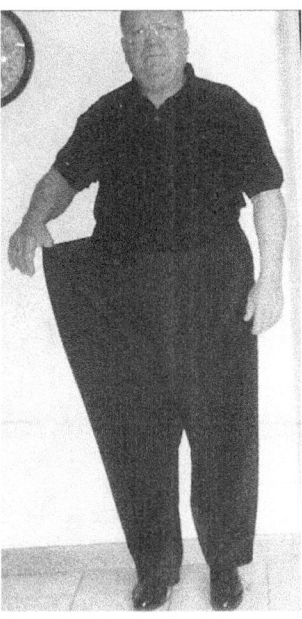
Walter AFTER

principles of exercising and nutrition, I have learned that it is necessary to put both together for any lasting results," he says.

Although his family and friends were unaware Walter had started the Onion program, they sure noticed as weight began falling off him. "My friends, some of them going all the way back to when we were in school, were amazed that something worked, that I was able to stay with it." Walter's kids are thrilled. In return, their happiness motivates him to continue the "slow, but steady" loss. "My goal is much more than 100 pounds, but I am grateful for what I've lost," he says.

Walter's life reflects his new freedom. Gaining better health and physical strength, he moves about with ever-increasing ease. Come September, Walter will enjoy an activity he's greatly missed. The avid outdoorsman will return to tromping around the woods, elk hunting in Colorado.

Firefighter's Stats

Below is a note that I found on my desk. To date, I am not sure which firefighter's wife shared this with me.

My husband is a professional fire fighter for the city. A requirement for his job is to have a complete physical each year. He uses a weight-loss program provided by the city. So my husband is not an "Onion," but he has changed the way he eats to support my change of [nutrition]. In other words, he eats what I eat. What is really cool is the person comparing his stats between this year's physical and last year's was prompted to ask him if he had changed what he eats.

For me, it was that aha moment when I knew all those long hours were making a difference.

Another note confirmed that the past few years of my life have been the best journey anyone could experience. An email from one of my guy Onions reads:

Lisa,

*Thank you so much. I have lost a total of 50 pounds as of today. I am going to try to keep it off by myself and train at home. So far, so good. I would like to lose another 30 pounds. I feel so much better than I did and do so much more than in the past. I am sure that it has done nothing but help my health also.
Thank you very much. What a lifesaver you are. Thank you again from the bottom of my heart.*

After 8 Weeks in "Man Camp"

Take a look at the great results another Man Camp Onion is producing! Matt has changed his nutrition and training, and he is inspiring us with his dedication. Here's what Matt lost in just eight weeks:

- ❖ 43 pounds
- ❖ 23 inches
- ❖ 4.2% body fat

With a Guy Onion, we see exactly how the layers peel.

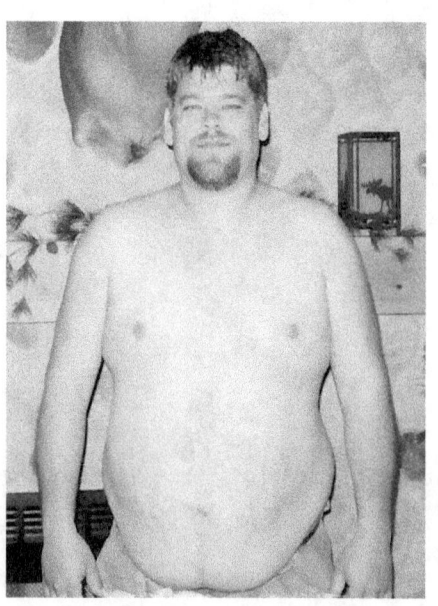

Matt BEFORE

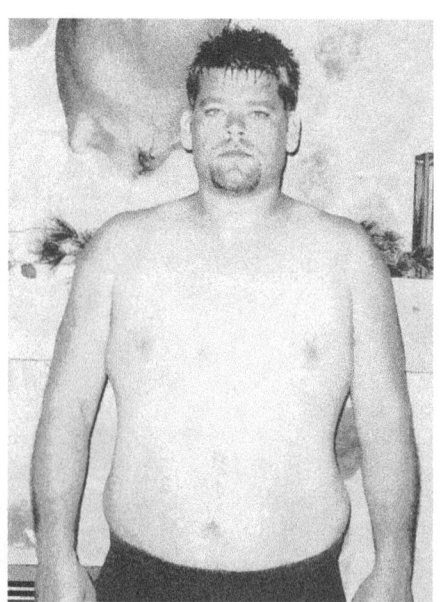

Matt AFTER

Circle of Influence

THEY DID IT... SO CAN YOU!

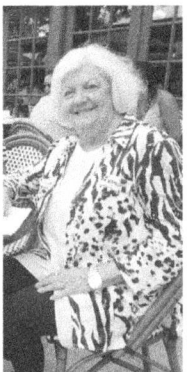

Becky - Age 77
Lost 54 lbs / 56" / 10% body fat

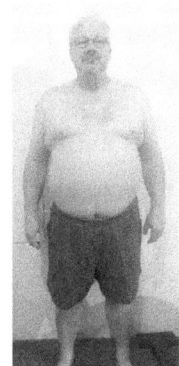

Dan - Age 61
Lost 77 lbs / 33" / 9% body fat

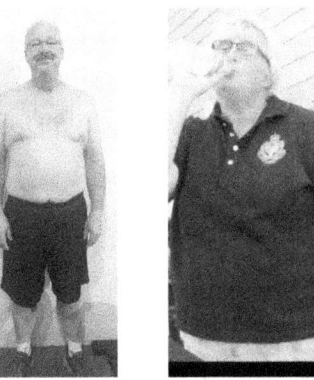

Angie - Age 52
Lost 82 lbs / 81" / 16% body fat

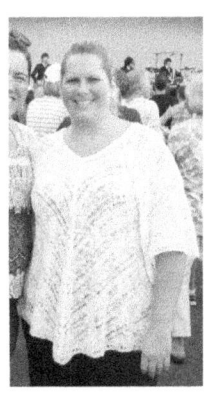

Darlene - Age 50
Lost 57 lbs / 40" / 6% body fat

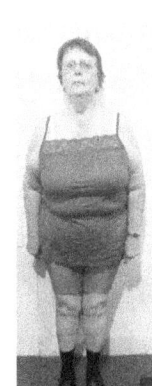

Gloria - Age 78
Lost 52 lbs / 48.5" / 9% body fat

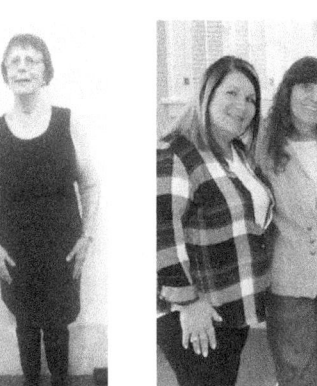

Laura F. - Age 48
Lost 46 lbs / 33" / 8% body fat

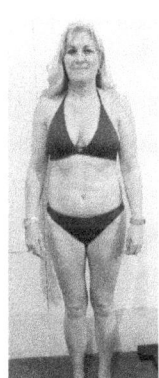

Laura R. - Age 57
Lost 22 lbs / 28.5" / 6% body fat

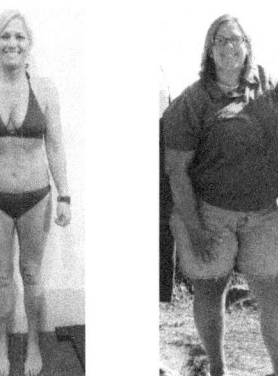

Marianne - Age 59
Lost 54 lbs / 33.5" / 7.5% body fat

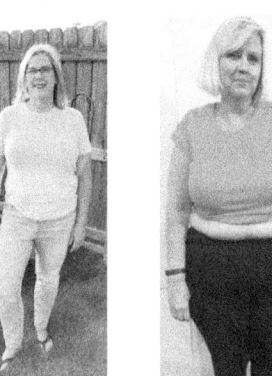
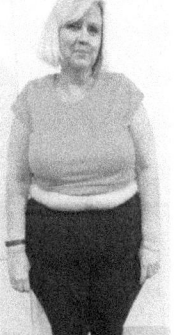
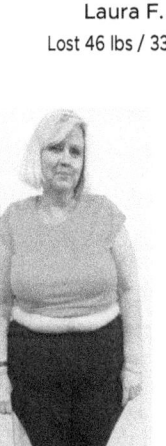

Sharon - Age 60
Lost 75 lbs / 65" / 11% body fat

13. Inspiration to Change

IF YOU ARE THINKING about picking up the challenge of working through the eight-week camp, but you feel unsure of your ability to make the lifestyle changes needed to peel, I have a few stories to tell you. They inspired me, and I'm sure they will inspire you. Let's start with Kerrie.

Kerrie's Story

Change begins when you start to identify where you are making mistakes. For Kerrie, that change started with passing up her daily trip to Dunkin Donuts. She realized that her goal of finishing the entire box of Munchkins, before she arrived at work, was not working for her. Before we go any further, take a look at what a box of doughnuts might do to you and what happens when you make a few changes.

My original goal was to help as many women as possible to obtain that 26-percent body fat benchmark. That is the number where the risk factors for health issues are no longer working against us. Kerrie did it. She went all the way. It took a year to reinvent herself. She went from 46 percent fat to 24 percent. Incredible.

I have come to the conclusion that I may not help everyone reach that 26-percent benchmark; however, I can guide most clients to change their overall level of fat by at least 10 percent. Remember, the eight-week camp record is 8-percent reduction. The average is more like 4-5 percent. If you

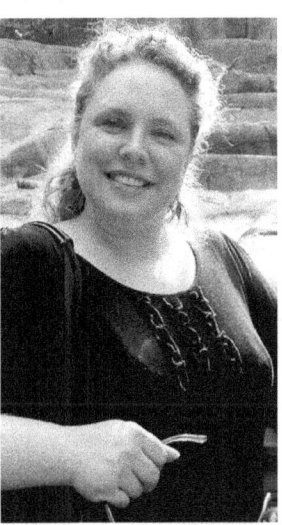

Kerrie BEFORE

232 /// The Fork Is Mightier Than the Gym

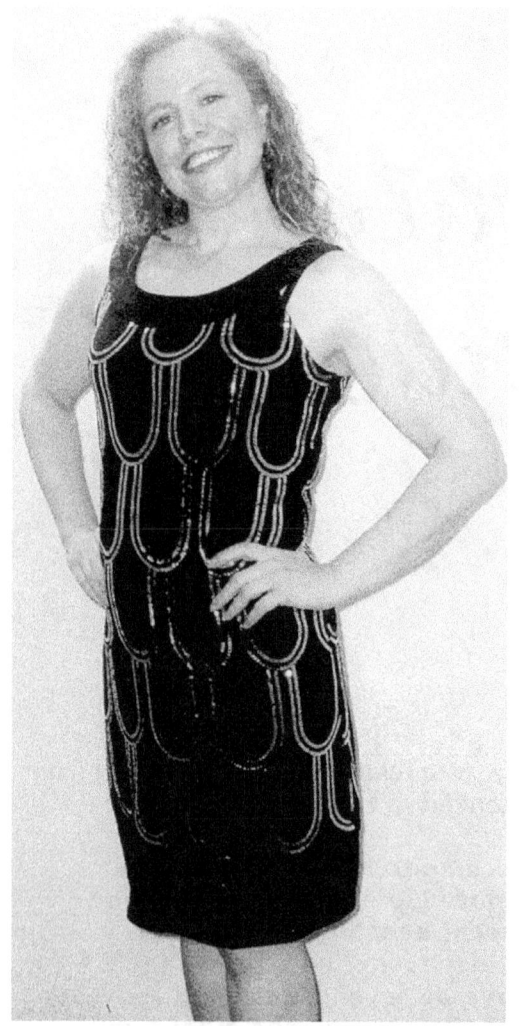

Kerrie AFTER

DATE	10/11/09	5/2/10	10/31/10	FINAL
R. ARM	14"	11.5"	10.5"	-7"
BUST	43"	36"	34.5"	-8.5"
WAIST	38"	30.5"	28.5"	-9.5"
ABS	46"	38"	34"	-12"
HIP	47"	38"	36"	-11"
THIGH	29"	23"	21"	-16"
WEIGHT	205	153.5	135	
FAT MASS	82.6	49.1	34.1	
% FAT	41	32.8	25.3	
LEAN MASS	118.9	104.4	100.9	
FAT TO GO	57.6	24.1	9.1	
			Lbs. Lost	66.5
			Inches Lost	64

Kerrie's Results

take the eight-week plunge and repeat it, you should be well on your way to repairing that engine of yours.

Kerrie's journey was such an inspiration because she not only finished the eight-week program but she realized along the way that she needed to work on her mind as well as her physical fitness and nutrition. She utilized a great tool she'd picked in one of her many self-help journeys. She shared the theory from Zarvos Consulting.

This theory says you have to want change more than you want your current behaviors. It identifies several levels of commitment, which go something like this...

1. I don't care about changing.
2. I wish. I hope I can change.

(We have all had that thought!)

3. I'll try to change.
4. I'm committed to change unless... Sounds like another excuse I have used!
5. I am committed to change 100 percent; whatever it takes.

"Whatever it takes" is the moment you see clients getting in their cardio workout at 5 A.M. or 11 P.M. because that was the only time option left. Onions are usually caregivers. Caregivers are so busy taking care of everyone and everything else that they may have become an Onion, because are not committed to themselves first, or even second, or third. Their personal needs seem to come last. Or maybe they do not want the results bad enough. What are you committed to? Do you have a vision for the future that is more exciting than where you are at right this moment? What is your urgency factor, and is that urgency for you or for someone else?

From all these wonderful stories shared from our community, I hope you find inspiration to change and find you are ready to change. Now you have the tools to change.

Transformations

Last week, a new client shared with me what is going on in her home. She is on her eleventh week and is down 50 pounds, 48 inches, and 4 percent fat. Her change is getting a little tough. In our chat, I learned she had lost before, but she knew this time things had to be different. "Different?" I asked. I looked at her perplexed.

She said that yes, this time she needed to work on the mental changes as much as the physical changes. This time she must work on the emotional connection with food, and redirect the comfort that food had been playing. This time, she needed support from her family. She was the caregiver, but her husband's role in the family had needed to change—so her role could. My client was very open, and she shared that this process of transformation was difficult on their relationship. As she found, change can be very uncomfortable.

Change is exactly what this Onion transformation is all about. As one client put it, "We are changing future generations by going back to the basics, nutritionally."

Yesterday at Starbucks®, I sat down with my morning group. Here we were, a massage therapist, a nursing student, and me, a crazy blonde who thinks she can change the course of obesity. We were all sharing our angles on how we were going to save our society. I knew obesity has reached epidemic proportions, but the word *pandemic* was thrown out on the table, so I decided to look it up. The World Health Organization suggests a pandemic can start when three conditions are met:

1. The emergence of a disease to the population.

2. The agent infects humans, causing serious illness.

3. The agent spreads easily and is sustainable among humans.

If our society does not take up the banner of changing the course of obesity, we most certainly will fall into the pandemic definition. And the future will look bleak indeed.

Medical Stories

I thought my life purpose was to change the course of obesity. Little did I realize there would be so many stories with medical miracles. I understood that obesity had reached epidemic proportions. Type 2 diabetes is growing exponentially, cholesterol levels are too high, and most Americans don't feel good physically—we have no energy and our backs hurt. What could I do to change this?

It started with anewspaper ad. I announced that I was looking for 25 women who were ready to change their lives. The phone rang off the hook. If memory serves me correctly, I had over 150 calls and 40 reservations for the Free Seminar. I was certain I had found my way. On the day of the seminar, only six people showed up. I was devastated. How can this be? Sure, I knew heading to someone's house must have been odd, but only six out of 40 reservations?

It started with one living room, one elliptical machine (a.k.a. The Beast), a few free weights that anyone could buy at Wal-Mart®, K-mart®, or Target®, and a little courage to get this thing going. Originally, I imagined that when I taught the seminar, people would have a light bulb moment and change would begin to happen. I was so wrong. Little did I realize that

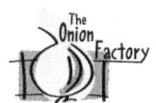

Once a body was well-fed and well-trained the fat just melted away.

even after a eight-week course, behavioral changes were not solidified. It would take eight weeks of changes and accountability before we could break old habits. After eight weeks of knowledge, support, and holding their feet to the fire, Onions truly started to peel.

By Camp Five, we were on a roll. Amazing results started to be typical. I am not talking about the loss of one or two pounds per week we had been led to expect. I am talking about major results—five pounds per week and, in some cases, a pound per day. It appeared that once a body was well-fed and well-trained using appropriate proportions of nutrition, the fat just melted away.

(I once had a client who had just taken off more than fifty pounds. One day at work, she was talking with a co-worker about her journey. The co-worker said, "I can't lose weight because I'm all muscle." My client responded, "I used to tell myself the same thing.")

Chris was the first Onion to replicate the pace I had set with my own weight loss of 100 pounds in nine months—just like birth. Once you have a pace setter, the level of expectation is created. It's easy to tell yourself that you cannot do something until you see someone older or bigger or with more medical challenges than you bring those results to the table. Change is simply about desire. By Camp Nine, the living room was busting at the seams. Parking was tough.

My children would tell you they had lost their privacy. The bathroom my Onions were using was "their" bathroom. My oldest son complained about my music selections and suggested if he heard the song "I will Survive" one more time, well, he was going to kill me. My youngest son inquired as to why I did not work with "hot" women. He was fourteen at the time.

I had an idea. (When I say I have an idea, the girls who have helped me grow this project get very nervous. In fact, if I say, "I have an idea..." they give me "the look." Here we go. You see, the idea usually includes boosting our performance to the next level so we can learn how to get more results.) I thought it was time to move out of the living room and create our first Onion Factory. Our community was downsizing and closing many of its factories, so I thought: *What a great idea! We could energize the community with a new spin on "factory." We would peel Onions and change the course of obesity at The Onion Factory*^{SM}.

For about a year and a half, we peeled many Onions at our first Factory, a three-car garage. Once you were inside, Onions said it did not feel like a garage. The first Onion Factory had bright colors, a little neon, mirrors, and energizing music to set the mood for change. But guess what? In time, we outgrew ourselves again. Many of the women had men in their lives who also needed to peel. I wanted to add case studies that were universal to men and women, so I needed a bigger garage.

Across the street sat a property with a huge garage, a lake, and a half-mile track around the lake. How perfect! It's a blur to me how the entire purchase came together, but it did, and we had a new 7,000-square-foot building to fill with Onion Factory components as well as a bathroom and a cooking school. We had loads of room to grow the Factory and peel more Onions.

My purpose in sharing our journey is this:

I saved writing the medical section of this guide until last because I wanted to

---

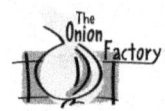

It's easy to tell yourself you cannot do something

until you see someone older or bigger

or with more medical challenges

bring those to the table.

make sure I had the proper case studies to share with you. I wanted to impress the medical community with the data, and I wanted the fitness industry to see how the opportunity of changing the course of obesity would all fit together and work. I was intimidated to write this section, let's call it stuck, until a few stories crossed my path. These stories allowed me to be able to simplify the prescriptive, and preventative, journey. And how amazing the results really are.

The following examples show how the body can repair itself and keep an overall level of health just by making a few simple changes. I'd like to tell you a few stories. Let's start with Cathy.

Cathy's Story

Remember my saying that in order to change your life, something dramatic may have to push you off the edge? Maybe it's a divorce, a special event such as a class reunion, or your son's or daughter's wedding. Perhaps it's a medical wake-up call.

It was a Thursday. Cathy had gone to see her doctor and the visit had rattled her cage. Her health had been deteriorating for some time because Cathy suffered from Type II diabetes and high cholesterol. During that Thursday appointment, Cathy's doctor handed her a business card with the doctor's home number on it, saying she would need dialysis by the weekend. Cathy's Type 2 diabetes was getting the best of her.

How could that be? She was a former tennis player, taught aerobics, and loved to run. Now she took 13 pills and four shots daily. Her A1C was 12.1 (normal is around 6.5, or lower), and her cholesterol was 280. Yikes! What is a girl to do?

In her words, "I was heading to Onion Camp!" Cathy had heard from a friend about what we were doing in the Onion Factory. She was ready to do whatever needed to be done in order to get healthy.

I guess I need to share a piece of important information. Remember that former life of mine— overweight and working in the fitness industry?

Well, Cathy was one of my aerobic instructors when we'd worked together in a fitness club. Our paths were meant to cross once again.

The episode that cinched the deal happened during a Disney family cruise. Unfortunately, Cathy spent a good deal of time getting sick over the deck rail. Not seasickness, but much more.

As I interviewed her, I listened intently because I had no idea what she went through with her health before deciding to make a few life-altering changes.

She said, "Lisa, I'm taking Byetta, which is the salvia from a gila monster, for my diabetes. I have a five-minute window to take it or I get violently ill." On that particular day, while on the Disney cruise, she missed her window of opportunity. One week after the cruise, Cathy started Onion Camp.

When Cathy walked in the door to start camp, she was eager to begin She started with 30 minutes on The Beast and would not stop until she burned 400 calories. Her fitness background was kicking in. She had drive and determination to get healthy again.

However, Cathy's fitness background did not always work in her favor. Her love of exercise actually got a tad obsessive so that

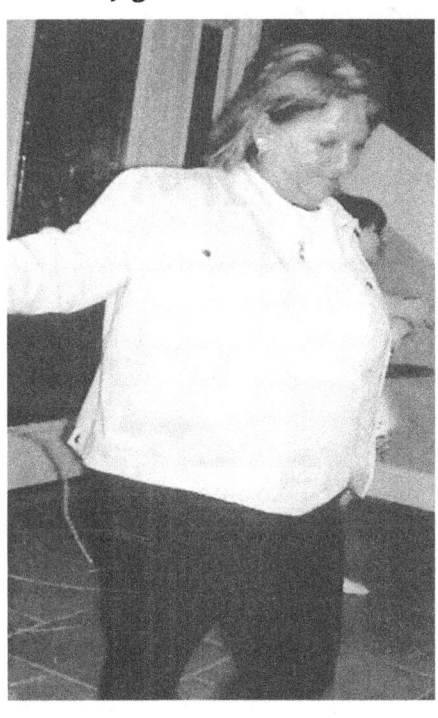

Cathy BEFORE

236 /// The Fork Is Mightier Than the Gym

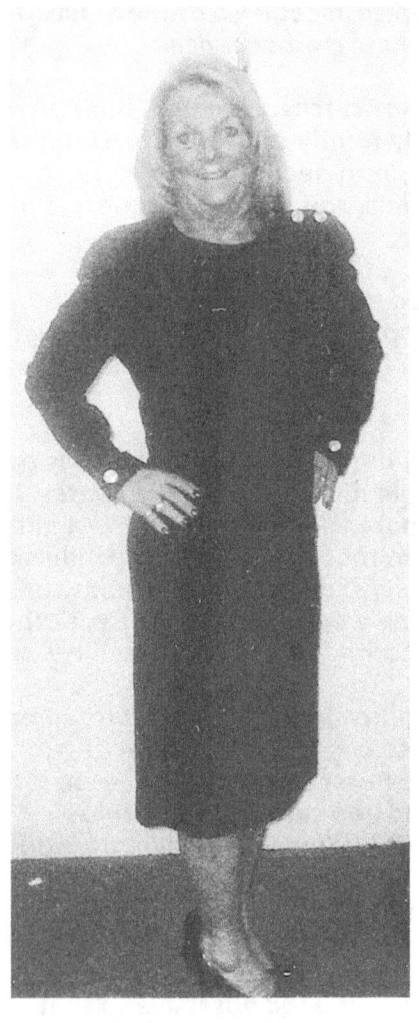

Cathy AFTER

Cathy's Results

DATE	8/27/08	12/4/10	FINAL
R. ARM	12"	10"	-4"
BUST	44"	35"	-9"
WAIST	38"	29"	-9"
ABS	45"	35"	-9"
HIPS	45"	36.5"	-8.5"
THIGH	24"	21"	-6"
WEIGHT	186	133	-53
% FAT	40	31.7	-10%
FAT TO GO	42.2	17.1	
		Lbs. Lost	53
		Inches Lost	45.5
		% Fat Lost	10.5

she got stuck. She stopped losing weight, even though she was training more than ever. How could that be? If you over-train and under-eat, that body of yours is going to protect itself and store some fat for a rainy day.

The solution? I locked her up in a weekend Onion Escape and threw away the keys. I got rid of the cell phone and ran the system by the books—proper protein, water, veggies, training, and rest. Now look how Cathy finished.

Sue's Story

Allow me to share Sue's journey. Two months prior to coming to camp, Sue had a stroke. Talk about a terrifying call to change!

After she recovered and with her doctor's permission, Sue signed up for Onion Camp. She was seriously committed to losing fat and gaining health. She did not allow her medical conditions, including high cholesterol, thyroid malfunction, and high blood pressure, nor the medications she was taking (Plavax, Lipitor, and Cynthroid), to get in her way.

In the beginning, she did not show big numbers lost on the scale. But check out her inches lost—26½" in her first eight weeks.

The scale only showed 15 pounds lost, but Sue continued transforming herself and went on to even greater results.

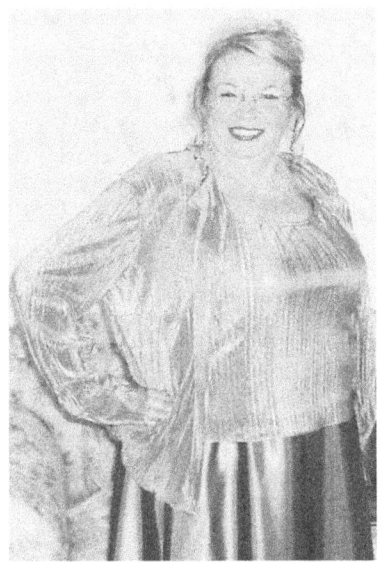

Sue BEFORE

DATE	5/6/07	10/17/07	11/19/08	FINAL
R. ARM	13.5"	11.5"	11"	-5"
BUST	44.5"	39"	37"	-7.5"
WAIST	40"	33"	30"	-10"
ABS	47.5"	40.5"	39"	-8.5"
HIPS	47.5"	40.5"	39"	-8.5"
THIGH	24.5"	21.5"	20"	-9"
WEIGHT	189	159	142	
FAT MASS	80.9	58.8	52.1	
% FAT	42.8	37.1	36.7	
LEAN MASS	108.1	100.2	89.9	
FAT TO GO	55.9	33.8	27.1	
Lbs. Lost				47
Inches Lost				48.5
% Fat Lost				6.1

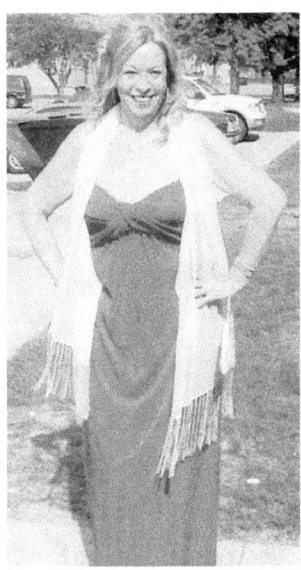

Sue AFTER

Wow! How is this for a before-and-after photo shoot? They both were taken at the Indy Senior Ball, exactly a year apart. Sue no longer looks like a senior in her sassy little red dress.

Harriet's Story

I could tell you many stories of clients I have worked with over the past years that peeled a layer or two in their senior years. But none of the stories are as fun as Harriet's. I will start right off the bat and tell you Harriet's self-proclaimed goal is to be a 78-year-old sex goddess. Just ask her. Her legs were incredible even before she came to Onion camp.

I want to show you what a little exercise and balanced nutrition can do at any age. After graduating the eight-week course in Onion camp, Harriet stayed on for a little extra polishing through personal training. What happened next is important to share, because I cannot say it enough times. When it comes to your nutrition, err on the side of protein. So many times I have seen fit girls and not-so-fit girls get stuck (in their goal to reduce weight-body fat percentage), because they are training too hard and not eating enough.

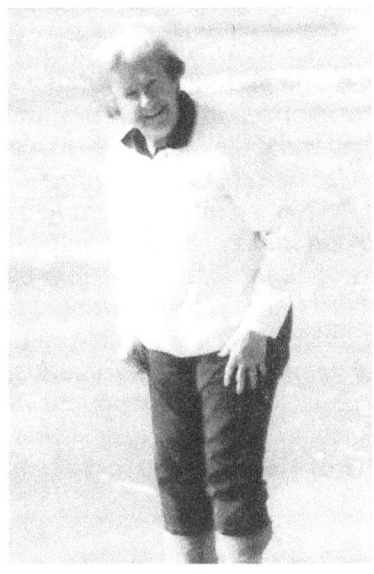

Harriet BEFORE

Remember, 80 percent of this journey is about solid nutrition. The body will naturally go into protection mode if you deprive it of enough

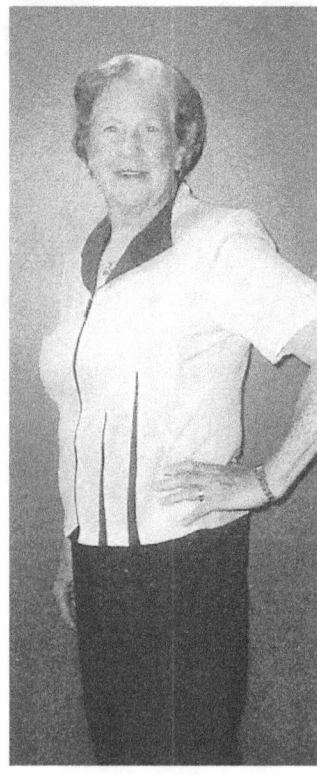

Harriet AFTER

	Wk. 1	Wk. 4	Wk. 8
R. ARM	13"	12"	11.5"
BUST	43.5"	41"	40"
WAIST	38"	36"	34"
ABS	45"	43"	41"
HIPS	46"	43"	41"
THIGH	25"	23"	22.5"
WEIGHT	187.5	180	167
% FAT	44.1	43.7	41.6
LEAN MASS	104	102	97.6
FAT TO GO	57.6	53.6	44.4

Harriet's Results

nutritious food. The body will store fat because fat is an insulator and the body prefers to be a little fatter. Until one day you wake up and realize, "Oh my gosh, what happened?"

Harriet hit this wall when she started personal training. Call it a plateau or just call it getting stuck, or call it what you want. Her protein intake was sufficient while she was doing a major muscle to minor muscle workout, but when we moved into total body training she needed to add more protein. It only took Harriet two weeks of no fat loss and little weight loss to convince her to kick in the additional protein.

Guess what happened in Week Three. Instead of losing one pound, she lost four pounds and 2.6 percent of her body fat while keeping her lean mass! I think one of the most perfect scenarios is when a prospective client is close to retirement and realizes that their prescription costs will severely impede the lifestyle they had imagined. Remember, it all goes back to that URGENCY factor. You must get to a point where you are ready to take responsibility for not just your appearance but your overall health as well.

Certainly, there are many illnesses that the only solution comes from a pill bottle. However, much of what ails this nation can be cured with a little activity and cleaning up our understanding of what is NORMAL, balanced nutrition when you are 30, 40, or 50 percent fat.

Don't ever forget. You are never too old to gain health by losing fat percentages and adding a little work out.

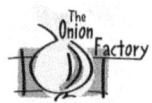

The body will go into protection mode if you deprive it of enough nutritious food.

14. Onion Camp

GET READY TO PEEL AWAY

25-40 POUNDS

IN 8 WEEKS.

SIT BACK, BUCKLE YOURSELF in, and get ready for eight weeks of reinventing yourself.

Nearly a quarter century into my journey, I am fairly confident that if you will follow my lead and learn from my mistakes, I can guide you to a victory line crossing of anywhere from 25-40 pounds lost and a few dress sizes smaller in 8 weeks. More importantly, you will lose anywhere from 4 to 8 percent of your body fat.

These result will be a better, healthier version of you and one that just may be in one of the plethora of clothes you have tucked away in your closet.

Getting Started

No more "would haves," "should haves," or "could haves." It's time. The good news is you will not be hungry. The bad news is you are going to have to carve out some time for prepping your food. This change all starts in the kitchen. I hope we have given you enough grocery ideas and recipes to help you until this new way of cooking is familiar. I also hope we have given you enough information for eating out and still staying in the box. Sure, you will have a little physical work and mental moments; however, the change is all about knowing what to buy, putting the food together, and making the time to feed your engine. Before you begin, here are few more food ideas to help you make good choices.

Breakfast Ideas

- Scrambled eggs or Eggbeaters® (Don't forget to dump the yolks.)
- Omelets
- Parfaits
- Hardboiled eggs (minus the yolks)

Add your favorite breakfast meat, but choose wisely. You'll need to pick a macronutrient such as berries, sliced tomatoes, or a V8 juice. This kindles your campfire.

Some people think it's fashionable to skip breakfast, but remember: You must eat in order to peel the fat!

Lunch Ideas

- Tuna Salad
- Chicken Salad
- Egg Salad
- Caesar Salad
- Your favorite turkey burger
- Your favorite soup

Dinner Ideas (Our Recipes)

- Meatloaf
- Baked Tilapia
- Lasagna
- Stuffed Peppers
- Beef Tips
- Spaghetti
- Chicken Broccoli Alfredo

Add a salad and your favorite veggie and you're good to go!

Snack Ideas

- Asparagus Wraps
- Cucumber Rounds
- Portabella Pizzas
- Low-Fat Mozzarella Sticks
- Sliced Tomato

Weight Training Works

Before you start Onion Camp, I'd like to encourage you to make working out work for you. Most Onions did not have a love affair with working out before they made the decision to improve. If Onions loved working out, they would not have grown into an Onion. There is nothing fancy about the Onion world, we just teach the basics. We teach balance. A little of this, a dab of that, and before you know it your new behaviors create a new you.

Lifting weights is fun. What was not fun is when we tried cardio, we tried lifting, and we did not see results. Okay, maybe lifting and doing cardio is not necessarily fun, but I promise you this. The results are! There is no better feeling in the world than putting your clothes on in the morning, and they fit. Yes, there is a better feeling, when the old ones in your closet are too big!

I use a few philosophies in weight training. They are major-to-minor muscle training, circuit, and body parts (body specific). Those are the top three that come to my mind. You are going to start with the Onion routine, which is largest to smallest muscle training. Each week you are going to challenge yourself to lift a little more weight. Weight lifting is progressive. You need to keep challenging the muscle. Actually your goal is to breakdown the muscle. Want to know why? Because the next day when the muscle is repairing itself, the source your body will use is some of your reserve tank. Guess what? We win the battle of the bulge when we allow our muscle to help us burn fat.

During weeks 5, 6, and 7, you are moving to the next level. I am going walk you through back, biceps and shoulders, then legs, and my favorite, chest and triceps.

We all know the first place fat goes on a woman is her underarm. You are in trouble when you wave, stop waving, and your loose skin keeps waving for you. Yikes! We hate it. The inner thighs go next. When they rub together and make your pants create little balls, perhaps that is a clue it's time to do something.

WEEK ONE

I want you to start on a Sunday. Take that day to shop, prep, and get all your ducks in a row. The first week is a little tough. You might even prepare your loved ones that you may be a little short fused the first week.

We are going to detoxify you. Get all the white sugar and white flour out of your system. Ouch! Once we do this, you might be tempted to go back to your old favorites, but you will not crave them as much. You will need a little willpower this week, but you will soon start feeling better and then the results will motivate you to fight for some more results.

Review your grocery list. Find the recipes that sound good to you and make a simple food plan for the week.

On the following page is a nutrition guide for tracking your daily food intake. Remember to feed your engine every 3 hours. Non-eating will feed your fat cells!

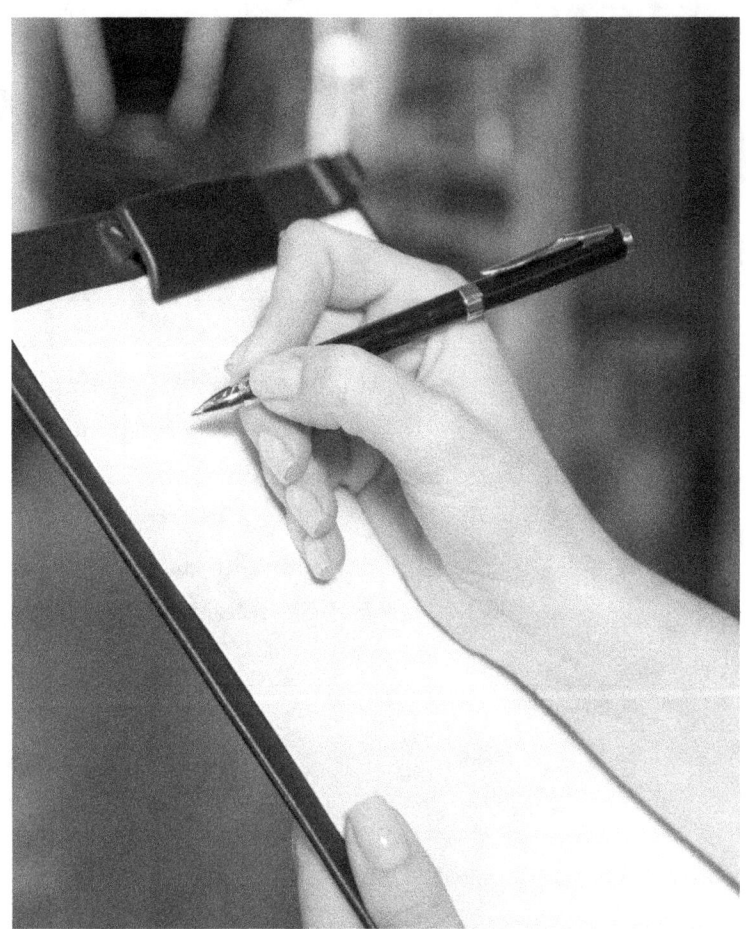

First-Week Tips

- For the first 8 weeks, stick to the berries, only one cup a day. I recommend using berries with your morning meal. If you are a sugar addict, then you may save this sweet treat for later in the day when you feel tempted.

- Read the section on salad dressings. NOW. Most mistakes about dressings are made by not taking account of their fat grams.

- Eat "grass of the lands" (green leafy stuff). Get 10 cups, spread throughout the day. Think of this as the kindling to keep your campfire lit. "Grasses of the lands" are also good for mindless nibbles.

- This week, focus on 30 minutes of cardiovascular training each day.

- Avoid caffeine.

- Write down what you do (eating and exercising) so you can learn along the way.

- Document your measurements at your starting point. Note your weight and your measurements at 6 points. (See chart on following page.) Try to get a body-comp measurement if you can buy or borrow a comp meter.

Nutrition 101

DAILY OVERVIEW GUIDE

	Protein (75 gms)	Carbohydrates		Fat (30 gms)	Water
		Simple (24 gms) "Sugars"	Macros (150 gms) "Veggies"		
Breakfast	20	8	50	10	
Snack	10	-	25	-	
Lunch	20	8	50	10	
Snack	10	-	25	-	
Dinner	20	8	50	10	
Snack					
TOTALS	80 GRAMS	24 GRAMS	200 GRAMS	30 GRAMS	

Cardio Time/Calories Burned: _____/_____ **Weights:** Yes   No

Make copies of the blank chart on the following page. Use it to track your first week until your weigh-in, so you can review your food selections.

Nutrition 101

DAILY OVERVIEW GUIDE

	Protein (75 gms)	Carbohydrates		Fat (30 gms)	Water
		Simple (24 gms) "Sugars"	Macros (150 gms) "Veggies"		
Breakfast					
Snack					
Lunch					
Snack					
Dinner					
Snack					
TOTALS					

Cardio Time/Calories Burned: _____/_____   Weights: Yes   No

Measurements

Date	#1	#2	#3	#4	#5	#6	#7	#8	Goal
Right Arm									
Bust									
Waist									
Abs									
Hips									
Right thigh									

Weight

% Fat									
Lean mass									
Fat to Go									

Beginning Weight and Measures

The buck stops here, so to speak. You will need an inexpensive tape measure. If you need to, ask a family member or close friend to help you measure the sections listed below and to tally up the numbers. Measure to keep track of your progress.

Right arm – Fullest part
Bust – Fullest part
Waist – First indentation; think empire waistline. As you peel, this area will stay consistent. Keep in mind; this is not necessarily where you wear your pants.
Abs – Three inches below your navel
Hips – Have your assistant turn you to the side and measure the fullest part.
Thigh – Fullest part

Keep in mind, you are looking for your ugly version; so do not suck everything in.

Have a great week!

Computing Your Weekly Weight and Body Composition

To help you make weekly adjustments and make sure you are only burning fat mass and not sacrificing lean, I highly recommend you invest in the body comp machine I suggested on page 55. Compute the numbers and analyze your progress by starting with your weight. Use your machine to find out this week's body fat percentage. Compute the numbers like this.

> *Example: 200 pounds x 39% fat = 78 pounds of fat.*
>
> *Subtract what you need for insulation (25#) =*
> *53 pounds*
>
> *The remainder is "Fat to Go" (the risk factor)*
>
> *To find your lean mass, subtract your fat pounds from your current weight.*

Multiply your current weight times your current percentage of fat.

When you're on your game, you want all of the pounds lost to be from FAT. If you find that you have lost some of your lean mass, it could mean one of three things:

1.) You did not consume enough water

2.) You did not consume enough protein

3.) You trained over your heart rate and/or pushed too hard

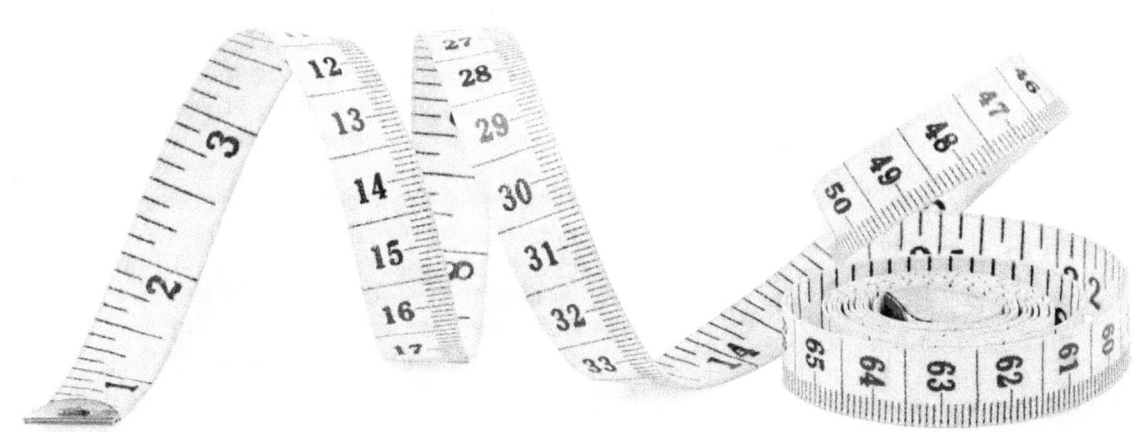

WEEK TWO

First things first. It's time for your first weigh and measure. Use Column #2 on the previous page. How did you do?

You add a little cardio, drink a little water, and learn to lift a little weight and watch the results begin! On game, this should mean 3-5 pounds of fat lost per week and 3-5inches. You might get stuck around week four. If you didn't quite make that target, it's OK. Keep your head in the game, and keep focusing on better choices and the results will kick back in. Your body just needs a moment to adjust itself.

Making Better Food Choices

Speaking of better choices, this is a good time to get a clear focus on better food choices, so let's take an extra moment to master an Onion Factory^{SM} understanding of the "goods," the "bads," and the "uglys." This change you desire is as easy as the KISS formula.

Eighty percent of the results you are looking for are going to begin with understanding balanced nutrition. For each day, this means:

> X amount of protein
> 10 cups grasses of the land
> 30 grams of fat
> 24 grams of sugar

Frequently, I will be asked if this Onion thing is like the Atkins Diet®. Limiting carbs seems to be the latest buzz. But 225 grams of carbohydrates per day (the Onion Factory^{SM} model) is nothing like Atkins®.

Perhaps the one similarity is that both systems address the deficiency in protein intake, which feeds the muscle. I have just taken that thought one step further and created loads of recipes around low fat, heart-healthy protein options.

So let's take another look at carbohydrates. I am going to make it easy for you.

The GOODS: Complex Carbohydrates (a.k.a Grass of the Land)

Know this. You are never going to get to 150 grams. Well, maybe if you really try; however, 150 grams is a lot of food. That is great if you love to eat. However, it's difficult if you find yourself being a non-eater, or a person who has relied on one meal a day. Let's face it not eating might be easier. But NON-EATING got us to where we are.

There are loads of great foods you can lean on. Probably the negative thought about eating loads is normally what you wanted to eat loads of went to your tushie. Now you will need to eat loads from items, which have nutritional value. Hopefully, you will find in our recipes that we were able to flip those grasses of the lands into fun food. Our goal is to teach you an entire new view of what normal eating looks like.

Remember, on your best game you are going to set aside the carbohydrates from the filler section, and you are going to graze more from the grasses of the lands. That adds another 50 grams of additional complex carbs for you to play with. You will never go hungry; however, you may miss a few of your old favorites until you find a few new ones.

The BADS: Sugars

The more sugar you eat, the more you crave. Stay away from the sugar bowl, and lean on fruit for your sweetness. In the first 8 weeks, keep it to berries. When you get closer to your goal, you will be able to lean on a larger variety of fruit. Even too much fruit will get in the way of your results. Why would you want to slow down your results?

When you are flipping labels, the good news is sugars are listed under the carbohydrates. Pay attention. You might be shocked to realize that ½ cup of green beans has 2 grams of sugar. Don't worry about counting the small amounts of sugar in the leafy greens for now, it will get too confusing. I just wanted you to know that SUGAR is everywhere.

Review the sections: Tomato Soup vs. Cream

of Chicken and Pasta sauces. Both sections will help you make sense of all this.

The UGLYS: Fillers
(your engine is already full)

I truly believe that this mess we are in stemmed from a food pyramid that suggested we make the base of our nutrition breads, pasta, rice, potatoes, and grains. Oh my! I guess we did exactly what we were told. Now what are we to do? Well, we are going back to basics.

If you do not see results quickly, you are going back to your old behaviors, and that is not going to work. So take a leap of faith with me. Review the results that we have been able to obtain. Learn the new Onion Food Pyramid. And eat away. It's that simple. No worries. We will bring a few of your old favorites back when you are closer to you goal.

Muscle Anatomy

I'd like you to see the anatomy of your muscles, so you will know exactly what muscle you are working on in our Onion training routine.

Week 2 Training

Let's add a little weightlifting to this week.

Basic Onion Routine

There is NO value in showing clients what they cannot do, so I've found it more enjoyable when you start slow, learn good form, and grab heavier weights as you are comfortable. That old saying, "No Pain, No Gain," has some truth. But as beginners, I am not so sure it is necessary to train at that level until you are ready. Just have fun! Learn about your muscles. Included in this guide is a basic anatomy chart. The chart will help you make sense of why you are lifting and how to properly isolate the muscle.

If you are still pondering: "Why do I need to lift weights?" or, "Which is more important, lifting weights, or getting my cardio in for the day?" Well, they are both very important.

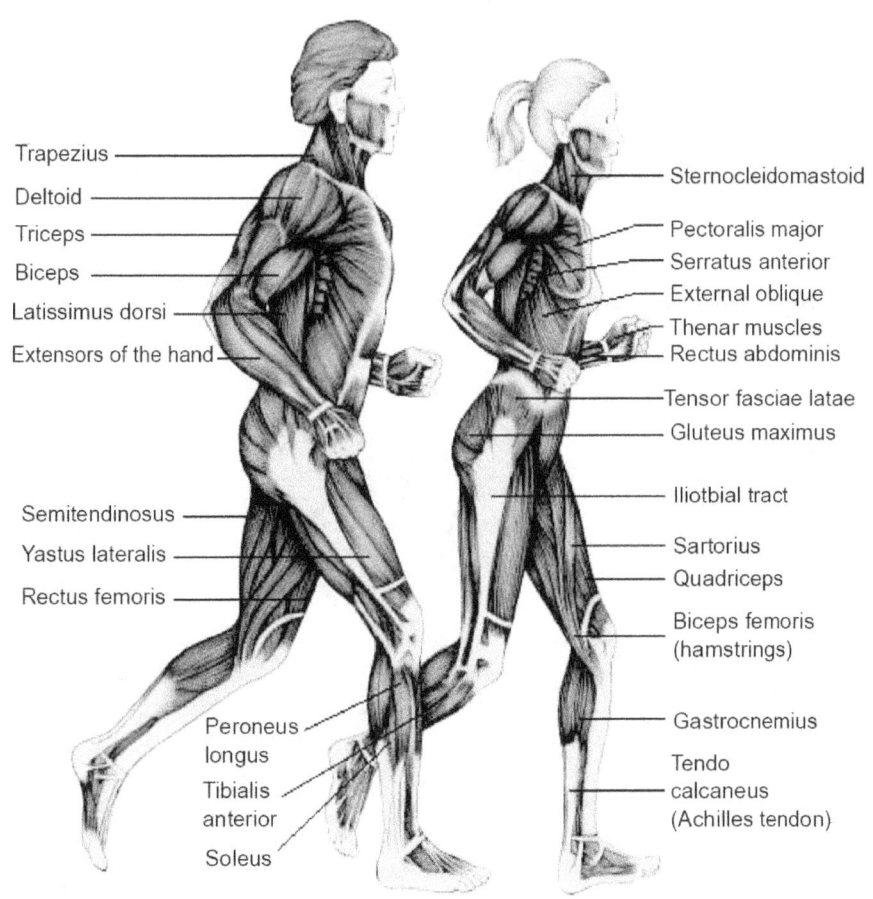

Your cardio days will be important for burning off your reserve tank; however, the days you lift will help you prevent the aging process by stimulating your muscle fibers, and you will burn fat (stored calories) the day you lift weights and the next day as your body rebuilds.

During weight lifting, once you are comfortable with the lifting process, your goal will be to break down muscle fibers. By breaking them down, you are asking the muscles to rebuild and restore. During this rebuilding process, your body will naturally lean on your reserves as long as your nutrition is balanced.

If you do not eat properly, then the body will have no choice but to lean on its own muscle for the nutrients it needs to rebuild. If I have said it once, I have said it a thousand times. Err your nutrition intake on the side of lean protein, not fats and sugars.

Think about it. Why in the world would you want to eat too many fats and sugars?

I start with Part 2 because, if I started with the legs, my clients would not come back! Beginners need a few weeks to build up endurance and confidence before I teach them how to flex the largest muscle group, the legs!

Part 2 is done with free weights. The sequence is easy to remember if you think, "**Great Big Loser**":

    G = Goal Post (Shoulder Press)
    B = Biceps
    L = Liberty (Triceps)

The Onion training routine has 4 parts:

1. Legs

2. Shoulder Press
    Bicep Curl
    Triceps
    X-tra Credit

3. Bust

4. Abs and obliques (muffin tops)

It's Test Time

Yes, it's time to take your first test! It's easy, because you can go back through the book and find the answers if you don't remember them. Do your best:

1. What is your target heart range (THR)?

2. What are the two places you can use to check your THR?

3. List two methods for checking your THR.

4. How many seconds do you count? Then multiply by what?

5. List training options you can use to move your heart rate into your fat-burning zone.

6. Why do you need to check your THR?

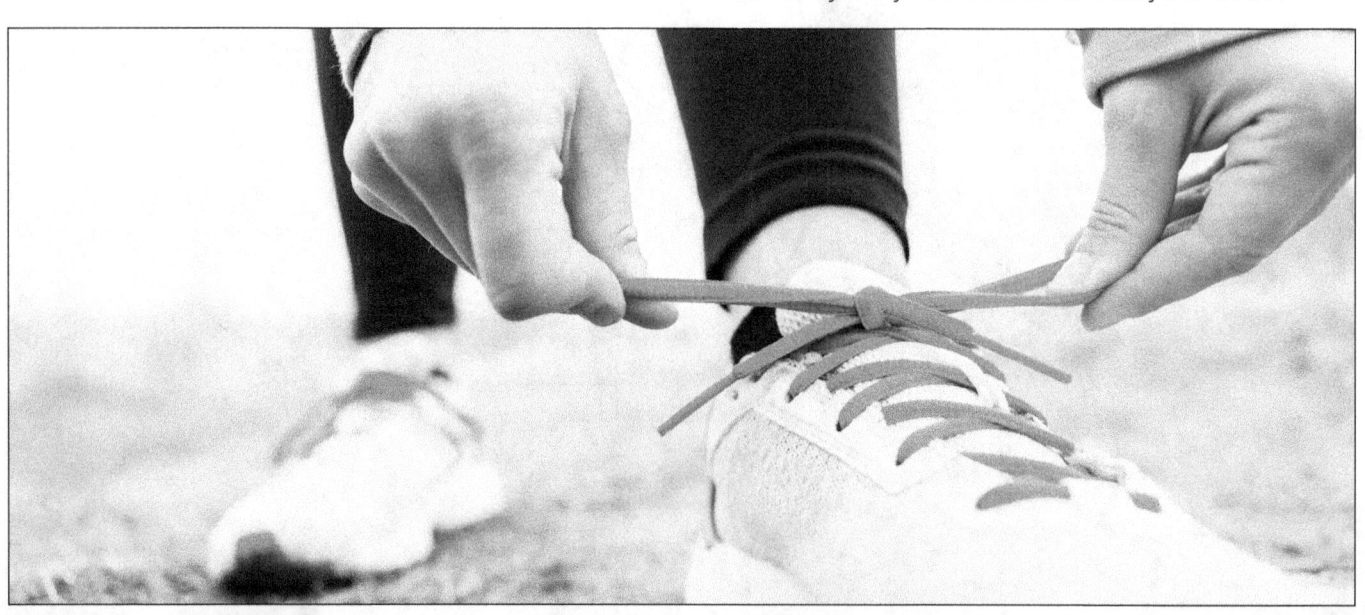

WEEK THREE

Grab your scale and tape measure and let's see how the week went!

As a trainer, one tool I have is *making adjustments*. Adjustments are as simple as suggesting a client drink a little more water, eat a little more frequently, grab a little more rest, and yes, eat more protein. Of course, a little less fat intake, and a little less sugar overload, goes a long way in having a great week of results.

I am following the outline of *The Fork Is Mightier Than the Gym* plus making weekly adjustments until I can help you lose 1 Percent of fat per week. In the past 25 years, I have seen plenty of people gain and lose 25 pounds, over and over. I have seen clients lose 25–40 pounds in eight weeks and still be close to, or exactly the same percentage of fat. That is not going to work in the big picture. I have no desire to help you be a fatter version of a smaller you.

I desire this to be a journey of changing the percentage of fat you are! Guess what? When you reduce your percentage of body fat, all the rest of the puzzle such as your cholesterol levels, energy levels, and high blood pressure levels will fall into place, including fitting into your skinny jeans.

How is your cardiovascular training going? Let's tweak your knowledge just a tad. Cardio needs to become a daily habit. Think of it this way. Would you go a day without brushing your teeth? I hope not. Well, then, think of cardio training as your way of preventing plaque building in your heart. Do it everyday and try to burn 400 calories. As you are plugging away, remember that one pound of fat is 3,500 calories stored, and you are just trying to use up your reserve.

Week 3 Training

I desire your primary focus to be on changing your eating habits, making your cardio routine a part of daily life, and growing a love affair for lifting weights. Your goal during the first month will be to lift weights twice a week.

This week, I want to add two exercises to your routine. The first will firm up the pectoral muscles of your bust.

Bust Exercise

1. Lie on your back on the floor.
2. Grab 5-lb weights for starters.
3. Put a weight in each hand and hold them horizontal to your chest.
4. Lift weights up over your chest.
5. Bring weights back to the floor.
6. Don't touch the floor with the weights and don't tap them at the top.
7. Raise your butt in the air and exhale as you bring the weights together. Try two sets of 15 repetitions.

Cardio Goals on the Elliptical Machine

- Stay in your target heart rate (THR) range.
- Build your endurance to 30 minutes.
- Keep your strides at 120/minute or more.
- Increase the machine's resistance from 1 to 20.
- Keep increasing the resistance so you burn more calories per minute. The goal is 11 calories per minute or more.

Abs

Your abdominal muscle and calf muscles are the only muscles you can train (work out) every day. All others need a day of rest in between. Did you get that statement? You need a day of rest in between!

The basic ab exercises are called 3-packs. I may never get you to a 6-pack stomach; however, I can surely help get you definition in three basics spots: the upper abdomen, lower abdomen, and mid section. One of the top three questions I get in the Factory is how can I get great abs? Guess what? You get great abs by having great nutrition. The abs work and sits ups will just make sure that what is under those additional layers of fat is tight and toned. Until you peel the fat layers away, you will not see the fruit of your labor.

ABS: Position 1

1. Lie down on the floor.
2. Cross your arms over your chest.
3. Bend your knees.
4. Look behind you.
5. Crunch forward slightly.
6. Do 15 repetitions. You will feel this in the upper part of your abdominal wall.

ABS: Position 2

1. Raise your legs off the floor to a 45-degree angle.
2. Crunch again for 15 repetitions. You will feel this in your lower abdominal wall.

ABS: Position 3

1. Put your feet back on the floor.
2. Cup your hands together over your chest.
3. Crunch forward for 15 repetitions. You will feel flexion in your midsection.

And you are finished for now!

X-Tra Credit

Choose 3-lb or 5-lb free weights. You will do 1 set of 12 repetitions for each.

HORIZONTAL ROW

Assume a standing position with soft knees and arms straight out in front of you. Now row backwards. You are working the area behind your neck, the trapezius.

DELT FRONT

Now lower your arms to your legs and pull back up level. Keep weights together, but not touching. Start with 5-lb weights but drop lower if necessary. (At first, you may need no weights.)

REAR DELT

This is one of my favorites because it is a key to a great appearance. If you work at a desk or at a computer, this muscle, posterior deltoid (see muscle chart) has probably shortened, causing a slouchy posture. Start with your chest out, arms at your side, then bring the weights up level.

X-Tra Credit

For extra credit, let's introduce a little shoulder work. I am passionate about shoulder work, because I think good posture is slimming. When we slouch, we are being lazy with our core and lazy with our muscles. If you do not use your muscles, you will lose them. Hence, *atrophy* (aging) which is the deterioration of muscle.

That's it quick and simple. This is a major muscle to a minor muscle, largest to smallest, weight training. With this routine, you are going to lift 2–3 times per week during the first four weeks.

It's Test Time

It's time for a test. This one is easy. The answers have been often repeated in the book so far.

1. What is fat?
2. Under what percentage of fat does the AMA recommend you stay to avoid heart disease?
3. What mass allows you to increase or decrease your metabolic rate?
4. What four components make the Onion Factory effective?
5. List the three categories of carbohydrates.
6. List as many lean protein options as you can.

WEEK FOUR

Let's tally it all up. Are you on course? Do you need to tighten your belt on your selections? If so, start now!

Week Four's class seems to be most clients' favorite. This is the moment when acceptance begins. I want you to take a moment a re-read the section on bean, pear, apple, and hourglass body shapes. I want you to start understanding your genetics, your body style, and your behaviors. I also want you to understand you are on a journey of inventing a better you. This will be a lifelong journey. You will have many temptations and distractions along the way. It's way easier to not eat, to not pay attention, and to sabotage your efforts. I believe week four is defining. I hope your results are motivation enough to continue to make new behaviors.

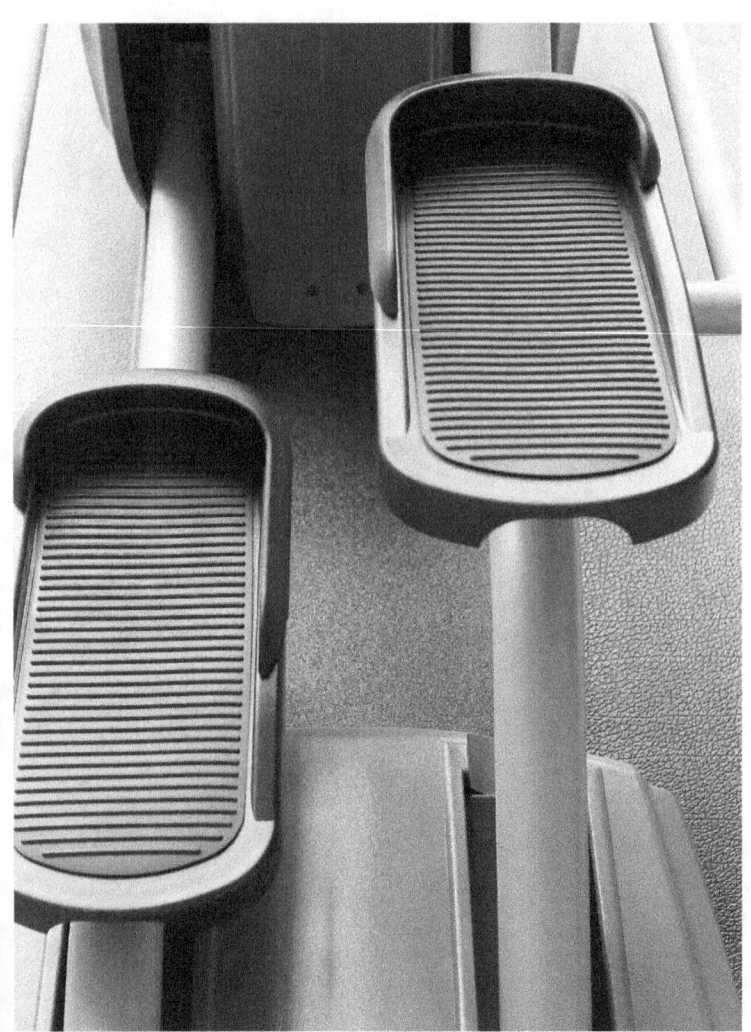

Making Adjustments

I felt such a sense of urgency to share this story that I asked my next client if I could bump her session in with the client after her. She said, "No problem." I ran to the house to write this story about Carolyn. I felt strongly about sharing her story, because you will see the importance and reward from making adjustments.

Carolyn had just finished her fourth week of camp. She felt a little frustrated; because last week, the scale did not give her the numbers she felt she had worked for. I have tried to express in the 8-week camp and in this guide that the scale will tell you nothing. The only thing we obtain from the scale is a beginning benchmark that will enable us to determine how much lean mass and how much fat mass one has from week to week. Burning fat is the mission, because fat is where all the issues with risk factors begin.

This week, Carolyn made the adjustments I had suggested. She increased her water intake and added a little relish tray to her food plan and paid attention to the proper protein additions on her training days. After a week of adjustments, we put her on the scale and discovered she had lost two pounds. Two pounds are more rewarding than her zero pounds last week. However, the results were far greater than the scale would measure.

Sure, her doctor was happy. And sure, her clothes were fitting much differently. But what really happened was she lost more than a percentage of fat, which represented three pounds of fat. Three pounds, not from water, or muscle, but from fat. Most importantly, her body burned 10,500 calories – three pounds – from her reserve tank in one week! That meant her body was regulated. Her body was getting enough water, protein, veggies, and not too many fats and sugars.

Carolyn is a 62-year-old woman who in her first four weeks of camp still has not gotten up to 400 calories per session on The Beast. She burns about 200 calories per session. So how did she burn up 10,500 calories of stored energy? Well, she got her body balanced, so it could burn fat. Call it anabolic, or a furnace, or just burning fat like crazy. It feels great!

Total Hip Workout

1. With the chair on your right, slowly lift your left leg. Try a set of 15.

2. Stand straight, don't wiggle or wobble, and push that leg behind you for 15 repetitions.

3. Turn facing the chair as straight as possible. Keep your center solid.

4. Move your right leg away from your body, toes forward, for 15 repetitions.

5. Make a quarter turn to your right. Take your right leg out in front of you and make a pendulum sweep in front of you for 15 repetitions.

Cliff Notes Version:
- Up = flexion, working your hip flexors
- Back = extension, working your hip extenders
- Out = abductors (outer thighs)
- Over = adductors (inner thighs)

The basic Onion routine looks like this:

- Legs—total hip workout
- GBL—(shoulder, biceps, triceps) with X-tra credits (additional shoulder work)
- Bust and Abs exercises

Week 4 Training

We are going to add legs to your Onion routine. At this point, you have all the tools to complete a beginner major muscle to minor muscle workout (largest muscle to smallest). The reason behind that training principle is that if you fatigue the smaller muscles first, you will not have the strength to fatigue the larger muscle later. Then you will not get the results you desire. We are doing all this work, specifically, for results.

The next sequence is very important. If you have done any knee or hip rehab, then you may have already tried this one. I love the total hip workout. The sequence is important; therefore, when we add the more advanced moves in later, your tendons and ligaments will be able to keep up with the workout load of the quadriceps, hamstrings, and glutes, a.k.a. the front of the leg, the back of the leg, and your rear.

First, if you have a chair, grab it. Place the seat away from you, so you may hold on to the back of the chair. It's that simple.

Continue to be progressive with how much weight you are using is the key. A rule of thumb is whatever poundage you utilize above your head; you can usually pull a little heavier when the movement is below your head, such as biceps. Anytime you do the shoulder work, you will notice the muscle fatigue quickly.

Emotional Health

Let's jump to another track. How are you feeling about yourself?

Use the chart on the following page over the next two weeks to find some insights into your feelings. Each day, write a sentence or a word that describes how you are finding the person within.

Reinventing Yourself:
How Do You Feel Today?

Week_____ to Week_____

Monday:

Tuesday:

Wednesday:

Thursday:

Friday:

Saturday:

Sunday:

Fourth-Week Tip

Find a quiet spot today, even if it's in your bathroom. Take a few moments to reflect upon your weight loss. Whether you are happy with your results or not, give thanks for the blessing of how much you have already changed. Good weeks are just ahead.

It's Test Time

Yes, it's that time again. See how many answers you can get without looking through the book.

1. List as many protein options as you can think of.

2. What body type do you have?
   a. bean
   b. pear
   c. apple
   d. hourglass

3. What does Body Composition measure?

4. How much rest is needed after you train a muscle group?

5. How many calories does one pound of muscle burn each day?

6. How many calories does one pound of fat burn each day?

7. Which type of mass takes up the least amount of space?

WEEK FIVE

Welcome to your second four weeks!

The first four weeks were about building a foundation. This is the point where you are either going to move forward with your new knowledge, or you are going back to your old ways. Peeling an Onion (creating a new you) is not the most enjoyable part of this journey. The enjoyment comes when you begin to get a little validation for all your efforts. I wish we did not need a pat on the back for something we should already be doing, however, we're human. A little vote of confidence goes a long way. Since you are not here with me in my studio in Anderson, let's have a heartfelt get-in-your-head moment.

Remember when I said 80 percent of the results you are looking for would come from your nutrition? Well, 100 percent of the results you desire and the change you need comes from your brain. Either you want this and you are ready to do the work, or you don't. It's that simple.

This could be a great week. Grab your tape measure and scale. Are you seeing a couple of pounds lost?

Let's review what is between your ears. The choices you face each month, each week, each day are these:

- ✓ Is this going to be a day you lose?
- ✓ Is this going to be a day you maintain?
- ✓ Is today going to be a day you gain?
- ✓ Or will this be a day you blow it and sabotage it all?

A great thing about the Onion system is you can eat almost anything you desire. You just need to understand how your food choices are going to plug into the equation for the day. You need adequate protein, enough veggies, and not too much fat and sugar. I kid you not. Losing 15–20 pounds per month is that easy. How do I know? Because I have more than 600 case studies to prove how to peel like an Onion.

Frequently, I am asked which is a tougher client to make a difference with? A client who has put on 50 pounds over 10 years, or one who has put on 50 pounds over the past six months? Both scenarios are tough because 50 pounds is 175,000 calories in your reserve tank that your need to burn up. But check this out, 50 pounds put on over 10 years is simply 50 calories per day too much, and/or 50 calories too few of activity.

A client who has put on 50 pounds over a shorter period—let's say six months—has overindulged 1,000 calories per day. I would suspect this client has been taking out their frustration in food. I usually find the frustration is loss, sadness, or just a case of the blues. The great part is either scenario is fixable. You can be in control.

Let's go back to basics and review how you need to eat.

Breakfast

- 20 grams of protein
- 1 cup of grasses of the land
- try not to use more than 10 grams of fat

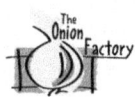

Week 5 is the point where you are going to move forward with your new knowledge, or go back to your old ways.

3 hours later: Snack time

- 10 grams of protein
- 1 cup grasses of the land
- as little fat as possible.

Hint: Two hardboiled eggs (minus the yolks) equal 14 grams of clean protein. Not glamorous, but it's easy. Your glamorous experience comes later when you get to show off a new outfit.

3 hours later: Lunch

- 20 grams of protein
- 2–3 cups grasses of the land
- try not to use more than 10 grams of fat.

3 hours later: Snack time

- 10 grams of protein
- 1 cup grasses of the land
- as little fat as possible.

Hint: If you need a grab-and-go option, try 17 turkey pepperoni slices (4 grams fat and 9 grams of protein) or a light cheese stick (2.5 grams fat and 8 grams of protein).

3 hours later: Dinner

- 20 grams of protein
- 3–4 cups grasses of the land
- try not to use more than 10 grams of fat.

You need to supplement your protein intake according to your weight and activity level for the day. Review the protein section; make sure you are getting enough protein. Add a relish tray to your day if you mindless eat. Try Walden's Farms® Dressing for a dip or sample the dressing (dip) recipe in this book.

Week 5 Training

By the second half of your 8-week journey, my goal is to give you a little more challenge. I would like to give you a little more information on the fitness basics, too. You have cardiovascular training, which is primary for the most important muscle, your heart. Cardio training is also a great way to burn off stored calories. Remember, the only mass you are trying to burn up is fat mass! If you push too hard, you may sacrifice your muscle. Don't do that. You will need all the muscle you have to maintain a solid metabolism. In fact, if done properly, you can build muscle and prevent aging by taking care of your muscle. Honor your muscle. Don't feed the fat.

I am going to expose you to a few advanced training ideas. If you have a weight-lifting background, you are more than welcome to test a few of those routines now. If the terms look foreign, stay with the basic Onion routine. Check our site online for advanced weight training protocols (www.onioncamp.com).

The Benchmark: How Sore Are You?

I have a little saying at the Factory:

One Day Sore = Good Job!

Two Days Sore = Great Job!

Three Days Sore = We kicked your butt. You're bound to see results!

Four Days Sore = NO EXTRA CHARGE!

Back, biceps, and shoulders

Lower Back Stretch
One-Arm Dumbbell Row
Horizontal Row

Bicep Curl
Hammer Curl
21's
Shoulder Press
Delta Front
Side Delts

I want you to try two sets of 15. Later you will want to bump it up to three sets of 12 repetitions. I placed a base line starting point for you to try. If you find that when you get close to the end the lift is still pretty easy, then increase the weight. The desire poundage goal is that when you get to the last couple of lifts, it is a bit of a struggle.

WEEK SIX

Grab your tape measure and scale. Chart your progress. How are you doing? Are you seeing inches lost?

By this week, you should be in the groove with your grocery shopping and preparing weight-loss worthy meals and snacks. If you aren't getting the weight loss and inches lost that you expected, go back over your nutrition and see if there are any weak spots. Are you eating and drinking enough? Are you getting enough protein to keep up with your weight training? Look for hidden sugars that might have kept you off your game. Are you sneaking in filler carbohydrates? You only have two more weeks. I know you can stay in the box until graduation, and perhaps beyond!
Take a few moments and review the Basic Onion Routine.

Week 6 Training

Take a deep breath. Today is leg training, everyone's favorite. You will be training your largest muscle group.
Remember the phrase, "No Pain, No Gain"? You probably thought to yourself that this is exactly why you do not want to work out. Who wants to be in pain?

What if I told you it was a good pain, or a beneficial pain? Then might you be convinced? I think by Week Six, you will begin to appreciate knowing you did a good job with your efforts in weight training.

The benchmark will be, How sore did you get? You may respect your lifting efforts and benchmarking the workout by how sore you are.

It feels really good as your body begins to tighten up. Keep it up. You can do this.

- ✓ Total Hip
- ✓ Chair Squats
- ✓ Front Lunges
- ✓ Squat Thrust
- ✓ Leg Lifts
- ✓ Butt Blasters
- ✓ Side Lunges
- ✓ Calf Raises

Something to Think About

Are you over your body-fat composition range because of one of the following reasons?

a. You did not have the knowledge of how to eat, or what to eat?

b. You needed to increase your activity level and work at an accountable level?

c. You struggle with cravings or food addictions?

d. Food fills your emotional and personal voids?

e. All of the above?

Are you working on a plan to solve the issues you've marked above? Find a safe person to confide in about your struggles.

It's Test Time

Once again, let's see how well you do on these questions *without* referring to the book.

1. How does your body react when you starve it?
2. How often should you feed your body's "engine"?
3. How are all carbohydrates processed?
4. What food source stimulates your appetite?
5. What food source helps you maintain your blood sugars and appetite?
6. What does *satiate* mean?
7. Which of these do you crave?

    a. salty foods

b. sweet foods

   c. warm/cold foods

   d. rich foods

   e. spicy foods

8. What are some alternative choices to satiate your cravings?

9. How are you feeling this week? Are you seeing results in your weight and inches lost? Are you eating every three hours?

WEEK SEVEN

I shared earlier in this guide that I had no desire to be the guru of supplements. I just wanted to learn how to be as healthy as possible, and then share what I have learned along the way with you. I love the idea that we have the ability to fix what ails many of us by simply eating well and getting the proper nutrients. If you are finding that you are enjoying the way you feel as much as the way you are beginning to look, then I highly recommend you reread the segment on nutrition.

A quick reference, which is free, is an online source called My Daily Plate. This site is a great support system while you learn what to eat to get the results you are looking for. I think I have shared enough tools with you that you can navigate your way around a label. Now, you just need time to practice and make your own adjustments along the way.

If you have not added the following items into your daily routine you might reread these sections and reconsider using these:

- A good multi-vitamin
- Biotin
- CLA

Week 7 Training

This week, let's do my favorite workout, chest and triceps!

- ✓ Push Ups
- ✓ Liberties
- ✓ Pec Fly
- ✓ Triceps Throwbacks
- ✓ Chest Presses
- ✓ Skull Crushers

Don't be surprised if, after this equence, drying your hair the next day is a little awkward. Don't worry; it's a good thing. The more frequent you challenge these body parts, the better you will get.

On the following chart (p. 262), circle the emotions you are feeling this week. Where did they come from? Why are you feeling this way? How can you use the emotions to strengthen your resolve?

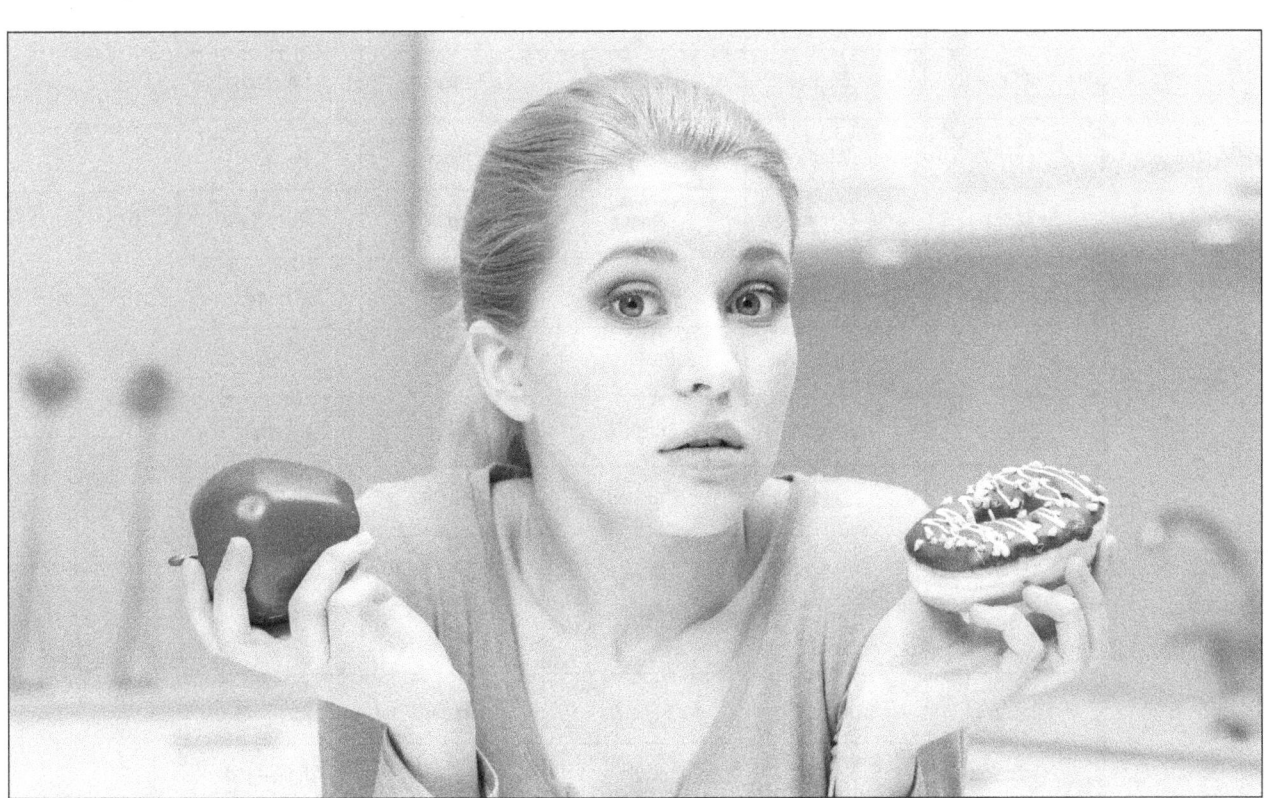

Compassionate	Cold	Holy	Despondent	Embarrassed
Watched	Suspect	Important	Disappointed	Judged
Needed	Unneeded	Rejected	No Good	Care For
Protected	Secure	Hopeless	Light	Lost
Inadequate	Disgusted	Used	Stopped	Cornered
Risky	Virile	Put Down	Inferior	Childish
Indifferent	Seen	Guilt	Ignored	Unseen
Cuddled	Despised	Startled	Childlike	Sunny
Timid	Loved	Bold	Unnoticed	Overloaded
Humiliated	Withdrawn	Serene	Grieved	Poor Me
Avoided	Relieved	Cloudy	Lonely	Powerful
Tough	Confident	Pitiful	Bright	Let Down
Babied	Spiritual	Repaid	Despondent	Close
Stepped On	Weak	Alone	Calm	Quiet
Left Out	Grateful	Foolish	Ashamed	Hopeful
Jittery	Empty	Forced	Trapped	Dejected
Funny	Whole	Shy	Gloomy	Pleasant
Cocky	Content	Tender	Joyous	Peaceful
Captivated	Unhappy	Wounded	Hurt	Martyred
Impish	Attracted	Positive	Complete	Fulfilled
Clumsy	Buoyant	Longing	Heavy	Sprightly
Stingy	Lively	Crushed	Alarmed	Horrified
Dour	Refreshed	Brave	Washed Out	Carefree
Icy	Beaten	Frantic	Turned Away	Satisfied
Frightened	Walked On	Tranquil	Irritated	Annoyed
Ridiculed	Humble	Powerless	Jealous	Challenged

WEEK EIGHT

We are close to putting all this change together. Wherever you land with your results, I want you to consider a few things. What if you continued making these changes for another eight weeks? What do think the results will look like then? I want to review the mindset of change. Change that may take a year! I want you to review the question, "what if" change was just one pound this month and two next month, and so on. Then, in one year, you will have peeled 78 pounds. Results can be that simple. All this is just making better choices each day, understanding the nutritional formula, and not allowing your head to get in the way of the results that I know you truly desire.

If you choose to continue with Onion Camp, and I hope you do, go back to Week Four and pick it up there. When you finish Week Eight, return to Week Four and keep the cycle going until you reach your goals.

Week 8 Training

Let's upgrade that Onion routine, so you will have the flexibility to perform a major muscle to minor muscle training two times per week (three if you have the time); however, if you have the time, I would prefer you select the body part training sequence.

Okay, here comes the fun part. Complete your measurement chart. You may be amazed when you add up how many inches you've lost. Keep up the good work. Remember, if you have more pounds and inches to lose, go back and pick up at Week Four.

Graduation Rant: About Those Filler Carbs

We end our 8-week course with a final rant about carbohydrates. Carbs are where most Onions make their mistakes. We also end the course with a pizza party. Why? Because we celebrate with food, pizza is fun, and a pizza party gives us an opportunity to share a little more valuable information. You learned on page 41 how various kinds of carbs stack up. I am talking here about the filler carbs in these food items, not their fat or protein content.

One slice of pizza has about 50 grams of the wrong kind of carbs per slice. I am pretty sure most of us eat at least 2 slices of pizza and, at some point in our life, maybe even the entire pizza. With the consumption of 2 slices, you have indulged in over one hundred grams of filler carbs (you know, the kind that go directly to your "assets"). In maintenance mode, we budget about 46 grams of filler carbs per day. If you are not burning off via physical activity any filler carbs that you consume over that amount, guess what happens. It's stored as FAT.

In the 1990s, low-fat eating was the method of choice. We purchased air-pop popcorn makers, ate rice cakes and fat-free anything. We thought that as long as a food item had no fat, we were good to go. Little did we

---

Eighth-Week Tip

On Sunday, grill a few pounds of chicken on your George Foreman or stick a few pounds of chicken in your Crock Pot. This will save you time during the week, and there are tons of recipes in which you can use chicken. Check Chapter 11 for a few good ideas.

realize that a large bag of popcorn has about 75 grams of the wrong kind of carbohydrates. Heck, yeah, popcorn has no fat (unless we add butter), but popcorn also has a day-and-a-half's supply of filler carbs.

Also during that "fat-free" era, a Panera's® bagel and cup of coffee were considered a great way to start the day. Little did we realize that a bagel has about 59 grams of fillers, and where was the protein?

My personal favorite of those days was Fazoli's®. I have always worked retail store hours, so I often found myself leaving the office after 8:00 P.M. without having planned my food consumption in advance, and I was hungry. Fazoli's® is a fast, affordable option; and while you wait for your main course, they start feeding you—breadsticks, no less! What more could a fluffy girl want? So as I waited, I had one, maybe two breadsticks as my appetizer. Almost everything on Fazoli's menu is heavy on the filler carbs, then they give you breadsticks on top of that. If you dine in, a Fazoli's team member walks around, offering you even more.

I am pretty sure that the average person would not even think about eating six slices of bread; however, I am pretty sure that most of us have enjoyed an order of breadsticks, usually six to an order. Yet a breadstick has about the same amount of filler carbs as a slice of bread. We think it's OK to consume an order of breadsticks, but our brains know better than to let us eat six slices of bread. Now you have the correct numbers and can begin having a more sensible relationship with your food choices. (Maybe take a pass on Fazoli's!)

Then there are potatoes. In the past, potatoes were taboo in my book. Fifteen years into peeling Onions, with a better understanding that this is a mental journey as much as it is a nutritional and physical one, I have a new spin on the potato.

While a MEDIUM potato has approximately 26 grams of fuller carbs, a potato can go a long way toward making you feel full and satisfied in the winter months. Our Onion Factory℠ taco salad is one of our most popular retail food items, but it does not always satisfy in winter. I have found that if you take your 4-ounce serving of taco meat (preferably

Eight-Week Upgraded Onion Routine

		ADD
Layer 1	• Total Hip	• Lunges
		• Chair Squats
		• Leg Lifts
Layer 2	• Shoulder Press	• Hammer Curl
	• Bicep Curl	• Tricep Throwbacks
	• Liberties	
Layer 3	• X-Tra Credit Bust	• Chest Press
Layer 4	• 3-Packs	• Sit Ups
		• Throw Downs
		• Standing Abs

	Calories	Carbs	Fat	Protein
Large slice pizza	447	52	18	20
Large popcorn	664	75	13	13
Panera's® bagel	290	59	1.5	10
Breadstick	150	28	2.5	5
Medium baked potato	110	26	0	2
Oatmeal ¼ cup dry	150	27	3	5
Cheerios® 1 cup	120	22	2	4

90/10 lean), place it on a baked potato, add your shredded lettuce, salsa, 2% cheddar cheese, light sour cream, and green onions, that baked potato will go a long way toward satisfying your hunger in the winter months. So mentally, it's a great choice. That loaded potato is a perfect weight maintenance item and, quite frankly, maintenance mode is often trickier than weight-loss mode. If that loaded baked potato helps you build a better menu because you feel satisfied, then it's a "win" in my book!

Oatmeal (*sigh*). I blew it one season with oatmeal and I knew better! We had a spate of cold weather and I was being lazy with my menu planning. In hindsight, my protein was probably off (under) and that mistake did not help with my other food choices. Remember, if you are craving carbs (including sugar), review your protein intake before you blow it.

Each night, I would make ½ cup of oatmeal in the microwave. (NOTE: The recommended serving size is ¼ cup, but that is simply not enough.) I would add Walden Farms® Pancake Syrup, which is a great guilt-free substitute for regular maple syrup. In hindsight, that may have been the move that convinced my brain that the oatmeal was OK. I would add a smidge of fresh cream because I knew that skim milk has more sugar than regular milk, and when it tastes bland you end up using more product. The oatmeal was a warm, delicious comfort food and I slept like a baby. I also packed on 15+ pounds, which I later had to clean up. Remember, keep an eye on the gains of 5, 10, or 15 pounds so you never have to clean up the 50, 75, or 100+ pounds again.

I just saved to my photos a post from Pinterest. This post claimed that Cheerios® has ¾g of soluble fiber, 12 essential vitamins and minerals, which can help to lower cholesterol and it's made with a natural sweetener, honey. Your brain instantly says, "Great choice!" So you buy the product because you want to be healthy, and advertisers know this.

Let's take a closer look. One cup of Cheerios® has 22g of the wrong carbs if you are fluffy. When you add milk, you add 12g of sugar, which is also a carb. You will start your day with 34g of carbs which metabolize as sugar, and sugar makes you crave more sugar. (Again, where in the heck is the protein to start your day?)

We moms bought into the idea that a Baggie of Cheerios® is a great healthy snack pack for our little ones. We didn't realize we were starting our children early with the desire, habit, and craving for a filler carb.

The last thing I have to say about Cheerios® and the power of advertising is this: The Pinterest post demonstrates the manufacturers' desire to promote and sell more product. General Mills® has done a fabulous job of convincing us that pulverized oats made into the shape of a solid torus is a healthy choice. In the Pinterest post, they give four reasons why their product is a heart-healthy breakfast.

First, it contains soluble fiber. Experts say that soluble fiber MAY lower the risk of heart disease. (I believe that the first and most important factor in heart disease is excessive layers of unwanted fat you are carrying on your body. The primary goal of this book is to help you get rid of them.) As a quick refresher, here is a list of the top 20 foods that are sources of soluble fiber:

- Black beans
- Broccoli
- Nectarines
- Flaxseed
- Lima beans
- Turnips
- Apricots
- Sunflower seed
- Brussel sprouts
- Pears
- Carrots
- Hazelnuts
- Avocado
- Kidney beans
- Apples
- Oats
- Sweet potatoes
- Figs
- Guavas
- Barley

Broccoli, brussel sprouts, and turnips are the most important sources of soluble fiber if you are fluffy—NOT Cheerios®. In maintenance mode, you can bring back to your diet some of the other sources such as lima beans, kidney beans, apples, avocadoes, and carrots. But pay attention if you gain five pounds or more. That's a wake-up call to lay aside the carbs and fibers so you can clean up this excess weight and don't have to clean up more.

The Cheerios® box says this food has 12 essential vitamins and minerals. Trust me, there are plenty of other foods that will give you these nutrients without adding 20g of filler carbs to your daily consumption.

Cheerios® is made with HONEY. Oh, my gosh, I think I could write an entire book on this topic. Honey is organic, so honey is healthy. Right? Consider this:

    1 Tbsp of honey has 17g sugar

    1 Tbsp of sugar has 12.6g sugar

A recipe made with honey actually has more sugar grams than if it was made with refined white sugar! Yes, I realize there are other benefits to honey; however, we are on a mission to fix fluffy, and the science of the numbers is what we have worked with over the past fifteen years. We have found that the math matters; you only have so many grams to work with each day. If you prefer to get your sugar grams from honey, that is fine; but please do not let advertisers convince you that their product is healthier because it's made with honey. It can sabotage your weight-loss goals.

You only have 24g of sugar per day to work with. After that, the extras are stored as fat. (Unless, of course, your workout plan helps you burn off the extra sugar you consume.) I have always wondered why anyone would want to drink a large glass of orange juice on the way to a workout, realizing that you'll be lucky if your exercise session burns off the extra sugar grams you just consumed. I would much rather let my workout session burn off the storage tank of excess fat I already have. That is why we go to the gym in the first place!

Congratulations!

YOU HAVE MADE IT THROUGH EIGHT WEEKS OF THE ONION CAMP. PAT YOURSELF ON THE BACK AND SEND ME YOUR BEFORE AND AFTER PICTURES AT WWW.ONIONCAMP.COM

Q and A

I have a love-hate relationship with questions. I realize we are taught that no question is a dumb question. And that might be true. However, because I have been sifting thru rubbish and dieting myths for 20 years,

I find a few of the questions to be truly out there. Since we are all on the same page, we will address the top few.

1. Can I eat after 6:00 pm?
Why not? As long as you are not eating beyond your baseline nutritional needs. The nothing-after-6 concept could not work for a third shift person. It was crazy.

2. Are protein bars okay?
What do you think they are stuck together with? Fillers! If you were going to pick between a candy bar and a protein bar, well then obviously a protein bar is a better choice. At the end of the day, both are loaded with sugar, carbs, and fat. Read the labels.

3. Can I eat sugar-free Jell-O?
Is it weight-loss worthy or does it add nutrition is the real question. This one is unique. While it is weight-loss-worthy, Jell-O has no nutritional value. I often find that women who satisfy their cravings with Jell-O forget to eat their baseline nutritional requirements, because, they are no longer hungry. If you have met all your protein and veggie needs, it will not impede your weight-loss goals, but you are just feeding a craving. Try exchanging the Jello with a protein drink.

4. Do I count sugar alcohol?
I have found through fifteen years of case studies that as far as weight loss goes you must count sugar alcohol as sugar; consume no more that 24 grams per day.

5. How does gum work into the puzzle?
I was working with a client who was stuck. No results! Her cardiovascular training was online and she was lifting her weights. We reviewed her food. Everything thing look okay, but she was still stuck. I thought it was some innocent mistake such as too much creamer, or too much salad dressing. One day, out of the blue, we began talking about gum. She chewed 20 pieces of Juicy Fruit every day. Each piece had 2 grams of sugar. She was getting nearly a two-day supply of sugar from her gum. Her exercise efforts on "the beast" were just burning off her stored sugars. If you are going to chew gum, select a sugar-free. But remember, if your body is processing too much artificial stuff then it cannot perform its job of getting rid of fat as efficiently.

6. Do I really need to drink all that water?
Dehydration slows down your metabolic rate. Your body cannot tell the difference between thirst and hunger, so at times you may graze when you really only needed to hydrate. Often, fatigue may be due to dehydration. So, don't skimp on the water.

7. You don't really mean I have to eat even when I'm not hungry, do you?
Yes, feed your lean muscle mass not your fat cells. Not-eating feeds your fat cells.

8. That little bit of mashed potatoes won't hurt me, right?
This statement usually comes from a person who is not really attempting to change their current level of health. Yes, one bite might hurt you, because, you may not be able to stop. Focus on what you can eat at that moment rather than on self-discipline until you get over the hump and see loads of results.

9 Surely a skinny latte is weight-loss worthy, right?
Low-fat milk contains twelve grams of sugar. Read the labels!

10. What if I just eat a smaller portion?
Has eating smaller portions worked for you?

11 Isn't fast food cheaper?
We all know eating healthy is expensive, right! What can you do with a $1.00? Double cheeseburgers are fast and easy. They taste really good, but they go directly to your assets! What you get for that $1.00 is 60 grams of fat; Artery clogging fat at that! For a dollar you could buy a dozen small eggs, a half-pound of ground turkey, a half-pound of chicken breast, or a 16-ounce bag of frozen veggies. Sure you need to cook them. You might need a little extra time to do the prep work. But it is healthy.

12. When can I eat normal again?
Oh my gosh! This question blew my mind! I seriously could have not put this guide together without the help of the women in my community and questions such as this one. The questions they ask are exactly what you at home might be thinking. I may have never known what to answer unless I had made the commitment to build the data, the stories, the case studies and the questions.

I was working with one of my favorite Onions, and she seriously looked up at me and asked the question, "When can I eat normal?" What is normal? Hopefully, you are gaining an understanding that the elements in this guide are normal, basic nutrition.

What we were doing before this guide, and what we have been doing for the past few decades, was abnormal. I mentioned earlier, as we, women, moved into the workforce, family nutrition was sacrificed. While we may be superwomen, we could not keep up with everything. Drive thrus and pre- packaged food became the mainstay for a busy week. Family dinners were a thing of the past generations. We ate on the fly. Life was so busy, and we stopped paying attention. Even worse, we forgot what to do in the kitchen, or perhaps never learned in the first place. Hamburger and fries for dinner use to be the exception not the rule. When did chicken nuggets really come into play as a meal replacement?

15. Vitamins and Minerals

IT FEELS SO WONDERFUL when you begin feeding your body well and choosing the foods that allow you to become the new healthy person you desire. These foods contain essential vitamins for your good health.

Some vitamins can only be digested and absorbed with the help of fat. Vitamins A, D, E, and K are fat-soluble. When we followed an eating plan with no fat or extremely low fat, we were losing hair, feeling listless, having a poor complexion, and so on. This all changes when you learn how to feed your body with food that has genuine nutritional value.

I highly recommend *Prescription for Nutritional Healing,* by Phyllis Balch. At this point in your journey her book may be a little overwhelming and advanced. However, it is a great reference book. I utilized her book to create a user-friendly snapshot explaining the benefits, deficiency ailments, and sources for vitamins A, D, E, and K. I hope this information expands your horizons with the knowledge of the health possibilities with correct eating.

I've never had a burning desire in my belly to be the guru of vitamins and minerals. Quite frankly, I am not very disciplined at taking a daily pill. Onions ask me frequently about taking a daily vitamin, I quickly respond, "Well, they can't hurt. If you take more than your body requires you will just discard them in the powder room."

I would like to think we get all the nutrition we need from the fruits and vegetables God provided for us, but we neglect to eat all of our fruits and veggies. I have evidence of that, provided by several years of analyzing what Onions ate the week before they came to camp. Horribly! In addition, studies illustrate how our soil is becoming more and more depleted. Anything we can do to help ensure our intake of proper nutrients cannot hurt, so select a well-balanced multivitamin.

I speak frequently about vitamins A, D, E, and K, because these vitamins are fat-soluble. I realized pretty early in my 23-year fitness career that when we were on the fat-free bandwagon we girls experienced several health repercussions. We suffered from listlessness, our hair falling out, mood swings, and more. Of course we noticed these things! Do you know why? Because we lacked the proper amounts of vitamins A, D, E, and K which require fat in the digestive system to be absorbed. When we incorporated a fat-free diet, we depleted our bodies of these essential vitamins. Someone along the way told us fat-free was the answer to weight loss so we jumped on board.

Allow me to give you a list of weight-loss worthy foods which provide you with the needed nutrition, and why you need these fat-soluble vitamins.

Vitamin A

Benefits

Prevents night blindness and other eye problems	Prevents some skin disorders such as acne.
Enhances the immune system.	May help to heal gastrointestinal ulcers.
Important in the formation of bones and teeth.	Protects against colds and influenza.
Protects against infections of the kidneys, bladder, and lungs	Acts as an antioxidant, helping to protect cells against cancer.
Slows the aging process.	A well-known wrinkle eliminator.
Protein cannot be utilized by the body without Vitamin A.	

Ailments Caused by Vitamin A Deficiency

Dry Hair or Skin	Insomnia
Fatigue	Reproductive Difficulties
Sinusitis	Pneumonia
Frequent Colds	Other Respiratory Infections

Sources of Vitamin A

Animal Liver	Fish Liver Oils	Green/Yellow Fruit	Apricots
Asparagus	Beet Greens	Broccoli	Cantaloupe
Carrots	Collard Greens	Dandelion Greens	Mustard Greens
Turnip Greens	Kale Greens	Spinach	Sweet Potato
Garlic	Papayas	Peaches	Pumpkin
Red Peppers	Green/Yellow Vegetables		
Red/Yellow Veggies			

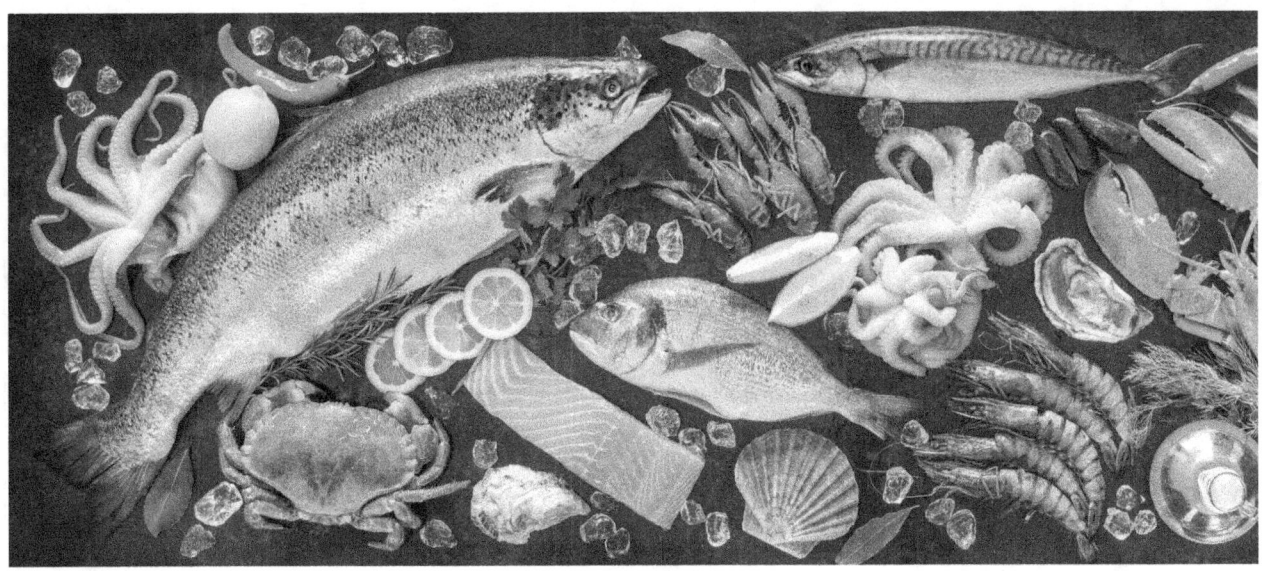

Vitamin D

Benefits

Important for normal growth and development	Important in the prevention and treatment of breast and colon cancer, osteoporosis, and hypocaldemia
Enhances immunity	Necessary for growth
Necessary for thyroid function	Necessary for normal blood clotting
Protects against muscle weakness	Involved in regulation of the heartbeat

Ailments Caused by Vitamin D Deficiency

Rickets in children	Diarrhea
Insomnia	Vision problems

Sources of Vitamin D

Vegetable Oil	Fatty Saltwater Fish	Dairy Products
Eggs/Egg Yolks	Butter	Cod Liver Oil
Dandelion Greens	Halibut	Liver
Milk	Oatmeal	Salmon
Sardines	Sweet Potatoes	Tuna

Vitamin E

Benefits

Improves circulation	Necessary for tissue repair
Promotes normal blood clotting	Reduces scarring
Reduces blood pressure	Aids in preventing cataracts
Reduces leg cramps	Maintains healthy nerves and muscles
May slow progression of Alzheimers	Protects against approx. 80 diseases
Antioxidant important in the prevention of cancer and cardiovascular disease	

Ailments Caused by Vitamin E Deficiency

May result in damage to red blood cells	Infertility
Menstrual problems	Linked to colon and breast cancer

Sources of Vitamin E

Cold-pressed vegetable oils	Dark green leafy vegetables	Legumes
Nuts	Seeds	Whole grains
Brown rice	Cornmeal	Eggs
Kelp	Milk	Oatmeal
Organ meats	Soybeans	Sweet potatoes
Watercress	Wheat	Wheat germ

Vitamin K

Benefits

Controls blood clotting	Converts glucose to glycogen
Involved in bone formation and repair	Slows bone loss

Ailments Caused by Vitamin K Deficiency

Nosebleed	Hemorrhage
Excessive bruising	Gastrointestinal disorders

Sources of Vitamin E

Leafy vegetables	Asparagus
Green tea	Coffee

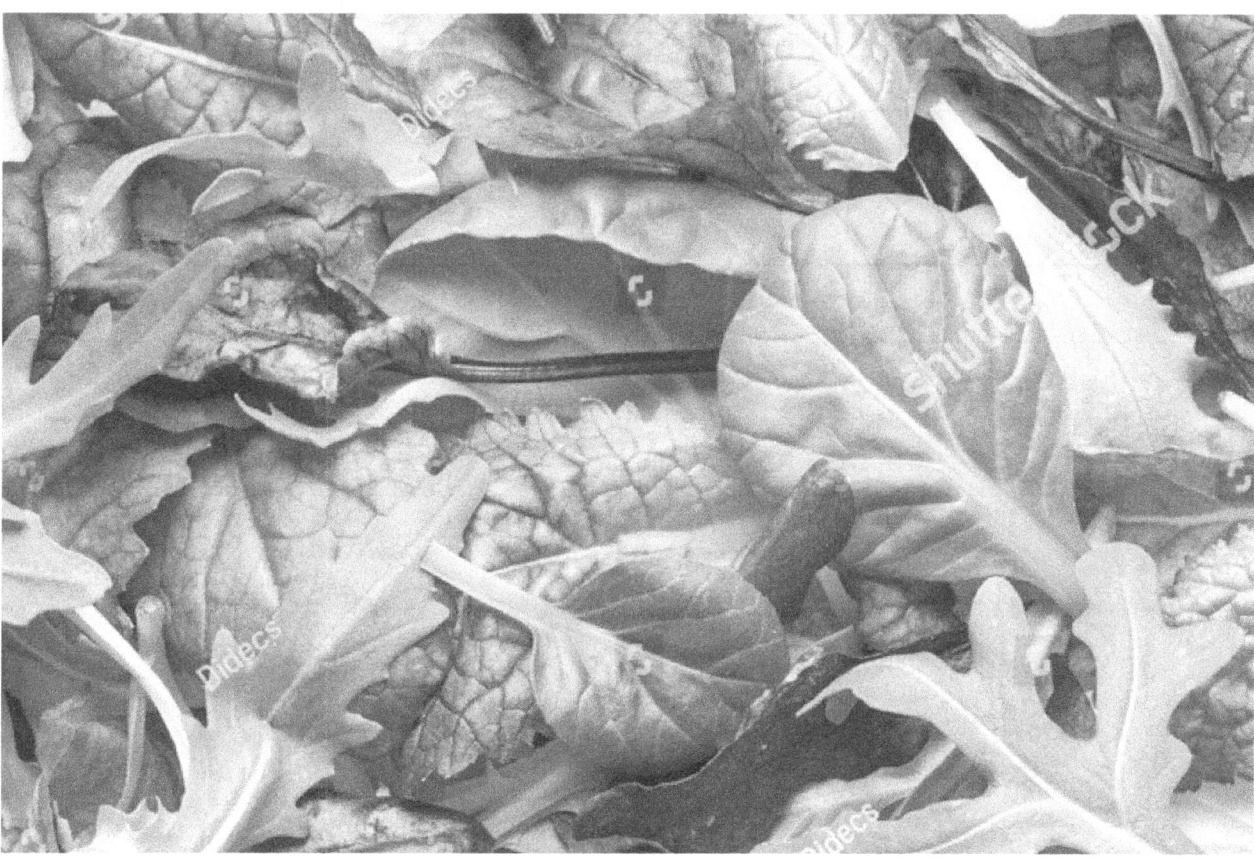

We are programmed to believe we get Vitamin C only from orange juice. Orange juice is loaded with sugar, almost as many grams of sugar as a Coke or a Pepsi. We thought we had to eat bananas for potassium. Bananas are healthy, but they are not weight-loss worthy. We thought we needed milk for our daily recommended allowance of calcium.. Not!

Take a careful look at the following charts. You'll see that all of these food sources allow you to obtain your Vitamin C, potassium, and calcium with weight-loss worthy foods.

Vitamin C

Benefits

Required for tissue growth	Repairs adrenal gland function
Important for healthy gums	Protects against cancer
Protects against infection	Enhances immunity
Promotes wound healing	Produces anti-stress hormones

Sources of Vitamin C

Asparagus	Broccoli
Brussel sprouts	Kale
Lemons	Mustard
Greens	Green peppers
Radishes	Spinach
Strawberries	Tomatoes
Turnip greens	Watercress

Potassium

Benefits

Healthy nervous system	Regular heartbeat

Sources of Potassium

Fish	Poultry	Vegetables
Garlic	Winter Squash	Yams

Calcium

Benefits

Blood clotting	Strong bones	Regular heartbeat
Helps prevent colon cancer	Needed for muscle growth	Prevents leg cramps
Healthy nervous system		

Sources of Calcium

Salmon	Asparagus	Broccoli
Cabbage	Collard greens	Dandelion greens
Kale	Parsley	Tofu
Turnip greens		

You can obtain your daily requirement of vitamins and minerals from a wide selection of food options. In addition, foods such as garlic and kale will aid proper nutrition.

Much of the nutrition in your new mindset will begin with an assortment of vegetables and a few fruits that you may have been neglecting in your past nutritional choices. Most of the options I offer you are green veggies, because most of them are unlimited, except for:

- Peas (high in sugar)
- Avocados (high in fat)
- Olives (high in fat)

These items are great nutritionally but difficult to manage in a weight-loss regimen.

As you make your changes, I would much rather you focus on what you *can* eat versus what you cannot. Fruits are tough, because they are processed as sugar, fructose. A bodybuilder on their best game would not utilize much fruit. These are ones you can work into the nutritional equation.

Berries	Serving	Sugar
Raspberries	1 cup	6 grams
Strawberries	1 cup	9 grams
Blueberries	1 cup	12 grams
Blackberries	1 cup	15 grams

If you must, eat a 6.5-ounce serving of Del Monte® fruit naturals grapefruit, no sugar added, or half a grapefruit, or half an apple. Even better... take the Del Monte® grapefruit and add half a cup of fat free cottage cheese for a quick, delicious breakfast.

We have researched the glycemic index (a tool to determine the rate at which carbohydrates are burned off) of fruits and vegetables. Remember, you want to choose the carbohydrates that burn off quickly, rather than veggies like potatoes and corn, which go directly to your assets. Unlimited options include green, leafy veggies, and cruciferous (broccoli family) ones. I always hated the portion-control mindset. We've selected and created a whole bunch of eye-pleasing and mouth-watering recipes from the unlimited options. We in the Onion world focus on what we can eat!

I do not want this guide to overwhelm you with the idea that you need to run out and purchase a cabinet full of vitamins and supplements. A good multivitamin will do the job.

Supplements

I mentioned early in this guide that I learned a lot from my bodybuilding friends. Body-builders know their stuff. They know how to protect and grow lean muscle. Exactly what those of us who have struggles with our weight need. After several years of case studies, and with a burning commitment to change the course of obesity, I vehemently assert that we need to think like a body-builder to succeed. Anyone who has struggled with his or her weight needs to think just like a bodybuilder. We are reinventing our bodies. And after we peel away the layers of fat, we have the opportunity to sculpt what is left. We need to learn how to protect the lean mass (muscle) and burn off the fat, not just try to lower that number on the weight scale. We need to learn how to feed our muscle tissue versus feed our fat cells. We need to change our nutrition and activity choices and move to a 26 body fat percentage and prevent premature death.

Along with a good multivitamin, I would like for you to consider the following supplements:

- L-Carnitine or Acetyl L Carnitine
- Omega 3, 6, and 9 essential oils
- CLA
- Biotin

These supplements are exactly what my trainer shared with me. In the beginning, I struggled to take supplements. I worked hard at trying to get everything I needed through good food choices. Luckily, I had a large base of medical professionals as clients, and we would discuss the pros and cons of the four mentioned above. I was comfortable with Biotin because I had taken this supplement in the past for great hair and nails. I hated to recommend items I did not utilize; however, I also needed to shut down the amounts of lean mass my clients were losing due to improper nutrition. Around Camp Nine, we began using all four of these supplements. I immediately saw fat loss increase and lean mass loss decrease. In essence, the supplements acted like an insurance policy in case a client missed a beat in feeding their muscles through their daily nutrition.

I asked an RN Onion why she chose to take CLA instead of L-Carnitine. I received the following email, which did a great job of explaining the difference between the two. This makes a lot of sense.

To further expand upon my answer to why I chose CLA over L-Carnitine: L-Carnitine seems more recommended for cardio-intensive workouts (we all know how I feel about cardio).

L-Carnitine makes sperm swim faster, not really a need, in my book. Finally, it didn't seem to have as many benefits as CLA, and the dosing was vague. CLA dosing is very clear. There are multiple reasons to take CLA:

- *helps dissolve body fat*
- *preserves muscle tissue*
- *helps fight autoimmune disorders (I have one)*
- *decreases the chance of developing Type II Diabetes (a fear of mine, truthfully)*
- *good for thyroid patients (that's me too) by increasing metabolic rate*
- *lowers cholesterol*
- *decreases chances of developing arthrosclerosis (that is what killed my dad)*
- *CLA is the most important of the 3 essential fatty acids that the body doesn't make and that we need. (you cannot safely eat enough meat to get the amount your body needs)*

So, in looking at the above lists, I think it's clear why I made the choice I did.

Joanne

Essential Fatty Acids

One of the things I have loved about the past few years has been the opportunity to share light-bulb moments with my clients. When something makes sense, the process of change seems easier. My top three thoughts are:

- *Diet.* Why didn't we realize the first three letters told us DIE?

- *Artificial sweeteners.* Hmm, why did we think anything artificial would be good for us?

- Last but not least—*essential fatty acids.*

How come we did not think we needed fat when the label clearly says some are "essential"? We need Omega 3, Omega 6, and Omega 9. Out of all the supplements I have shared with Onion campers, I had the most resistance to the three Omega acids. Usually, local health food stores will recommend a fish oil supplement for the Omega fatty acids. Guess what? They do not taste that great. I am sitting here on Labor Day sifting through scads of information about essential fatty acids. And one phrase stands out above all the rest: "essential to human health." Bingo. Let's dig a little deeper.

Omega 3

Benefits

Reduces blood clotting and inflammation	Inhibits abnormal heart rhythms
Lowers trigyceride levels (a risk for cardiovascular disease)	May lower blood pressure
May reduce risk of heart attacks and cancers	May reduce risk of some cancers

Sources

Salmon	White albacore tuna	Mackerel	Anchovies
Sardines	Walnuts	Flaxseed	Canola oil
Soybean oil	Tofu	Dark green leafy vegetables	

Omega 6

Benefits

Reduces bloating and pain of PMS	Maintains healthy skin, hair, and nails
Helps hormonal and emotional balance to prevent inflammation	Works with Omega 3
Plays a crucial role in brain function and development	Plays a crucial role in growth

Sources of Omega 6

Poultry	Eggs
Avocados	Nuts
Most vegetable oils	

Omega 9

Benefits

Promotes healthy inflammation response	Lowers cholesterol

Sources of Omega 9

Olive oil	Salmon
Sardines	Crab

As I was collecting ideas, articles, and research, a connection struck me. A deficiency in Omega 3 is linked to depression. Allow me to explain.

Back in the 90's, I was a wellness counselor for a local facility. I met with prospective clients about joining the facility. In the 90's, I kept seeing an increase in the medical section of the interview; everyone and their mother were taking anti-depressants. Well, guess what? We had spent the 80's eating fat-free and our bodies were screaming at us!

Bodybuilder Friend

Along the way, I learned so much from my bodybuilding friends. I spent 20-some years in the fitness industry. I managed and consulted for several million-dollar facilities, but in all those years, I had blinders on to the bodybuilding world. I guess it was because I operated health and wellness facilities, and I guess, because I desired so much for the facilities to be user friendly to the client who needed it most, the beginner. Or just because I am bullheaded and stubborn and I needed to figure it out the hard way. I felt that a bodybuilder's look was so far out of reach, and so very intimidating, that I just did not pay enough attention.

Until one day when that world was smack-dab in front of me. I fell for a bodybuilder, and I discovered a few of the missing pieces of the weight loss and weight management world. Specifically, I listened to him and began to understand the value of protein, and how it feeds the muscle. I also started to see the value of certain vitamins, amino acids, and minerals to guide us along the way.

The two supplements that I feel are very important are Biotin and CLA. As girls, we have known about biotin for a very long time. Biotin is a water-soluble vitamin. Biotin used to be known as vitamin K. Biotin is a member of the B-class vitamin family, it plays a key role in the metabolism of proteins, fats and carbohydrates. Biotin plays a major role in the growth and maintenance of hair, nails, and bone. Biotin helps the body better use food for energy. Symptoms of biotin deficiency may include hair loss, dry skin, fatigue, short attention span, mental depression, birth defects, and nausea.

Now let's talk about CLA. What a cool story this is! CLA is short for Conjugated Linoleic Acid. CLA is research proven to build muscle, reduce body fat, and induce an optimum cellular environment for improved health. It is available naturally in foods such as milk, cheese, beef, and lamb. Getting enough CLA in your daily nutrition from the above sources would be difficult due to the amount you would need to consume and the high levels of fat from the sources. The great news is you can buy CLA in pre-measured soft gel capsules. You may also find CLA in protein drinks.

Weight-Loss-Worthy Fruits and Vegetables

Artichokes	Aids digestion	Lowers cholesterol	Protects your heart	Stabilizes blood sugar	Guards from liver disease
Blueberries	Combats cancer	Protects your heart	Stabilizes blood sugar	Boots memory	Prevents constipation
Broccoli	Strengthens bones	Saves eyesight	Combats cancer	Protects your heart	Controls blood press.
Cabbage	Combats cancer	Prevents constipation	Promotes weight loss	Protects your heart	Helps prevent hermorrhoids
Cauliflower	Combats prostate cancer	Combats breast cancer	Strengthens bones	Banishes bruises	Resists heart disease
Flax	Aids digestion	Battles diabetes	Protects your heart	Improves mental health	Boosts immune system
Fish	Protects your heart	Boosts memory	Combats cancer	Supports immune system	
Strawberries	Combats cancer	Protects your heart	Boosts memory	Calms stress	
Tomatoes	Protects prostate	Combats cancer	Lowers cholesterol	Protects your heart	
Water	Promotes weight loss	Combats cancer	Helps prevent kidney stones	Smoothes skin	

Prevention Is the Key

In case it takes you awhile to indulge in the *Prescriptive Healings* guide, let me tickle your fancy with some knowledge that might motivate a change in your choices.

Cruciferous Options

If you knew you could reduce the risk of cancer simply by making a few alterations in your daily nutrition, would you? I hope the answer is yes! The world of cruciferous options intrigues me. Why are these vegetables cancer preventative? Cruciferous veggies contain photochemical, vitamins and minerals, and fiber. All are important to your overall health. I selected the ones most common in our recipes:

Kale	Collard greens
Brussel sprouts	Broccoli
Turnips	Rutabagas
Radishes	Horseradish
Cabbage	Watercress

If you like sushi, you know about wasabi, and it is also cancer preventative. So eat more sushi!

The more I've learned about the body and the more I've discovered the nutritional deficiencies we are facing due to the lack of balanced nutrition, the more I am paying attention.

As you know by now, my path was to find out how I could eat for the rest of my life, not starve. My goal was to learn how to feed myself without gaining weight, to feel better, and to prevent health issues as I age. I have always desired to know more about food as a source of preventative options before searching for prescriptive options.

Sure, we all understand we should take a daily vitamin. I was the girl who always thought if we ate well-balanced, then we should be able to obtain all the proper vitamins and minerals from the food we ate.

Let's face it, if we really took an honest look at the way society has been eating for the past couple of decades, our essential vitamin and mineral intakes has some serious flaws.

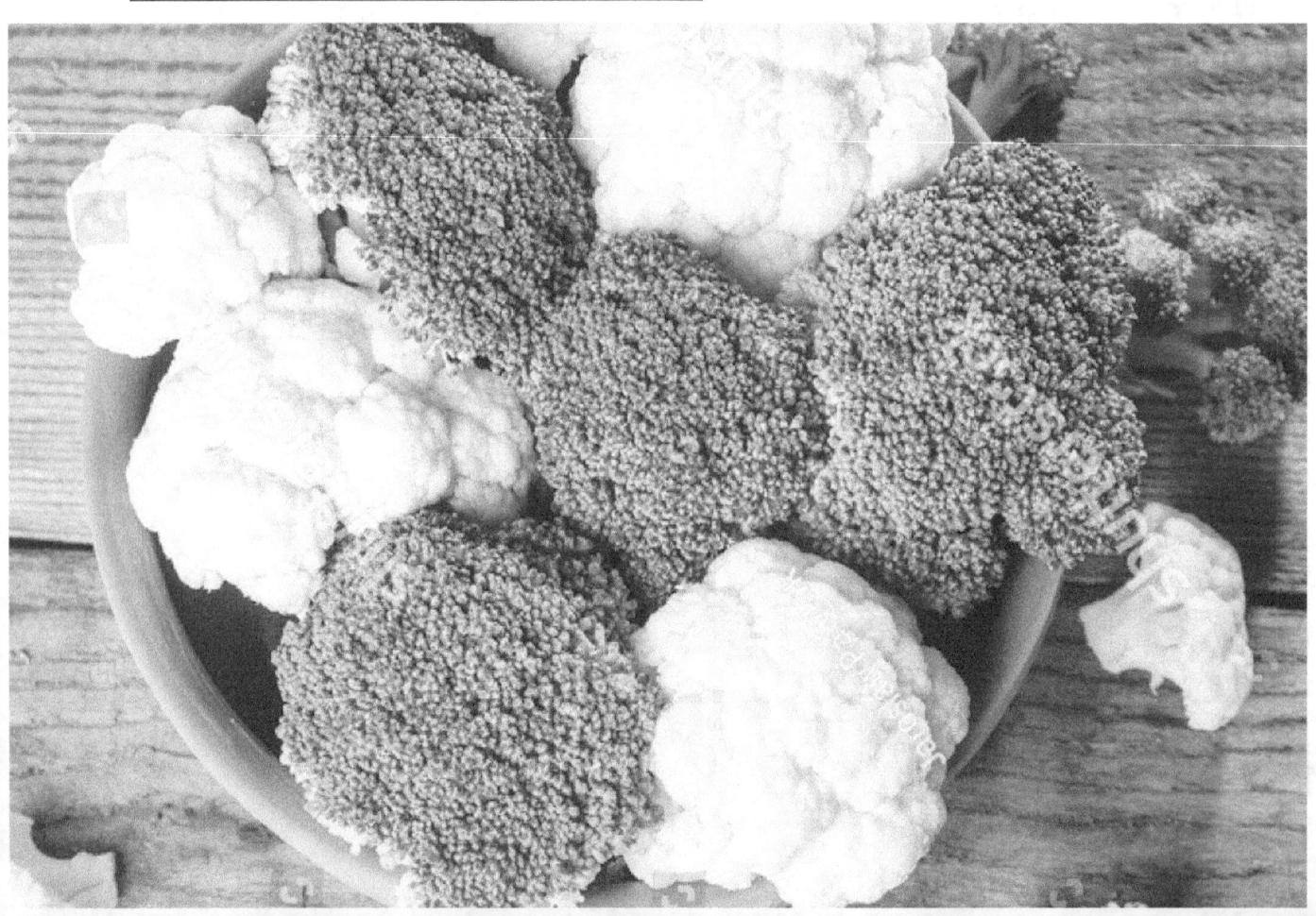

16. Living in Maintenance

PEELING IS AN EVOLUTION of change. Change takes perseverance, persistence, and patience. The good news is that maintaining your newfound results will not be as difficult as it was to peel away the extra layers of fat. Once you have made it to maintenance, the next step will be managing your results and paying attention to your behaviors.

Once you get to maintenance, you have already made the needed changes. You have pushed aside the fillers, because you realized your storage tank was already full. You have made the decision to take better care of yourself. Good for you. Keep making those choices, and be careful not to slip back to old habits, which grew you into an Onion.

In maintenance, it will be time to bring back the slow burning carbs, the fillers a.k.a. breads, pasta, rice, potatoes, corn, carrots, bananas, and peas. Adding these back into your daily nutrition will be very strategic. Let me explain. If you have gained a love affair with your exercise routine and plan to train at the same pace you did in peel mode, and if you do not bring back the starchy carbs such as breads, pastas, rice, potatoes, bananas, peas, and corn, then you will continue to lose. While obesity is not an attractive look, neither is an anorexic look appealing. Refer back to your body fat percentage section, so you may reevaluate what percentage will be a comfortable landing spot for you.

In maintenance, it is now about maintaining your new level of cardiovascular training and balancing your nutrition accordingly. If you pull back on your exercise efforts, then you will need to pull back on intake of fillers. If you decide to increase your exercise or activity levels, then you will need to also add to, and adjust, your nutritional intake. Bottom line. You are now in control. Stay focused. Stay in control.

The toughest part of maintenance is life. Life is about temptations, and food temptations surround us. A favorite Onion of mine looked at me and said, "I see candy everywhere." Our social events revolve around celebration, and celebration usually is an open invitation to party with food.
By the time you have reached maintenance, you will have worked through the attachment of the filler, feel-good foods. You will have

worked through the voids in your life, or maybe you are still working through those voids; however, you have figured out that food cannot fill the empty places. I know it will be a constant battle to manage the new you and the emotions that were wrapped around food.

If you grew into an Onion because of your lack of knowledge, then your maintenance journey will be far simpler. You may even slip, occasionally, but I assure you, you are now armed with the accurate tools to create and maintain the "you" that you truly desire to be. From the process of change comes an amazing validation of increased energy levels, an improved self-confidence, longevity, and you will enjoy a better quality of life.

The difficult part about maintenance is once you begin to open the door to foods of the past and lean on old habits, it may take you a minute, and it may be difficult, to find that happy balance between what your crave and what you know to be the proper choice. You will need to pay attention to what things trigger you to make choices that are not weight-loss worthy. You will need to find a form of accountability. It may be your skinny jeans that keep you in check. Or, it may even be an ugly picture of you taped on the refrigerator door to remind you that if you go back to your old habits, you will surely find the old you.

My goal was to learn how to eat for the rest of my life, not how to learn how to eat well for three days and, then, go back to my old ways. I had been doing that, and it was not working. I had grown myself into a 300-pound girl. Sure, we all still would love to be able to go to that social event and indulge in a few of the wonderful treats that are laid out in front of us; however, we can no longer open the gates to continued indulgence and expect different results.

If you are like me and truly want to get a handle on your weight management, then the Onion System is the perfect fit for you, because this is a journey about eating. Eating more food than you may have eaten in the past. Once you are satisfied with all the new ideas in the kitchen, your weight management will be much easier. You will have learned how to eat a lifetime, a healthy, nutritionally valuable weight loss, and weight maintenance food.

Once you reach your personal goals, you may decide to take a night and enjoy past habits such as a slice of pizza (hopefully not the entire pizza). You might get a bucket of popcorn and enjoy it at the movies. You may even make the decision to go out for that greasy cheeseburger and French fries (and order that Diet Coke® to go along with it, so you believe you are making better choices).

The Fillers

Once you get to the point with your body fat percentage that you are ready to land, you will be ready to bring back some of the foods that were on hold during your peel. I will go ahead and warn you.

If these items got you in trouble in the past, they can do the same in the future, unless you are aware of the nutritional values and choose wisely. I have found that once you bring these selections back into your nutrition, you will crave more and more of them, and you will become tired.

Let's take a look at how you could manage these selections.

Once you begin to open the door to your past,

it may be difficult to find a happy balance

between what you crave and

what you know to be a healthy food choice

If you decide to indulge in one piece of pizza, go ahead. But understand that you have used all your filler carbs and half your fat allotments for the day. You had better work out well on that day, or you might end up gaining. Look what happens if you have two slices.

Large pizza	Calories	Carbs	Fat	Protein
2 slices	894	102	36	40

One of the biggest mistakes I see is; where is the nutrition? Might I suggest you give our pizza recipe a try? And make it for the family. You will be surprised that everyone will, most likely, enjoy it—especially the Mexican version.

If you were in that *fat-free mindset*, you might have selected the potato, the oatmeal, or the Cheerios, because, yes, the fat grams are good. However, you must factor in the amount of carbs and understand your baseline amount is about 46, or you may have found you did not get the desired results, or you may have even gained. Especially if your bowl of cereal looked more realistic, which most likely equates to two cups. Plus, you dumped milk (12 grams of sugar) in the bowl.

If you were in that *calorie-counting mindset*, you might have thought that you could manage 290 calories for that bagel. The bagel would be worth it and not get in your way. At second glance, you can see that 51 grams of filler carbs is already over your daily allotment with rolls, potatoes, and corn. While you are ready to add back some of your favorite foods, be aware of each bite you put in your mouth. Then make it work!

Cardio Seven Days a Week

If you continue to perform cardio training everyday, you will continue to burn 400 calories per day, and you will continue to lose. At this point, you will need to eat more! I know during this entire journey eating may have been a struggle, not eating, or eating once a day was so much easier. But those behaviors grew our society into the shape we are in today. Feeding your engine the proper nutrition is the journey you have been on to lose, and it will be the same journey to continue those results. But now, you need to find the right balance.

Let's take that 400 calories and break it down. Four hundred calories can be consumed a few different ways. If you select the additional calories from fat, that would equate 44 additional grams of fat. The challenge with fat is that your choices need to come from fat that has nutritional value, not artery-clogging fat such as animal fat, but fat such as avocados, nuts, canola oils, etc. Each gram of fat equates to 9 calories. By now you understand that all that extra weight we were carrying was stored calories, stored energy waiting for us to utilize it.

If you choose to add carbohydrates, the magic number is 100 grams per day. Each gram of carbohydrate equals 4 calories. If you choose to utilize the extra calories in carbohydrates, please keep in mind the ones that burn off slow and the ones which burn off quickly. With carbohydrates you will also need to consider your activity needs. If you begin more intensive training like running or walking a mini-marathon, then carbohydrates will play a huge part in energy storage.

Last but not least, let's review the option of adding extra protein. In this case, you would need an additional 100 grams. Each gram equals 4 calories like a carbohydrate. The great thing about protein is that protein feeds our muscles. Choose lean proteins rather than high-fat selections.

We looked at increasing your nutritional needs to balance your maintenance weight. You also need to factor in the days you weight-train. In most of the weight-training workouts I've evaluated, the calories burned ranged from 400 calories per workout to as much as 1,000 calories for a vigorous legs workout. How do I know? I strapped on the handy Polar heart-rate monitor and let it do the computing for me. A heart-rate monitor is one of the best tools available to insure you are burning fat, not just burning time.

Overtraining?

It is amazing to me that even though we grew into an Onion over a period of time, as we

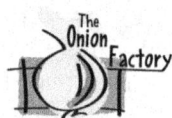 *No matter how well you follow the plan, your body will let go of the fat in its own time.*

start making a few modifications, we all want immediate results. On weight-loss, reality TV shows, we sometimes see unbelievable numbers pop up after a week of excruciating training. Why can't we achieve those numbers?

The psyche of weight loss you will need to accept is this: no matter how well you follow the plan, your body will change and let go of the fat in its own time. Fat loss is not an exact science. It is, however, the ultimate test of one's patience and discipline. Hence, the reason why I put step four, the psychology of the Onion system, last is because it is the most difficult part of the equation.

Have you ever heard the term, "overtraining"? Overtraining is a level of training that is simply too much for your body. Surely those on TV were sacrificing some of their muscle mass.

Results Are Typical

Have you ever seen a weight-loss client lose seven pounds of fat in one week? Impossible, my thoughts exactly. However, our Onion program can provide a loss of 3–5 pounds of fat per week. I did the math and collected fifteen years of data. In my case studies, I have seen some amazing things happen.

After I saw seven pounds of fat lost in a week, I sat down with a few local doctors. I shared with them the Onion formula and the process of peeling. Then I reviewed what seven pounds of fat-loss in one week equated to. An astounding 24,000 calories in the reserve tank were utilized. How can that be? How are we doing it? Let me show you what the numbers look like: Seven pounds of fat-loss equals 24,500 calories spent. Let's review the numbers. Three to five pounds of fat lost per week are possible, because here is the math per day (see chart below):

Add it all up, and it is 1,700 calories burned off your storage tank per day. Multiple it by seven, and there you have it: 11,900 calories. Divide it by 3,500 calories for each pound lost, and you get 3.5 pounds of fat loss per week. It's simple. Do the work—get the results. I turned the paper around to them and with my perplexed but

How to Get Results!

Calories burned	400 on the "Beast" (cardiovascular training) takes care of the heart
Weight lifting routine	400 calories burned and prevents atrophy
BMR—caloric difference	500 calories burned (yours may be more or less than this number)
Proper hydration	200 calories burned and a real no-brainer
Nutritional value	200 calories burned, eating six small meals a day

excited look, I asked, "How are we losing more than this?" They suggested that the metabolic increase must play a bigger role. The seven-pound loss confirmed a couple of theories. Let me explain.

Let's look again at the states anabolic, catabolic, and the one you are most likely familiar with metabolic. An anabolic state is difficult to explain but when you are there you know you are there. I asked girls, when they have had a big week of fat loss, if they can feel the anabolic state? The best way I can describe it to you is you are hungry, and your furnace is burning fat like crazy.

Have you ever been to a Chinese buffet where you ate, and ate, and ate, and a few hours later you were hungry again? Part of that reason is a Chinese buffet, normally, has a lot of veggies and lean protein to select from. Even if you do consume more rice than you should, your body had to work to digest and process the stir-fry and the other items on the buffet. This digestion is unlike the process of digesting a pizza, or a burger and fries, which are mostly fat. Those foods just sit there and we are not hungry for the rest of the day.

Anabolic also means your hydration is online; you are consuming enough protein, so your muscle is not sacrificed, and you have consumed enough whole foods (green leafy veggies). You are forcing your body to perform most efficiently. Hence, you are burning fat off like a fire. The thermal value of digestion, how beautiful!

Catabolic, on the contrary, is where your body goes into storage mode. Not being hungry is a sign you may be in a catabolic state. Actually, catabolic is protection mode, because you are starving the body, or overtraining it. The first three letters of catabolic says it all, cat. What do cats do all day? They sleep, they are lazy, and they store. Well, occasionally, they may catch a mouse if one is around.

Over the past few decades, diets have taken our caloric intake as low as 800 calories per day. I have even heard of some liquid programs that were as low as 500 calories per day. In these cases, individuals were dissuaded to exercise. Well, no wonder. Their caloric intake was so low they had very little energy. Guess what? Your body adjusts to lower calories. Your metabolism slows down to preserve itself from going after all of your lean muscles' mass. All of these stories and case studies further prove the theories of why dieting has not worked. You already know in your heart, as you read this, they do not work. You have tried it. And you are still trying. So let's review eating.

If you drink juice, your body has to do very little to digest and process. When you select whole foods such as broccoli, brussels sprouts, cabbage, asparagus, spinach, cauliflower, etc., you are forcing your body to work, to digest. Many times over the past few years when a client was stuck, or at a set point, I would stir up their metabolism by suggesting they increase their water intake and add an additional cup, or two, of the abovementioned vegetables. Clients usually fall short, anyway, of their 10 cups per day. So a little more can never hurt. Make your body work for you.

I love adding broccoli to get the digestive system going. I love broccoli for so many reasons. Broccoli is a cruciferous vegetable, one of a select few known to be a cancer preventative. A serving of broccoli has the same amount of protein as an egg, but without the fat. Remember, protein feeds the muscle! Broccoli takes a lot of work for your body to process. Yes, on this journey be prepared to add back all those veggies we neglected. There are more vegetables and fruits in this plan than potatoes, corn, and bananas. The downside to adding back all these forgotten vegetables? You may feel a little gassy. A little Beano goes a long way.

Let's talk about metabolic, metabolism, and calories. We were trained to count calories and to cut back our eating to lose weight. Now you are realizing, what weight did we actually lose? And did all that dieting mess with our metabolism? The answer is yes! Here are a few holes. Your metabolic rate is the number of calories your body requires when it is at rest. I am asked all the time, when I share the benchmark metabolic number, "Is that good?" The number is not necessarily good or bad. Your metabolic rate is just your metabolic rate. Just do me a favor; protect it, and then increase it by adding lean mass. Do not sacrifice any more lean mass all for a number on the scale.

Clarification

As I am nearing the final stages of my thoughts, I need to clarify the word *obese*. I hate it! I gave up on the word diet a long time ago. When someone says diet, it resonates in me like fingernails raking down a chalkboard. I spent so much time searching for the next diet out there; the answer to why I could not look and feel the way I wanted to. I need to set the record straight on the word obesity. It's pretty much up there with diet. The word *obesity* is such a negative imprint. To think that you or I are obese is self-deflating to anyone's ego and aspirations.

Let's take the word a step further in understanding. The word obesity suggests that our ratios are off. If you are more than 30 percent fat, you are considered obese. The word obese represents a percentage. The numbers equate risk factors. Risk factors you can indeed change. You may be amazed when you learn the high body fat percentages of some who, by society's standards, may look okay. The numbers do not lie, and the numbers are a form of accountability.

Accountability gives us the knowledge, via a number, to make adjustments—adjustments such as more water, less fat, more protein, less sugar, more cardio, and more strength training. The numbers teach you how to change the course of obesity on your specific course, your path.

17. Fallen Onions

IF WE COULD SORT THROUGH THE REASONS WE KEEP

SABOTAGING AND CELEBRATING OURSELVES WITH FOOD,

THE JOURNEY WOULD BE FAR SIMPLER.

REMEMBER WHEN I MENTIONED that if you go back to you old habits, your old results are sure to come back? It's NO different for my clients in the factory. Temptations and distractions will always get in your way. You must learn how to manage them. Find what works for you.

I hope this guide has given you awareness of unhealthy nutrition and the knowledge of how to make the change to weight-loss worthy nutrition. I trust this guide has given you every tool you need to make a better you. I hope you grow a love affair with your workouts, or, at least, an appreciation of your increased energy levels and of just feeling better.

As you are learning, food plays such a critical role in our life. Onions are the segment of society that leans on food to fix voids in their life. And I am not talking about leaning on broccoli. I'll wager if you are an Onion, you have been nurtured with goodies. So we develop a bond with food and a feeling of being okay when we are nurtured with food.

The psychology part of this guide was one of the toughest to put together. If we could sort through the reasons we keep sabotaging and celebrating with food, the journey of change would be far simpler.

I knew this story, which needed to be told, would not be complete until I shared what happens if you fall and cannot get back up. Recently, I sent an email asking for fallen Onions to please stand up. I was looking for girls who were ready to roll up their sleeves again and tackle their darkest adversary, food. And obesity. There, I said it, that nasty word. Why would anyone risk premature death, why be tired, why have bad knees because you are carrying 50, 75, or 100 pounds too much. I have no idea why. I just know a lot of us fall into that category.

I was totally amazed when the majority of the girls who showed up were girls I'd already written stories about. I thought once I'd taught them how to eat, what to eat, and why to eat, the rest would be easy. I was wrong.

This is tough. You gotta be mentally tough. You must desperately desire change for change to happen. You must jump back up in the saddle when you have fallen off. Never give up. You can get there. Look what happened in the first four weeks with these "fallen Onions" who decided to try again: If you are a fallen Onion, be encouraged by the success you see here.

	Pounds Lost	Inches Lost	% Fat Lost
Deb	34	31"	2%
Susan	24	27"	3%
Donna	19	14.5"	1%
Connie	15	18"	2.3%
Tami	12.5	17.5"	2%
Traci	12	22"	2.4%
Debbie	12	5"	3%
Christi	11	19.5"	1.8%
Rose	11	6"	--

A Note
Of Gratitude

*I appreciate the wonderful people
who trusted this program
and lost inches, pounds, and fat percentages.
They have made me so proud
of their accomplishments.*

*I'm also proud of the fact that The Onion Factory[SM]
is evidence-based, not an untested theory.
To date, we have graduated
more than fifteen hundred men and women.
They now have the foundation
to peel away their layers.*
—Lisa Cook

Thank You
for the opportunity to help you change your life.

www.ingramcontent.com/pod-product-compliance
Lightning Source LLC
Chambersburg PA
CBHW081151290426
44108CB00018B/2507